Computational Intelligence in Biomedical Imaging

Kenji Suzuki
Editor

Computational Intelligence in Biomedical Imaging

Springer

Editor
Kenji Suzuki
Department of Radiology
University of Chicago
Chicago, IL, USA

ISBN 978-1-4614-7244-5 ISBN 978-1-4614-7245-2 (eBook)
DOI 10.1007/978-1-4614-7245-2
Springer New York Heidelberg Dordrecht London

Library of Congress Control Number: 2013952918

Printed on acid-free paper

Springer is part of Springer Science+Business Media (www.springer.com)

I dedicate this book to my wife, Harumi Suzuki, for her support, encouragement, and love, and to my daughters, Mineru Suzuki and Juno Suzuki, for their love.

Kenji Suzuki

Preface

Medical decision-making is a crucial element in medicine and in patients' healthcare; yet, it is a complex task that is often difficult even for experienced physicians. Biomedical imaging offers useful information on patients' medical conditions and clues to causes of their symptoms and diseases. Thus, biomedical imaging is indispensable for accurate decision-making in medicine. However, physicians must interpret a large number of images. This could lead to "information overload" for physicians, and it could further complicate medical decision-making. Therefore, computer aids are needed and have become indispensable in physicians' decision-making such as detection, diagnosis, and treatment of diseases. Computational intelligence plays an essential role in computer aids for medical decision-making, including computer-aided detection and diagnosis, computer-aided surgery and therapy, medical image analysis, automated organ/lesion segmentation, automated image fusion, and automated image annotation and image retrieval.

As medical imaging has been advancing with the introduction of new imaging modalities and methodologies such as cone-beam/multi-slice computed tomography (CT), positron-emission tomography (PET)-CT, tomosynthesis, diffusion-weighted magnetic resonance imaging (MRI), electrical-impedance tomography, and diffuse optical tomography, new computational intelligence algorithms and applications are needed in the field of biomedical imaging. Because of its essential needs, computational intelligence in biomedical imaging is one of the most promising, growing fields. A large number of researchers studied in the field and developed a number of computational intelligence methods in biomedical imaging. However, there has been no book that covered the state-of-the-art technologies and recent advances in the field.

This book provides the first comprehensive overview of state-of-the-art computational intelligence research and technologies in medical decision-making based on biomedical images. This book covers the major technical advances and research findings in the field of computational intelligence in biomedical imaging. Leading researchers in the field contributed chapters to this book in which they describe their cutting-edge studies on computational intelligence in biomedical imaging.

This book consists of three parts organized by research area in computational intelligence in biomedical imaging: Part I deals with decision support, Part II with computational anatomy, and Part III with image processing and analysis. As mentioned earlier, computer aids have become indispensable in physicians' decision-making. This books starts with the research on decision support systems. In these systems, accurate segmentation and a precise understanding of anatomy are crucial for improvement of the performance of decision support systems. Part II covers this important topic, called "computational anatomy." Image processing and analysis are fundamental components in decision support systems as well as in biomedical imaging. Part III deals with this indispensable topic.

Part I contains four chapters provided by leading researchers in the research area of decision support.

In Chap. 1 in the decision support part (Part I), Drs. Cheng, Wee, Liu, Zhang, and Shen describe a computerized brain disease classification and progression in MRI, PET, and cerebrospinal fluid by using machine-learning classification and regression techniques. Their study represents state-of-the-art brain research by use of machine-learning techniques.

Chapter 2 is on content-based image retrieval (CBIR) systems based on perceptual similarity for decision support in breast cancer diagnosis in mammography using machine-learning algorithms by Drs. El Naqa and Yang. The authors are ones of the pioneers who introduced and developed perceptual similarity in CBIR systems for mammography. They also describe case-adaptive classification in computer-aided diagnosis (CADx) for breast cancer. Their case-adaptive classification is useful for improving the performance of a classifier in CADx.

In Chap. 3, Drs. Firjani, Khalifa, Elnakib, Gimel'farb, El-Ghar, Elmaghraby, and El-Baz introduce computer-aided detection and diagnosis (CADe and CADx) of prostate cancer in dynamic contrast enhanced MRI (DCE-MRI) by using image analysis and classification techniques. The authors tackled this challenging problem with their cutting-edge techniques.

In Chap. 4, Drs. Arimura, Magome, Kakiuchi, Kuwazuru, and Mizoguchi describe a system for treatment planning in radiation therapy by use of image analysis techniques, including automated beam arrangement based on similar cases, segmentation of lung tumors using a support vector machine classifier, and a method for determining robust beam directions against patient setup errors in hadron particle therapy. This is one of the leading studies in the area of radiation therapy planning.

Part II contains four cutting-edge studies in the field of computational anatomy. Computational anatomy is a relatively new, yet promising, rapidly growing area in biomedical imaging because of its essential needs. Four leading groups working in this area contributed chapters to this part.

In the first chapter (Chap. 5) in the computational anatomy part (Part II), Drs. Linguraru and Summers describe automated multi-organ analysis in the abdomen in CT by using a graph cut technique. The authors are among the leading researches in this area. They also describe CADe of tumors from the segmented liver.

Chapter 6 describes computerized segmentation of the liver in MRI by use of a 3D geodesic active contour model with a level-set algorithm, as provided by Drs. Huynh, Karademir, Oto, and Suzuki. Their study tackled this challenging topic with cutting-edge techniques, and they accomplished highly accurate liver segmentation in MRI.

In Chap. 7, Drs. Hayashi, Chen, Miyamoto, Zhou, Hara, and Fujita present a quantitative analysis of the vertebral anatomy in CT by using image analysis techniques, including a population-based statistical analysis on volumetric bone mineral density. Quantitative analysis of anatomy and its use as a diagnostic aid are becoming more and more important, as diagnosis in radiology becomes quantitative.

Chapter 8 is on segmentation of the lungs in CT by use of multi-stage learning and level-set optimization, provided by Drs. Birkbeck, Sofka, Kohlberger, Zhang, Wetzl, Kaftan, and Zhou. The authors especially focused on lung segmentation in difficult cases of lung pathologies by using advanced machine-learning, in particular discriminative modeling, and pattern recognition approaches.

Part III contains six studies in the area of image processing and analysis in biomedical imaging. Image processing and analysis are fundamental, indispensable components of biomedical imaging, including decision support systems and computational anatomy. The studies presented may be used as a very important, necessary pre-processing, processing itself, or post-processing. Six leading groups working in this area contributed chapters to this part.

In the first chapter (Chap. 9) in the image-processing and analysis part (Part III), Drs. Chen and Suzuki describe a method for separating bones from soft tissue in chest radiography by means of a pixel/patch-based machine-learning technique called anatomically specific multiple massive-training artificial neural networks (MTANNs). The author group is a pioneer in this area. This technique solves the fundamental problem of overlapping structures with projection X-ray images. Separation of bones from soft tissue improves the diagnostic accuracy of radiologists as well as a computer. This technique is indispensable for image analysis of projection X-ray images.

In Chap. 10, Drs. Tasdizen, Seyedhosseini, Liu, Jones, and Jurrus describe a method for reconstruction of circuits of individual neurons and synapses in electron-microscopy images by using machine-learning techniques. This topic is highly challenging, because the purpose was to reconstruct individual neural circuits on a microscopic scale for individual neurons and synapses. The chapter contains the pioneering work of the authors in this area.

Chapter 11 is on the quantification of brain tumors in MRI by use of image analysis techniques, including pre-processing of images, segmentation of tumors, and feature extraction, provided by Drs. Verma, Cowperthwaite, Burnett, and Markey. The authors describe the quantitative analysis of brain tumors on MR images. Their results can quickly be translated into construction of CADe and CADx systems.

In Chap. 12, Drs. Tanaka and Sanada present a computerized analysis method for respiratory and cardiac functions in dynamic chest radiography by use of image analysis techniques. The authors are pioneers in developing a new modality, a dynamic chest radiography system, and its image analysis. Unlike ordinary chest radiography, dynamic chest radiography can acquire dynamic information on the lungs and heart. The authors successfully extracted respiratory and cardiac functions from the images.

Chapter 13 describes a novel method for adaptive noise reduction and edge enhancement in MRI and PET by use of independent component analysis, provided by Drs. Han and Chen. Noise reduction and edge enhancement are very important fundamental problems in biomedical imaging. The authors tackled these problems by using a novel approach, independent component analysis.

In Chap. 14, Drs. Ishida, Yamamoto, and Okura describe advanced subtraction techniques for CT and digital subtraction angiography (DSA) and CADe of lung nodules in CT. The authors used subtraction in useful ways to improve the accuracy and efficiency in reading CT and DSA images. They also describe a CADe system for detection of lung nodules in CT which they developed.

In summary, this book provides the first comprehensive overview of state-of-the-art computational intelligence research and technologies in medical decision-making based on biomedical images. It covers major technical advancements and research findings in the field. Leading researchers contributed chapters in which they describe recent developments and findings in their cutting-edge studies. In these studies, they developed new computational intelligence technologies to solve specific problems in biomedical imaging. Thus, readers can learn and gain knowledge from the book on recent computational intelligence in biomedical imaging. Readers will learn that the most advanced computational intelligence technologies and studies have reached a practical level, and that they are becoming available in clinical practice in hospitals. The target audience of this book includes graduate and college students in engineering and applied-science schools, medical students, engineers in medical companies, professors in engineering and medical schools, researchers in industry, academia, and health science, medical doctors such as radiologists, cardiologists, and surgeons, and healthcare professionals such as radiologic technologists and medical physicists. Professors may find this book useful for their classes. Students can use this book for learning about state-of-the-art research in the field of computational intelligence in biomedical imaging. Engineers can refer to the book during their development of new products. Researchers can use the book for their work and cite it in their publications. Medical doctors, medical physicists, and other healthcare professionals can use the book to learn about state-of-the-art studies on computational intelligence in biomedical imaging. Therefore, it is expected that researchers, professors, students, and other professionals will gain valuable knowledge from the book, use it as a reference, and expand the current state-of-the art technologies. I hope that this book will inspire readers and help to advance the field of computational intelligence in biomedical imaging.

Chicago, IL, USA — Kenji Suzuki

Acknowledgments

This work would not have been possible without the help and support of countless people. The author is grateful to the 14 leading research groups in the field of computational intelligence in biomedical imaging for valuable contributions to this publication, to all members in the Suzuki laboratory, i.e., postdoctoral scholars, computer scientists, visiting scholars/professors, medical students, graduate/undergraduate students, research technicians, research volunteers, and support staff, in the Department of Radiology at the University of Chicago, for their invaluable assistance in the studies, to colleagues and collaborators for their valuable suggestions, and to Ms. E. F. Lanzl for proofreading the book. Many of the authors of chapters in this book served as reviewers of manuscripts submitted by their peers. The author is grateful to all reviewers for their time and effort. The author is grateful to his mentors in the past decades for their guidance in his career. The author is also grateful to his wife, Harumi Suzuki, for her support, encouragement, understanding, patience, and love, and her parents and brothers for their understanding and support; his daughters, Mineru Suzuki and Juno Suzuki, for cheering him up, and the joys that they have brought to his life; and his parents, Souichiro Suzuki and Mitsuru Suzuki, and his brothers, Eiji Suzuki and Junji Suzuki, for their support, encouragement, and inspiration.

Contents

Part I
Decision Support

Chapter 1
Brain Disease Classification and Progression Using Machine Learning Techniques

Bo Cheng, Chong-Yaw Wee, Manhua Liu, Daoqiang Zhang, and Dinggang Shen

Abstract In the past two decades, many machine learning techniques have been applied to the detection of neurologic or neuropsychiatric disorders such as Alzheimer's disease (AD) and its prodromal stage, i.e., mild cognitive impairment (MCI), based on different modalities of biomarkers including structural magnetic resonance imaging (MRI), fluorodeoxyglucose positron emission tomography (FDG-PET), and cerebrospinal fluid (CSF), etc. This chapter presents some latest developments in application of machine learning tools to AD and MCI diagnosis and progression. We divide our discussions into two parts, pattern classification and pattern regression. We will discuss how the cortical morphological change patterns and the ensemble sparse classifiers can be used for pattern classification and then discuss how the multi-modal multi-task learning (M3T) and the semi-supervised multi-modal relevance vector regression can be applied to pattern regression.

B. Cheng • D. Zhang
UNC IDEA Group, Department of Radiology, Biomedical Research Imaging Center (BRIC), University of North Carolina at Chapel Hill, CB #7513, 130 Mason Farm Road, Chapel Hill, NC 27599, USA

Department of Computer Science and Engineering, Nanjing University of Aeronautics and Astronautics, Nanjing, China
e-mail: chengb@med.unc.edu; dqzhang@med.unc.edu

C.-Y. Wee • D. Shen (✉)
UNC IDEA Group, Department of Radiology, Biomedical Research Imaging Center (BRIC), University of North Carolina at Chapel Hill, CB #7513, 130 Mason Farm Road, Chapel Hill, NC 27599, USA
e-mail: cywee@med.unc.edu; dgshen@med.unc.edu

M. Liu
UNC IDEA Group, Department of Radiology, Biomedical Research Imaging Center (BRIC), University of North Carolina at Chapel Hill, CB #7513, 130 Mason Farm Road, Chapel Hill, NC 27599, USA

Department of Instrument Science and Engineering, Shanghai Jiao Tong University, Dongchuan Road #800, Shanghai 200240, China
e-mail: mhliu@sjtu.edu.cn

K. Suzuki (ed.), *Computational Intelligence in Biomedical Imaging*,
DOI 10.1007/978-1-4614-7245-2_1,

Background

Alzheimer's disease (AD) is the most common form of dementia diagnosed in people over 65 years of age. It is reported that there are 26.6 million AD sufferers worldwide, and 1 in 85 people will be affected by 2050 [1]. This becomes worse as life expectancy increases. With the aging of the world population, AD has become a serious problem and a huge burden to the healthcare system, especially in the developed countries. Recognizing this urgent need for slowing down or completely preventing the occurrence of a worldwide healthcare crisis, effort has been under way to administer and to develop effective pharmacological and behavioral interventions for delaying the onset and progression of the disease. Thus, accurate diagnosis of AD and progression of its early stage, i.e., mild cognitive impairment (MCI), is critical for timely therapy and possible delay of the disease.

A significant body of literature [2–4] suggests that pathological manifestation of AD begin many years before it can be diagnosed using cognitive tests. At the stage where symptoms can be observed, significant neurodegeneration has already occurred. Studies suggest that individuals with MCI tend to progress to probable AD at an annual rate of 10–15 % [5], compared with healthy controls who develop dementia at a rate of 1–2 % [6]. Compared with AD, MCI is more difficult to diagnose due to the subtlety of cognitive impairment, especially in high functioning individuals who are able to maintain a positive public or professional profile without showing obvious cognitive impairment.

Over the past decade, many machine learning and pattern classification methods have been used for early diagnosis of AD and MCI based on different modalities of biomarkers, e.g., the structural brain atrophy measured by magnetic resonance imaging (MRI) [7–10], metabolic alterations in the brain measured by fluorodeoxyglucose positron emission tomography (FDG-PET) [11, 12], and pathological amyloid depositions measured through cerebrospinal fluid (CSF) [8, 13–15], etc. Many existing methods use the structural MRI brain images for classification between AD/MCI patients and normal controls [16–18]. Neuroimaging measurements that are used include: regional brain volumes [19, 20], cortical thickness [21–23], and hippocampal volume and shape [24, 25]. Another important imaging modality for AD/MCI detection is FDG-PET [19]. With FDG-PET, some recent studies have reported reduction of glucose metabolism in the parietal, posterior cingulate, and temporal brain regions of AD patients [26]. Besides neuroimaging techniques, biological or genetic biomarkers are effective alternatives for AD/MACI diagnosis. Researchers have found that (1) the increase of CSF total tau (t-tau) and tau hyperphosphorylated at threonine 181 (p-tau) are related to neurofibrillary tangle, (2) the decrease of amyloid β ($A\beta_{42}$) indicates amyloid plaque deposit, and (3) the presence of the apolipoprotein E (APOE) $\varepsilon 4$ allele can predict cognitive decline or conversion to AD [8].

In addition to classification, several recent works begin to estimate continuous clinical variables from brain images by using pattern regression methods [27–31]. In all these methods, the classification or regression models are learned from the training subjects to predict the disease categories or stages on the test subjects. In the following, we will discuss AD or MCI diagnosis and progression from two aspects, i.e., pattern classification and pattern regression.

AD/MCI Diagnosis Using Pattern Classification Approaches

Advanced statistical pattern classification techniques have been actively applied to map neurodegenerative patterns during the early stage of the disease where only very mild symptoms are evident [17, 32–34]. In addition to determining group differences, pattern classification methods can be trained to identify individuals who are at risk for AD [17, 33, 35–38]. A recent study demonstrated that classification methods are capable of identifying AD patients via their MRI scans with accuracy comparable to experienced neuroradiologists [35].

Machine learning techniques are often used to design an optimal classifier to classify the test samples. So far, various classification models have been used for classification of different patterns between AD and normal controls. Among them, support vector machine (SVM) may be the most-widely used classifier, because of its high performance for classification of high-dimensional data [35, 39–42]. SVM is a supervised learning method that searches for the optimal margin hyperplane to maximally separate different groups. On the other hand, to enhance the robustness of classification to noise, sparse representation technique, which can be regarded as one of the recent major achievements in pattern classification, has been proposed and successfully applied to various classification problems, e.g., face recognition [43–45]. In sparse representation-based classification, the input test sample is coded as a sparse linear combination of the training samples across all classes via L_1-norm minimization, and then it evaluates which class of training samples could produce the minimum reconstruction error of the input test sample with the sparse coding coefficients. However, the discriminative features from neuroimaging data could lie in multiple low-dimensional subspaces of a high-dimensional feature space, which makes it difficult to build a single global classifier with high classification accuracy and robustness to noise. To this end, the ensemble learning methods are generally used to further improve the classification performance.

AD/MCI Progression Using Pattern Regression Approaches

Rather than predicting categorical variables as in classification, some recent studies begin to estimate the continuous clinical variables based on the cognitive tests from brain images [27–31]. Efforts have also been undertaken to develop regression techniques for relating clinical scores to imaging data [28, 46, 47], facilitating continuous monitoring of AD progression. This kind of research is important because it can help evaluate the stage of AD pathology and predict future progression. Different from classification that classifies a subject into binary or multiple categories, regression needs to estimate continuous values and are thus more challenging. In the literature, a number of regression methods have been used for estimating clinical variables based on neuroimaging data. For example, linear regression models were used to estimate the 1-year mini-mental state examination (MMSE) changes from structural MR brain images [28, 29]. High-dimensional kernel-based regression method, i.e., relevance vector machine (RVM), was also used to estimate clinical variables, including MMSE and Alzheimer's disease assessment scale-cognitive subscale (ADAS-Cog), from structural MR brain images [27, 30, 31]. Besides clinical variables, regression methods have also been used for estimating age of individual subject from MR brain images [48, 49].

In the practical diagnosis of AD, multiple clinical variables are generally acquired, e.g., MMSE and ADAS-Cog. Specifically, MMSE is used to examine the orientation to time and place, the immediate and delayed recall of three words, the attention and calculations, language, and visuoconstructional functions [50], while ADAS-Cog is a global measure encompassing the core symptoms of AD [51]. It is known that there exist inherent correlations among multiple clinical variables of a subject, since the underlying pathology is the same [30, 31]. However, most existing regression methods model different clinical variables separately and using supervised learning techniques, without considering their inherent correlations and using the unlabeled subject information that may be helpful for robust and accurate estimation of clinical variables from brain images. On the other hand, although multi-modal data are often acquired for AD diagnosis, e.g., MRI, PET, and CSF biomarkers, nearly all existing regression methods developed for estimation of clinical variables were based only on one imaging modality, i.e., mostly on the structural MRI.

The rest of this chapter is organized as follows. In section "Pattern Classification," we first study pattern classification methods for AD/MCI diagnosis and prognosis. Specifically, we will employ gray matter cortical thickness as morphological data and further use sparse representation to construct ensemble classifier for AD/MCI classification. Then, in section "Pattern Regression," we study pattern regression methods for AD/MCI progression, which includes multi-modal multi-task learning (M3T) and semi-supervised multi-modal relevance vector regression (SMRVR). In section "Results," we present experimental results on the ADNI dataset to validate the efficacy of all proposed methods. Finally, in section "Summary," we conclude this chapter.

Pattern Classification

In this section, we will discuss the pattern classification techniques for AD/MCI diagnosis and prognosis using the cortical morphological change patterns and also the ensemble sparse classification methods.

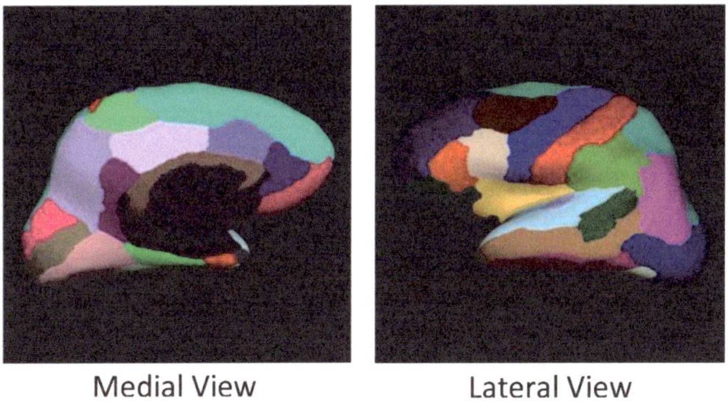

Fig. 1.1 Desikan–Killiany cortical atlas used for brain space parcellation. The medial and lateral views of the atlas are obtained from http://web.mit.edu/mwaskom/pyroi/freesurfer_ref.html

Classification Using Cortical Morphological Change Patterns

Cortical thickness estimation performed in vivo via MR imaging is an important technique for the diagnosis and understanding of the progression of neurodegenerative diseases, such as AD. Gray matter cortical thickness can be utilized as morphological data to address the AD/MCI classification problem via a less explored paradigm: Is the morphological changes in different cortical areas correlated, especially in relation to pathological attacks, such as AD? Correlative morphological information can be extracted from structural MRI to provide a new type of features for AD and MCI classification. ROI-based morphological information, i.e., gray matter (GM) and white matter (WM) volumes, and regional mean cortical thickness, is also utilized to provide extra information for better characterization of anatomical changes associated with AD. The correlative and ROI-based morphological features are integrated via a multi-kernel SVM to further improve classification capability.

Two types of features are extracted from the MR volume of every subject based on the Desikan–Killiany cortical atlas [52], which contains 68 gyral-based ROIs, 34 for each hemisphere. The first feature type is the ROI-based morphological features which contain the regional mean cortical thickness, cerebral cortical GM, and cortical associated WM volumes, while the second feature type is the correlative features which are obtained by constructing a similarity map signifying the relative mean cortical thickness between pairs of ROIs. The Desikan–Killiany cortical atlas is provided in Fig. 1.1.

The ROI-based morphological features, i.e., regional mean cortical thickness, cerebral cortical GM, and cortical associated WM volumes, are extracted in an automated manner using atlas-based FreeSurfer software suite (http://surfer.nmr.mgh.harvard.edu/Version 4.5.0). Then, the regional mean cortical thickness features, after normalized by their respective standard deviation, are combined with the regional cortical volumetric information to better describe morphological pattern of the brain. We utilize the same ROIs defined in Desikan–Killiany cortical atlas to extract the cerebral cortical GM and cortical associated WM volumes. We normalize the regional volumes of each subject by their respective intracranium volume (ICV) value to provide a more appropriate volumetric representation.

It is well known that AD/MCI and similar dementias exhibit subtle, spatially and temporally diffuse pathology, where the brain is damaged in a large-scale, highly connected network, rather than in one single isolated region [53, 54]. In view of this, we design an interregional description, which might be more sensitive in conveying the pathological information for accurate diagnosis of neurological diseases. Hence, we propose to use correlative derived from cortical thickness information between pairs of ROIs for AD/MCI classification. By using the Desikan–Killiany cortical atlas, a 68×68 matrix map is constructed with every element representing the similarity of regional mean cortical thicknesses between a pair of ROIs. The similarity map is symmetric with ones along its diagonal.

Specifically, for the i-th and j-th ROIs, the dissimilarity of the cortical thicknesses is defined as [76]

$$d(i,j) = [t(i) - t(j)]^2 \tag{1.1}$$

where $t(i)$ and $t(j)$ denote the regional mean cortical thickness of the i-th and j-th ROIs, respectively. Then, the similarity between the i-th and j-th ROIs is computed as

$$s(i,j) = \exp\left(-\frac{d(i,j)}{2\sigma^2}\right) \tag{1.2}$$

where $\sigma = \sqrt{\sigma_i + \sigma_j}$ with σ_i and σ_j denoting the standard deviation of regional cortical thickness of the i-th and j-th ROIs. This new feature type provides the relative morphological changes across different encephalic regions, instead of morphological changes in the isolated regions as used in the conventional methods. It is worth noting that the dissimilarity measure (1.1) and the similarity measure (1.2) can be replaced by other functions for similarity map construction. Due to symmetry, only the upper (or lower) triangular of the similarity map is used. For each subject, all similarity values of the upper triangular part of the similarity map are concatenated to form a long feature vector with 2,278 elements ($N \times (N - 1)/2$, with $N = 68$).

Due to high dimensionality of the correlative morphological features, we utilize a hybrid feature selection method, a combination of filter-based and wrapper-based approaches, to select the most relevant features for AD/MCI classification. Two filter-based approaches are initially used to reduce the number of features. In the first filter-based approach, only those features with their p-values smaller than the predefined threshold, measured via between-group t-test, will be retained for subsequent feature selection. Despite the reduction in dimensionality, the features retained by this simple approach may still inevitably be inter-correlated. Therefore, another filter-based approach, called minimum redundancy and maximum relevance (mRMR) [55, 56], is employed to further reduce the feature dimensionality. The mRMR model provides a balance between two aspects of feature selection, i.e., efficiency and broadness. Efficiency ensures that characteristics can be represented with a minimal number of features without significant reduction in prediction performance. Broadness ensures that the selected feature subset can be the maximally representative of original space covered by the entire dataset.

SVM recursive feature elimination (SVM-RFE) [57, 58] is finally utilized to further reduce the number of selected features by selecting a subset of features that are most favorable to AD/MCI classification. The goal of SVM-RFE is to find a subset of features that optimizes the performance of the SVM classifier. The basic principle of SVM-RFE is to ensure that the removal of a particular feature will make the classification error smallest. SVM with linear kernel is utilized to evaluate the discriminative power of the selected features. It is noteworthy that the hybrid feature selection is performed separately on each feature type (i.e., correlative and ROI-based features) to obtain an individual optimal subset for each feature type.

To classify a new test subject, the ROI-based features are firstly extracted from the subject's MR volumes. Then, the correlative features are constructed from the regional mean cortical thickness. Individual kernel matrices are constructed for each feature type based on the optimal features selected in the training process. These individual kernel matrices are then integrated to form a mixed-kernel matrix that will act as the input to the previously trained SVM classifier to determine the class where the new test subject belongs to. Specifically, in every experiment, the data is randomly divided into two sets, one for training set and one for testing set, with similar number of subjects for each class in each set. The experiment was repeated for 20 times to evaluate the performance of all compared methods by determining their mean classification accuracy, area under receiver operating characteristic (ROC) curve, sensitivity, and specificity. The average classification performance estimated using this approach tends to be more conservative than the traditional leave-one-out approach. It also ensures that the trained SVM models are validated with independent test sets for more precise estimation on how accurately they will perform in practice.

Ensemble Sparse Classification of Structural MR Images

Sparse representation has been successfully used in various applications where the original signal needs to be reconstructed as accurately as possible, such as denoising [59], image inpainting [60], and coding [61]. Recently, a sparse representation-based classifier (SRC) was proposed to harness the sparsity for discrimination [43]. The basic idea of SRC is that the test data is considered as a linear composition of the training data belonging to the same category if sufficient training samples are available for each class. In our previous work [62], a random

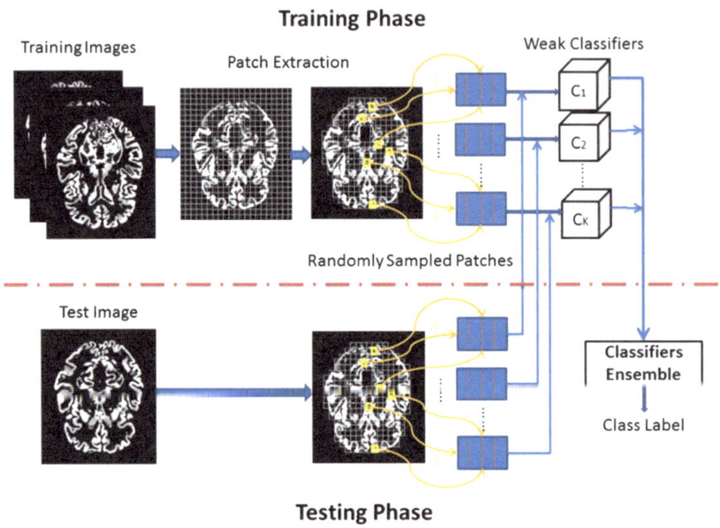

Fig. 1.2 The framework of the random patch-based subspace ensemble classification method

patch-based subspace ensemble classification framework was proposed to combine multiple weak classifiers built with the sparse representation-based classification method (denoted as RPSE_SRC). The proposed ensemble sparse classification framework is shown graphically in Fig. 1.2. It consists of three main steps: (1) patch extraction and random patch sampling; (2) design of individual weak classifier using SRC; (3) ensemble of multiple weak classifiers. We will detail each step in the rest of this section.

Although the proposed classification framework makes no assumption on a specific neuroimaging modality, for demonstrating its performance, the T1-weighted MR Imaging data are used in this work. Specifically, the MR brain images are skull-stripped and cerebellum-removed after correction of intensity inhomogeneity using nonparametric nonuniform intensity normalization (N3) algorithm [63]. Then, each brain image is segmented into three kinds of tissue volumes, e.g., GM, WM, and CSF volumes. All three tissue volumes will be spatially normalized onto a standard space by a mass-preserving deformable warping algorithm proposed in [64]. The warped mass-preserving tissue volumes are also called as the tissue density maps below. These spatially normalized tissue density maps are used as the imaging features for classification.

Patch Extraction

For simplicity, we uniformly divide the tissue density maps into patches of fixed size without overlapping. For accurate classification, the noisy voxels should be first excluded from the feature subspaces. On the other hand, the sampled subspaces for the individual classifiers should be as diverse as possible to give complementary information for effective ensemble. To balance the trade-off between accuracy and diversity, we perform the simple t-test on each voxel of the whole brain and select the relevant voxels with the p-value smaller than 0.05. The patch extraction is carried out based on these preselected relevant voxels. The patch pool for random sampling is composed of the patches in each of which more than 50 % voxels are the preselected relevant voxels. We randomly select a subset of patches from the patch pool and all the preselected relevant voxels contained in the sampled patches are concatenated into a feature vector for classification. Each random sampling defines a feature subspace for one weak classifier.

Sparse Representation-Based Classifier

After patch extraction, we construct an independent weak classifier for each randomly sampled subspace, using SRC method. SRC first encodes the test sample as a sparse linear combination of the training samples by L_1-norm minimization and then performs classification by evaluating which class produces the minimum reconstruction error with the sparse coefficients. Unless specially noted, all feature vectors are the column vectors and $\|\cdot\|_2$ represents the standard Euclidean norm, while $\|\cdot\|_1$ represents the standard L_1 norm. Suppose that there are N training samples represented by $\boldsymbol{X} = \left[\boldsymbol{X}^1 \ldots, \boldsymbol{X}^l \ldots, \boldsymbol{X}^C\right] \in \Re^{M\times N}$ belonging to C classes, where $N = N_1 + \cdots N_l + \cdots N_C$ and $X^l = \left[\boldsymbol{x}_1^l \ldots, \boldsymbol{x}_i^l, \ldots, \boldsymbol{x}_{N_l}^l\right] \in \Re^{M\times N_l}$ consists of N_l training samples of the l-th class with the i-th feature vector $\boldsymbol{x}_{\mathrm{i}}^{\mathrm{l}}$. In this study $C = 2$, but the proposed framework allows to include more classes such as MCI subjects. The SRC model can be summarized as [43]

1. Input: A matrix of training data $\mathbf{X} = \left[\boldsymbol{X}^1 \ldots, \boldsymbol{X}^l, \ldots, \boldsymbol{X}^C\right] \in \Re^{M\times N}$ for C classes with each column being a feature vector, a test sample represented by a column vector $\boldsymbol{y} \in \Re^M$, and an optional error tolerance $\varepsilon > 0$.
2. Normalize each column of $\mathbf{X}$ and the test sample $\boldsymbol{y}$ to have unit L_2 norm.
3. Compute the decomposition coefficient vector $\hat{\alpha}$ by solving the L_1-norm minimization problem by sparse coding

$$\hat{\alpha} = arg\ \min_\alpha \|\alpha\|_1, \quad \text{subject to} \quad \|\boldsymbol{X\alpha} - \boldsymbol{y}\|_2 \leq \varepsilon \tag{1.3}$$

4. For each test sample $\boldsymbol{y}$, compute the residual (i.e., the sparse reconstruction error) with the sparse coefficients $\hat{\alpha}^l$ associated with each class l

$$r_l(\boldsymbol{y}) = \left\|\boldsymbol{X}^l\hat{\alpha}^l - \boldsymbol{y}\right\|_2 \text{for}\, l = 1, \ldots, C \tag{1.4}$$

5. Output: The class label for the test sample $\boldsymbol{y}$ is assigned as the class with the minimum residual over all classes

$$\text{Label}\,(\boldsymbol{y}) = arg\ \min_l\ r_l(\boldsymbol{y}) \tag{1.5}$$

The L_1-norm minimization in Eq. (1.3) can be efficiently solved by using some L_1-regularized sparse coding methods such as those proposed in [65–68]. We can see that the classification of the test sample $\boldsymbol{y}$ depends on the residuals. There are two important terms in the above classification model. One is to characterize the signal sparsity by the L_1-norm constraint $\|\boldsymbol{\alpha}\|_1$. Another one is to characterize the signal fidelity by the L_2-norm term $\|\boldsymbol{X\alpha} - \boldsymbol{y}\|_2 \leq \varepsilon$ especially when the test sample $\boldsymbol{y}$ is noisy. Ideally, the sparse coefficients of $\|\boldsymbol{\alpha}\|_1$ are associated with the training samples from a single class so that the test sample can be easily assigned to that class. However, noise and modeling error may also lead to small nonzero sparse coefficients associated with multiple classes. Instead of classifying test sample based on the sparse coefficients, the classification made by Eq. (1.5) is based on how well the sparse coefficients associated with the training data in each class can reconstruct the test sample, which can better harness the subspace structure of each class. For each randomly sampled subspace, we construct a dictionary composed of all training samples to build an SRC. Finally, we get multiple SRCs based on different feature subspaces.

Ensemble of Weak Classifiers

The classifier ensemble is usually considered to be more accurate and robust than single classifier. Majority voting is one of the widely used methods for fusion of multiple classifiers. However, this method puts equal weight on the outputs of all weak classifiers for ensemble. In fact, the classifiers might have different confidences for a test sample. From Eq. (1.5), we know the classification of a test sample is performed in terms of the residuals with respective to the C classes, which also measures the similarity between the test sample and the training samples of each class. Smaller residual also indicates that the test sample is better approximated by the sparse representation of the training samples belonging to the corresponding class. We combine multiple weak classifiers by using the residuals instead of the class label output. In this way, if the residuals of a classifier corresponding to the C classes are close to each other, the classifier will have low contribution to the final ensemble, and vice versa. Suppose that we have K weak classifiers for final ensemble. Defining $r_l^k(\boldsymbol{y})$ as the residual of the test sample $\boldsymbol{y}$ obtained from the k-th weak classifier for the l-th class, the empirical average of the l-th residuals over the K classifiers can be calculated as follows

$$E_l(\mathbf{y}) = \frac{\sum_{k=1}^{K} r_l^k(\mathbf{y})}{K}. \quad (1.6)$$

Finally, the class label of test sample $\mathbf{y}$ can be assigned to the class with the minimum average residual

$$\text{Label}(\mathbf{y}) = arg\ \min_l E_l(\mathbf{y}) \quad (1.7)$$

Pattern Regression

In this section, we will discuss the pattern regression techniques for AD/MCI diagnosis and prognosis using M3T and SMRVR methods.

Multi-Modal Multi-Task Learning

A new learning method, namely M3T learning [69], is presented here to simultaneously learn multiple tasks from multi-modal data. It is worth noting that M3T is a general learning framework, and here we implement it through two successive major steps, i.e., (1) multi-task feature selection (MTFS) and (2) multi-modal SVM (for both regression and classification).

Multi-Task Feature Selection

For imaging modalities such as MRI and PET, even after feature extraction, the number of features (extracted from brain regions) may be still large. Besides, not all features are relevant to the disease under study. So, feature selection is commonly used for dimensionality reduction, as well as for removal of irrelevant features. Different from the conventional single-task feature selection, the MTFS simultaneously selects a common feature subset relevant to all tasks. This point is especially important for diagnosis of neurological diseases, since multiple regression/classification variables are essentially determined by the same underlying pathology, i.e., the diseased brain regions. Also, simultaneously performing feature selection for multiple regression/classification variables is very helpful to suppress noises in the individual variables.

Denote $\mathbf{X}^{(m)} = [\mathbf{x}_1^{(m)}, \ldots, \mathbf{x}_i^{(m)}, \ldots, \mathbf{x}_N^{(m)}]^T$ as the training data matrix on the m-th modality from N training samples, and $\mathbf{y}^{(j)} = [t_1^{(j)}, \ldots, t_i^{(j)}, \ldots, t_N^{(j)}]^T$ as the response vector on the j-th task from the same N training samples. Following the method proposed in [70], linear models are used to model the MTFS as below

$$\hat{t}^{(j)}\left(\mathbf{x}^{(m)}, \mathbf{v}_j^{(m)}\right) = \left(\mathbf{x}^{(m)}\right)^T \mathbf{v}_j^{(m)}, j = 1, \ldots, T; m = 1, \ldots, M \tag{1.8}$$

where $\mathbf{v}_j^{(m)}$ is the weight vector for the j-th task on the m-th modality, and $\mathbf{x}^{(m)}$ is the m-th modal data of a certain subject. The weight vectors for all T tasks form a weight matrix $\mathbf{V}^{(m)} = [\mathbf{v}_1^{(m)}, \ldots, \mathbf{v}_j^{(m)}, \ldots, \mathbf{v}_T^{(m)}]$, which can be optimized by the following objective function

$$\begin{aligned} \min_{\mathbf{V}^{(m)}} & \frac{1}{2}\sum_{j=1}^{T}\sum_{i=1}^{N}\left(t_i^{(j)} - \hat{t}^{(j)}\left(\mathbf{x}_i^{(m)}, \mathbf{v}_j^{(m)}\right)\right)^2 + \lambda\sum_{d=1}^{D^{(m)}}\|\mathbf{V}^{(m)}|_d\|_2 \\ &= \frac{1}{2}\sum_{j=1}^{T}\|\mathbf{y}^{(j)} - \mathbf{X}^{(m)}\mathbf{v}_j^{(m)}\|_2^2 + \lambda\sum_{d=1}^{D^{(m)}}\|\mathbf{V}^{(m)}|_d\|_2 \end{aligned} \tag{1.9}$$

where $\mathbf{V}^{(m)}|_d$ denotes the d-th row of $\mathbf{V}^{(m)}$, $D^{(m)}$ is the dimension of the m-th modal data, and λ is the regularization coefficient controlling the relative contributions of the two terms. Note that λ also controls the "sparsity" of the linear models, with the high value corresponding to more sparse models (i.e., more values in $\mathbf{V}^{(m)}$ are zero). It is easy to know that the above equation reduces to the standard l_1-norm regularized optimization problem in Lasso [71] when there is only one task. In our case, this is a multi-task learning for the given m-th modal data.

The key point of the above objective function of MTFS is the use of l_2-norm for $\mathbf{V}^{(m)}|_d$, which forces the weights corresponding to the d-th feature (of the m-th modal data) across multiple tasks to be grouped together and tends to select features based on the strength of T tasks jointly. Note that because of the characteristic of "group sparsity," the solution of MTFS results in a weight matrix $\mathbf{V}^{(m)}$ whose elements in some rows are all zeros. For feature selection, we just keep those features with nonzero weights. At present, there are many algorithms developed to solve MTFS; here, we adopt the SLEP toolbox [72], which has been shown very effective on many datasets.

Multi-Modal SVM

In our previous work [42], the multi-modal support vector classification (SVC) has been developed for multi-modal classification of AD and MCI. Following [41], in this paper, we derive the corresponding multi-modal support vector regression (SVR) algorithm as below. Assume that we have N training subjects with the corresponding target output $\{z_i \in \mathbb{R}, i = 1, \ldots, N\}$ and each subject has M modalities of data with the features selected by the above proposed method and denoted as $\mathbf{x}'_i = \{\mathbf{x}'^{(1)}_i, \ldots, \mathbf{x}'^{(m)}_i, \ldots, \mathbf{x}'^{(M)}_i\}$. Multi-modal SVR solves the following primal problem

$$\begin{aligned}
&\min_{\mathbf{w}^{(m)},b,\xi,\xi^*} \quad \frac{1}{2}\sum_{m=1}^{M}\beta_m\left\|\mathbf{w}^{(m)}\right\|^2 + C\sum_{i=1}^{N}\xi_i + C\sum_{i=1}^{N}\xi_i^* \\
&s.t.\ (1) \quad \sum\nolimits_{m=1}^{M}\beta_m\left(\left(\mathbf{w}^{(m)}\right)^T\phi^{(m)}\left(\mathbf{x}'^{(m)}_i\right)+b\right) - z_i \le \varepsilon + \xi_i; \\
&\qquad (2) \quad z_i - \sum\nolimits_{m=1}^{M}\beta_m\left(\left(\mathbf{w}^{(m)}\right)^T\phi^{(m)}\left(\mathbf{x}'^{(m)}_i\right)+b\right) \le \varepsilon + \xi_i^*; \\
&\qquad (3) \quad \xi_i, \xi_i^* \ge 0, i = 1, \ldots, N.
\end{aligned} \tag{1.10}$$

where $\mathbf{w}^{(m)}$, $\phi^{(m)}$, and $\beta_m \ge 0$ denote the normal vector of hyperplane, the kernel-induced mapping function, and the combining weight on the m-th modality, respectively. Here, we constrain $\sum_m \beta_m = 1$. The parameter b is the offset. Note that *ε-insensitive loss function* is used in the above objective function, and ξ and ξ^* are the two sets of slack variables.

Similar to the conventional SVR, the dual form of the multi-modal SVR can be represented as below

$$\begin{aligned}
\max_{\boldsymbol{\alpha},\boldsymbol{\alpha}^*} \quad & -\frac{1}{2}\sum_{i,j=1}^{N}\left(\alpha_i^* - \alpha_i\right)\left(\alpha_j^* - \alpha_j\right)\sum_{m=1}^{M}\beta_m k^{(m)}\left(\mathbf{x}'^{(m)}_i, \mathbf{x}'^{(m)}_j\right) \\
& - \varepsilon\sum_{i=1}^{N}\left(\alpha_i^* + \alpha_i\right) + \sum_{i=1}^{N}\left(\alpha_i^* - \alpha_i\right)z_i \\
s.t. \sum_{i=1}^{N}\left(\alpha_i - \alpha_i^*\right) = 0 & \quad \text{and} \quad 0 \le \alpha_i, \alpha_i^* \le C, i = 1, \ldots, N.
\end{aligned} \tag{1.11}$$

where $k^{(m)}(\mathbf{x}'^{(m)}_i, \mathbf{x}'^{(m)}_j) = [\phi^{(m)}(\mathbf{x}'^{(m)}_i)]^T\phi^{(m)}(\mathbf{x}'^{(m)}_j)$ is the kernel function for the two training samples on the m-th modality.

For a test sample with the selected features $\mathbf{x} = \{\mathbf{x}^{(1)}, \ldots, \mathbf{x}^{(m)}, \ldots, \mathbf{x}^{(M)}\}$, we denote $k^{(m)}(\mathbf{x}'^{(m)}_i, \mathbf{x}^{(m)}) = [\phi^{(m)}(\mathbf{x}'^{(m)}_i)]^T\phi^{(m)}(\mathbf{x}^{(m)})$ as the kernel between each training sample $\mathbf{x}'_i$ and the test sample on the m-th modality. Then, the regression function takes the following form

$$f(\mathbf{x}) = \sum_{i=1}^{N}\left(\alpha_i^* - \alpha_i\right)\sum_{m=1}^{M}\beta_m k^{(m)}\left(\mathbf{x}'^{(m)}_i, \mathbf{x}^{(m)}\right) + b \tag{1.12}$$

Similar to the multi-modal SVC, the multi-modal SVR can also be solved with the conventional SVR, e.g., through the LIBSVM toolbox, if we define the mixed kernel $k(\mathbf{x}'_i, \mathbf{x}'_j) = \sum_{m=1}^{M}\beta_m k^{(m)}(\mathbf{x}'^{(m)}_i, \mathbf{x}'^{(m)}_j)$ between multi-modal training samples $\mathbf{x}'_i$ and $\mathbf{x}'_j$, and $k(\mathbf{x}'_i, \mathbf{x}) = \sum_{m=1}^{M}\beta_m k^{(m)}(\mathbf{x}'^{(m)}_i, \mathbf{x}^{(m)})$ between multi-modal training sample $\mathbf{x}'_i$ and test sample $\mathbf{x}$. Here, β_ms are the nonnegative weight parameters used to balance the contributions of different modalities, and their values are optimized through a coarse-grid search by cross validation on the training samples.

After obtaining the common feature subset for all different tasks by MTFS as described above, we use multi-modal SVM, including multi-modal SVC and multi-modal SVR, to train the final SVC and regression models, respectively. Here, we train a model for each corresponding variable (task). Specifically, we train SVR models corresponding to the regression variables, and SVC models corresponding to the classification variable, respectively. It is worth noting that since we use the common subset of features (learned by MTFS during the feature selection stage) to train both regression and classification models, our models are actually performing the M3T.

Semi-Supervised Multi-modal Relevance Vector Regression

In this section, we will first extend the standard relevance vector regression (RVR) method to the multi-modal RVR (MRVR) and then introduce our proposed SMRVR method.

The main idea of RVR is summarized as follows. Specifically, RVR is a sparse kernel method formulated in a Bayesian framework [73]. Given a training set with its corresponding target values, such as $\{x_n,t_n\}_{n=1}^{N}$, RVR aims to find out the relationship between the input feature vector x and its corresponding target value t

$$t = f(x, \mathrm{w}) + \varepsilon \tag{1.13}$$

where ε is the measurement noise (assumed independent and following a zero-mean Gaussian distribution, $\varepsilon \sim N(0,\sigma^2)$, and $f(x,\mathrm{w})$ is a linear combination of basic functions $k(x,x_n)$ with the following form

$$f(x, \mathrm{w}) = \sum_{n=1}^{N} \mathrm{w}_n k(x, x_n) + \mathrm{w}_0 \tag{1.14}$$

where $\mathrm{w} = (\mathrm{w}_0,\mathrm{w}_1, \ldots,\mathrm{w}_N)^T$ is a weight vector. According to [73], we can obtain a sparse kernel regression model based on the weight vector w. Now we can extend RVR to MRVR for multi-modal regression by defining a new integrated kernel function for comparison of two multi-modal data x and x_n as below

$$k(x, x_n) = \sum_{m=1}^{M} c_m k^{(m)}\left(x^{(m)}, x_n^{(m)}\right) \tag{1.15}$$

where $k^{(m)}$ denotes the kernel matrix over the m-th modality, similar to the definition given above for the single modality case. This new integrated multiple-kernel can be expediently embedded into the conventional single-kernel RVR, and thus

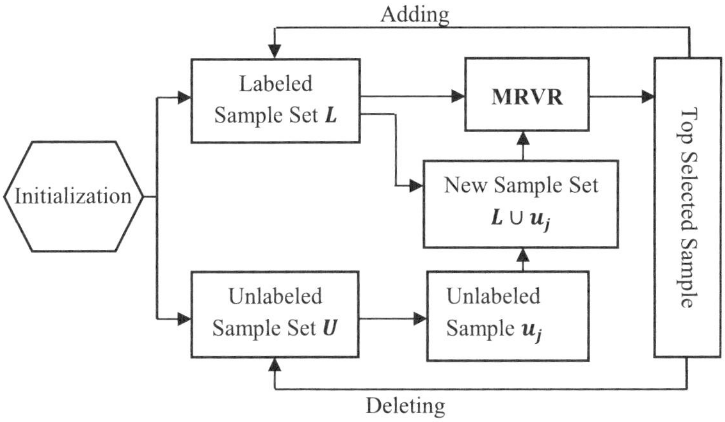

Fig. 1.3 The flowchart of selecting the most informative MCI subject

solved by the programs developed for the conventional single-kernel RVR. For c_m, we constrain $\sum_{m=1}^{M} c_m = 1$ and adopt a *coarse-grid search* through cross-validation on the training samples to find their optimal values.

The algorithmic procedure of SMRVR is detailed as below:

Step 1: Initialization of parameters (RVR kernel functions type, the nearest neighbors $\boldsymbol{k}$ used in KNN regression method, and the maximum number of iterations $\boldsymbol{T}$);

Step 2: For each modality data use k-nearest neighbor (KNN) regression method and current training set $\boldsymbol{L}$ of labeled sample [AD, Health controls (HC)] to estimate clinical scores of unlabeled MCI subjects $\boldsymbol{U}$; then average all estimated clinical scores (using all modality data) as the final clinical scores of unlabeled MCI subjects.

Step 3: For unlabeled MCI sample set $\boldsymbol{U}$, $\{(\boldsymbol{u}_j, t_j), j = 1, \ldots, u\}$ denote an unlabeled sample set with its corresponding target values. As shown in Fig. 1.3, we seek the most informative MCI subject and join it into $\boldsymbol{L}$. Specifically, for each sample $\{(\boldsymbol{u}_j, t_j), j = 1, \ldots, u\}$ in unlabeled MCI samples set $\boldsymbol{U}$, respectively, plus current training set $\boldsymbol{L}$, and train the MRVR with $\boldsymbol{L}$ as testing set. After that we compute the value of square root of mean square error (RMSE) for each sample $\boldsymbol{u}_j$. Finally, a sample with the top informative (i.e., minimum RMSE value) in $\boldsymbol{U}$ was selected and added into $\boldsymbol{L}$, and further deleted from $\boldsymbol{U}$.

Step 4: Go to Step 2 for running the next iteration;

Step 5: After reaching the maximum iterations $\boldsymbol{T}$, we can obtain the final MCI subsample set $\boldsymbol{U}'$, and use $\boldsymbol{L} \cup \boldsymbol{U}'$ as training set for training new MRVR.

Results

In this section, we will evaluate both machine learning-based classification and regression techniques (discussed above) for AD/MCI diagnosis and progression using single modality or multi-modality data.

Pattern Classification

Classification Using Cortical Morphological Change Patterns

Data used in the study were obtained from the Alzheimer's disease neuroimaging initiative (ADNI) database (http://adni.loni.ucla.edu). The ADNI was launched in 2003 by the National Institute on Aging (NIA), the National Institute of Biomedical Imaging and Bioengineering (NIBIB), the Food and Drug Administration (FDA), private pharmaceutical companies and nonprofit organizations, as a $60 million, 5-year public–private partnership. The primary goal of ADNI has been to test whether serial MRI, PET, other biological markers, and clinical and neuropsychological assessment can be combined to measure the progression of MCI and early AD. Determination of sensitive and specific markers of very early AD progression is intended to aid researchers and clinicians to develop new treatments and monitor their effectiveness, as well as lessen the time and cost of clinical trials. Readers are referred to www.adni-info.org for more information.

Five hundred and ninety-eight subjects who belong to one of the AD, MCI, or HC groups were analyzed in this study. These subjects were selected randomly for a ratio of AD vs. MCI vs. HC roughly as 1:1:1. All subjects received the baseline clinical/cognitive examinations including 1.5T structural MRI scan and were reevaluated at specified intervals (6 or 12 months). The baseline scans were used as the input data in our experiments. Table 1.1 shows the demographic information of the participants used in this study.

Table 1.1 Demographic information of the participants used in this study

	Diagnosis group		
Variables	HC	MCI	AD
Number of subjects (N)	200	200	198
Gender (M/F)	103/97	143/57	103/95
Age (mean ± SD)	75.8 ± 5.0	75.1 ± 7.1	75.7 ± 7.7
Education years (mean ± SD)	15.7 ± 3.6	15.5 ± 3.9	13.8 ± 4.8
Cognitive scores			
ADAS-Cog (mean ± SD)	6.1 ± 3.0	11.3 ± 4.4	17.3 ± 8.0
MMSE (mean ± SD)	28.6 ± 3.8	26.3 ± 4.1	21.8 ± 6.1
CDR (mean ± SD)	0 ± 0.1	0.4 ± 0.2	0.6 ± 0.5

HC health controls, *sMCI* stable MCI, *pMCI* progressive MCI, *AD* Alzheimer's disease

Table 1.2 Mean classification performance between integrated, correlative, and ROI-based features over 20 repetitions

AD vs. HC					
Features	ACC	p	SEN	SPE	AUC
Thickness	0.845	<0.0001	0.828	0.865	0.918
Volume	0.870	0.0002	0.852	0.897	0.936
Correlative	0.885	0.0002	0.846	0.917	0.954
Integrated	0.925	–	0.904	0.943	0.974
MCI vs. HC					
Feature	ACC	p	SEN	SPE	AUC
Thickness	0.749	<0.0001	0.733	0.764	0.830
Volume	0.770	<0.0001	0.746	0.793	0.853
Correlative	0.790	0.0001	0.757	0.823	0.886
Integrated	0.838	–	0.836	0.840	0.923

Thickness regional mean cortical thickness, *Volume* regional cortical volumes, *Correlative* correlative features, *Integrated* integration of the correlative and ROI-based features, *ACC* accuracy, *SEN* sensitivity, *SPE* specificity, *AUC* area under the ROC curve

The discriminative powers of the integrated and correlative morphological features were compared with three ROI-based features, i.e., regional mean cortical thickness and regional cortical volumes. The performance of the multi-kernel SVM using the integrated features was compared with the single-kernel SVMs using other feature types. For each comparison, performance of every compared method was validated through two different classification tasks: AD vs. HC and MCI vs. HC. The classification performance is summarized in Table 1.2.

It is clear that the regional mean cortical thickness performed the worst among all compared feature types in AD classification. However, when the correlative features were used, classification performance improved significantly. The proposed integrated morphological approach shows significantly better performance than all other feature types in all compared statistical measures. Promising classification results were achieved using the integrated features: 92.4 % (AUC = 0.974) and 83.8 % (AUC = 0.923) for AD and MCI classifications, respectively. High AUC value achieved indicates excellent diagnostic power and generalizability of the proposed framework to unseen dataset. In addition, our framework substantially improves the classification performance, particularly the sensitivity rate, compared to the ROI-based morphological feature-based classifiers. These results indicate that the proposed framework can be used to provide additional diagnostic information for early treatment of the disease. The provided p-values indicate how significant the integrated morphological features performed better than the other feature types in terms of classification accuracy for 20 repetitions.

Table 1.3 Demographic characteristics of the studied subjects from ADNI database (denoted as mean ± standard deviation)

Diagnosis	Number	Age	Gender (M/F)	MMSE
AD	198	75.7 ± 7.7	103/95	23.3 ± 2.0
HC	229	76.0 ± 5.0	119/110	29.1 ± 1.0

AD Alzheimer's disease, *HC* healthy control, *MMSE* mini-mental state examination

Ensemble Sparse Classification of Structural MR Images

We performed the experiments on the T1-weighted MR images of the baseline visit obtained from the ADNI database. MRI acquisition was done according to the ADNI acquisition protocol in [74]. The MR images from 427 ADNI subjects including 198 AD and 229 HC are used for evaluation. Table 1.3 presents a summary of the demographic characteristics of the studied population from the ADNI database. The processing of MR images was performed as described above, which included the correction of intensity inhomogeneity, skull-stripping, and cerebellum-removing. Furthermore, each MR image was segmented into three tissue types: GM, WM, and CSF, and was further spatially normalized into a template space by a mass-preserving registration framework [64]. After spatial normalization, the tissue density maps were smoothed using a Gaussian kernel to improve signal-to-noise ratio. Since GM density maps were more related to AD than white matter and CSF, we only used the GM density maps for classification in the experiments. For computational efficiency, we down-sampled the GM density maps as the classification features.

In the experiments, ten fold cross-validation is performed to evaluate the classification performance. For each time, one fold dataset is used for testing while the other folds are used for training. The training set can be split further into training part and validation part for parameter tuning. The final classification accuracy is the average of the classification accuracies across all ten cross-validation folds. In addition, we also compare the results with the SVM classifier that has been widely used for AD classification. In the experiments, the SVM classifier is implemented using LIBSVM toolbox [75], with a linear kernel and a default value set for the parameter C (i.e., C = 1).

Before we evaluate the ensemble classification performance, we test the performance using a single SRC in comparison with the SVM classifier. Both the SRC and SVM classifiers are tested on the selected voxel-wise features. To test the classification performances on varying number of relevant features, we perform the t-test on each voxel of the GM density maps. Then all voxels are ranked in ascending order according to their p-values of the t-test. Smaller p-value indicates larger group difference for the voxel-wise feature. We select different numbers of top ranked voxels in terms of p-values to construct feature vector as the inputs to SRC and SVM classifiers. The number of top ranked features varies from 200 to 24,000. Figure 1.4 shows the classification accuracies with respect to different numbers of top ranked features.

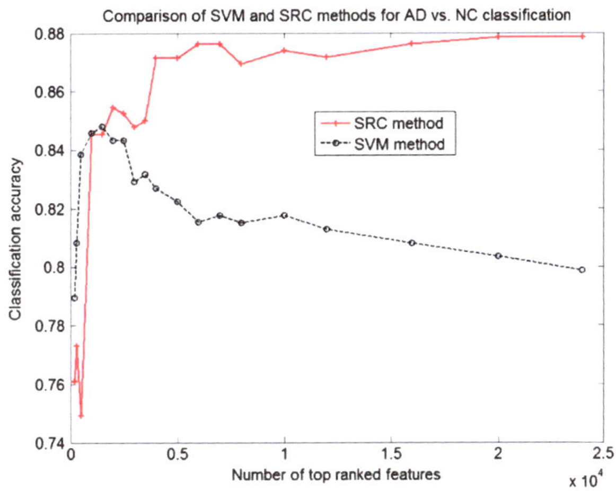

Fig. 1.4 Classification accuracies of SVM and SRC with respect to different numbers of top ranked features selected for AD classification

As can be seen from Fig. 1.4, SVM classifier performs better than the SRC method when the number of features is smaller than 1,500, but its performance degrades gradually and is inferior to SRC when the number of features is further increased beyond a certain number. In contrast, SRC can achieve better classification performance than SVM when more features are used. Since SVM classifier aims to maximize the discriminative power on the training data, the features with larger *p*-values will provide more irrelevant or noisy information which will reduce the discrimination capability. This explains why SVM achieves better performance with a relatively small number of top ranked features. On the other hand, SRC is based on combining the sparsity and reconstruction via sparse representation and thus can achieve high robustness to noisy features due to its reconstruction property. In general, to make the L_1-norm sparse coding computationally feasible, the feature dimensionality should be reduced to a subset of features. However, our experimental results show that SRC method continues to perform well when the feature dimensionality increases.

Next, we tested the random patch-based subspace ensemble classification framework with both SRC and SVM classifiers to construct the weak classifier. In general, there are three important parameters that are required to determine and affect the ensemble performance, which are, respectively, the patch size, the sampling rate (i.e., the ratio of sampled patches to the cardinality of patch pool), and the ensemble size (i.e., the number of weak classifiers for the final ensemble). In practice, these three parameters (i.e., patch size, sampling rate, and ensemble size) can be optimized in each fold with the training dataset to run the random patch-based subspace ensemble classification algorithm. Based on our experimental analysis, the effect of ensemble performance by the ensemble size is small if the number of weak classifiers is larger than 15. For simplicity, the ensemble size is

Table 1.4 Comparison of AD classification by five different classification methods

Methods	ACC	SEN	SPE	AUC
COMPARE	0.811	0.788	0.829	0.877
SVM	0.846	0.728	0.948	0.914
SRC	0.878	0.808	0.939	0.938
RPSE_SVM	0.855	0.755	0.942	0.924
RPSE_SRC	0.908	0.863	0.948	0.949

ACC ACCuracy, *SEN* SENsitivity, *SPE* SPEcificity, *AUC* Area Under the ROC curve

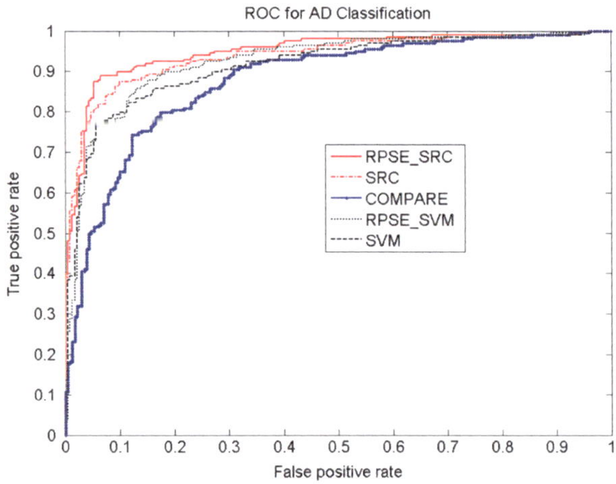

Fig. 1.5 ROC curves of five different methods for AD classification

fixed to 17 in our experiments. The other two parameters are optimized with the training dataset. Since the ensemble of different weak classifiers may produce different classification results, the ensemble classification accuracy is computed by averaging the accuracies of multiple independent runs (20 in our experiments). We also run the COMPARE algorithm [39] on the same dataset for comparison, by using its suggested parameters. Table 1.4 gives the comparison of AD classification in five different classification methods, which are COMPARE, single SVM classifier (SVM), single SRC classifier (SRC), random patch-based SVM ensemble (RPSE_SVM), and random patch-based SRC ensemble (RPSE_SRC), respectively. For single SVM and SRC classifiers, we report their best classification results in Table 1.4 among those on the different numbers of features selected by t-test as shown in Fig. 1.4. The ROC curves of these methods are shown in Fig. 1.5. We can see that single SRC method performs better than COMPARE and both single and ensemble SVM methods. Our method, RPSE_SRC, can further improve the classification accuracy by ensemble of multiple weak classifiers.

Table 1.5 Demographics of all used subjects

	AD ($N = 45$)	HC ($N = 50$)	MCI-C ($N = 43$)	MCI-NC ($N = 48$)
Female/male	16/29	18/32	15/28	16/32
Age	75.4 ± 7.1	75.3 ± 5.2	75.8 ±6.8	74.7 ± 7.7
Education	14.9 ± 3.4	15.6 ± 3.2	16.1 ±2.6	16.1 ± 3.0
MMSE (baseline)	23.8 ± 1.9	29.0 ± 1.2	26.6 ±1.7	27.5 ± 1.6
MMSE (2 years)	19.3 ± 5.6	29.0 ± 1.3	23.8 ±3.3	26.9 ± 2.6
ADAS-Cog (baseline)	18.3 ± 6.1	7.3 ± 3.3	12.9 ±3.9	9.7 ± 4.0
ADAS-Cog (2 years)	27.3 ± 11.7	6.3 ± 3.5	16.1 ±6.4	11.2 ± 5.7

AD Alzheimer's disease, *HC* healthy control, *MCI* mild cognitive impairment, *MCI-C* MCI converter, *MCI-NC* MCI non-converter, *MMSE* mini-mental state examination, *ADAS-Cog* Alzheimer's disease assessment scale-cognitive subscale

Table 1.6 Comparison of performances of five different methods on experiment 1

	Correlation coefficient		Classification accuracy	
Methods	MMSE	ADAS-Cog	AD vs. HC	MCI vs. HC
MRI-based	0.504 ± 0.038	0.609 ± 0.014	0.848 ± 0.026	0.739 ± 0.028
PET-based	0.658 ± 0.027	0.670 ± 0.018	0.845 ± 0.035	0.797 ± 0.023
CSF-based	0.465 ± 0.019	0.474 ± 0.013	0.805 ± 0.022	0.536 ± 0.044
CONCAT	0.658 ± 0.023	0.695 ± 0.011	0.920 ± 0.033	0.800 ± 0.024
Proposed M3T	0.697 ± 0.022	0.739 ± 0.012	0.933 ± 0.022	0.832 ± 0.015

The reported values are the correlation coefficient (for MMSE and ADAS-Cog regression) and accuracy (for AD vs. HC and MCI vs. HC classification), averaged on tenfold tests (with standard deviation also reported)

Pattern Regression

Multi-Modal Multi-Task Learning

In the following experiments, 186 ADNI subjects with all corresponding baseline MRI, PET, and CSF data are included. In particular, it contains 45 AD patients, 91 MCI patients [including 43 MCI converters (MCI-C) and 48 MCI non-converters (MCI-NC)], and 50 healthy controls. Table 1.5 lists the demographics of all these subjects.

Experiment 1: Estimating Clinical Stages (MMSE, ADAS-Cog, and Class Label)

We first estimate the clinical stages, including two regression variables (MMSE and ADAS-Cog) and one classification variable (i.e., class label with a value of "AD," "MCI," or "HC"), from the baseline MRI, PET, and CSF data. It is worth noting that the original multi-class classification problem is formulated as two binary classification problems, i.e., AD vs. HC and MCI vs. HC, as mentioned above. Table 1.6 shows the performances of the proposed M3T method, compared with three methods each using individual modality, as well as the CONCAT method (as detailed below). Specifically, in Table 1.6, MRI-, PET-, and CSF-based methods denote the classification results using only the respective individual modality of data. For MRI-based and PET-based methods, similarly as our M3T method, they contain two successive steps, i.e., (1) the single-task feature selection method using Lasso [71] and (2) the standard SVM for both regression and classification. For CSF-based method, it uses the original three features without any further feature selection and performs the standard SVM for both regression and classification. For comparison, we also implement a simple concatenation method (denoted as CONCAT) for using multi-modal data. In the CONCAT method, we first concatenate 93 features from MRI, 93 features from PET, and 3 features from CSF into a 189-dimensional vector, and then perform the same two steps (i.e., Lasso feature selection and SVM regression/classification) as in MRI-, PET-, and CSF-based methods. It is worth noting that the same experimental settings are used in all five methods as compared in Table 1.6.

As can be seen from Table 1.6, our proposed M3T method consistently achieves better performance than other four methods. Specifically, for estimating MMSE and ADAS-Cog scores, our method achieves the correlation coefficients of 0.697 and 0.739, respectively, while the best performance using individual modality is only 0.658 and 0.670 (when using PET), respectively. On the other hand, for AD vs. HC and MCI vs. HC classification, our method achieves the accuracies of 0.933 and 0.832, respectively, while the best performance using individual modality is only 0.848 (when using MRI) and 0.797 (when using PET), respectively. Table 1.6 also indicates that our proposed M3T method consistently outperforms the CONCAT method on each performance measure, although the latter also achieves better performance than three MRI-, PET-, or CSF-based methods in most cases, because of using multi-modal imaging data. However, CSF-based method always achieves the worst performances in all tasks and is significantly inferior to MRI- and PET-based methods in this experiment. Finally, for each group (i.e., AD, MCI or HC), we compute its average estimated clinical scores using M3T, with respective values of 24.8 (AD), 25.5 (MCI), and 28.1 (HC) for MMSE, and 14.9 (AD), 13.3 (MCI), and 8.3 (HC) for ADAS-Cog. These results show certain consistency with the actual clinical scores as shown in Table 1.5.

Experiment 2: Predicting 2-Year MMSE and ADAS-Cog Changes

In this experiment, we predict the 2-year changes of MMSE and ADAS-Cog scores and the conversion of MCI to AD, from the baseline MRI, PET, and CSF data. Here, we have two regression tasks corresponding to the prediction of the regression variables of MMSE and ADAS-Cog changes from baseline to 2-year follow-up, respectively, and one classification task corresponding to prediction of the classification variable of MCI conversion to AD, i.e., MCI-C vs. MCI-NC. It is worth noting that as in Experiment 1, only the baseline MRI, PET, and CSF data are used for all prediction tasks. We use the same subjects as in Experiment 1, except

Table 1.7 Comparison of performances of five different methods on experiment 2

Methods	(a) Correlation coefficient		(b) MCI-C vs. MCI-NC		
	MMSE change	ADAS-Cog change	Accuracy	Sensitivity	Specificity
MRI-based	0.419 ± 0.019	0.455 ± 0.037	0.620 ± 0.058	0.566 ± 0.069	0.602 ± 0.056
PET-based	0.434 ± 0.027	0.401 ± 0.046	0.639 ± 0.046	0.570 ± 0.067	0.623 ± 0.069
CSF-based	0.327 ± 0.018	0.425 ± 0.028	0.518 ± 0.086	0.454 ± 0.094	0.493 ± 0.089
CONCAT	0.484 ± 0.009	0.475 ± 0.045	0.654 ± 0.050	0.573 ± 0.062	0.651 ± 0.064
Proposed M3T	0.511 ± 0.021	0.531 ± 0.032	0.739 ± 0.038	0.686 ± 0.051	0.736 ± 0.045

The reported values are the correlation coefficient [for regressions of MMSE and ADAS-Cog change (a)] and accuracy, sensitivity and specificity [for MCI-C vs. MCI-NC classification (b)], averaged on tenfold tests (with standard deviation also reported)

for 19 subjects without 2-year MMSE or ADAS-Cog scores, thus reducing to totally 167 subjects with 40 AD, 80 MCI (38 MCI-C and 42 MCI-NC), and 47 HC that are finally used in Experiment 2. Table 1.7 shows the performance of the proposed M3T method compared with three individual-modality based methods and also the CONCAT method, which are the same methods as those used in Experiment 1. Here, for MCI-C vs. MCI-NC classification, besides reporting the classification accuracy, we also give other performance measures including sensitivity (i.e., the proportion of MCI-C subjects correctly classified) and the specificity (i.e., the proportion of MCI-NC subjects correctly classified).

Table 1.7 shows that, as in Experiment 1, M3T also consistently outperforms the individual-modality based methods and the CONCAT method, on both regression and classification tasks. Specifically, our method achieves the correlation coefficients of 0.511 and 0.531 and the accuracy of 0.739, for predicting the 2-year changes of MMSE and ADAS-Cog scores and the MCI conversion, respectively, while the best performance of individual-modality based methods are 0.434 (when using PET), 0.455 (when using MRI), and 0.639 (when using PET), respectively. In addition, the area under the ROC curve (AUC) is 0.797 for MCI-C vs. MCI-NC classification with our M3T method, while the best AUC using the individual-modality based method is 0.70 (when using PET) and the AUC of the CONCAT method is 0.729. On the other hand, if comparing Table 1.7 with Table 1.6, we can see that there is a significant decline in the corresponding performances. It implies that predicting future MMSE and ADAS-Cog changes and the MCI conversion is much more difficult and challenging than estimating the MMSE and ADAS scores and the class labels.

Semi-Supervised Multi-modality Regression

The ADNI dataset is used to test our semi-supervised regression method. Only the baseline ADNI subjects with all corresponding MRI, PET, and CSF data are

Table 1.8 Subject information (mean ± std)

	AD	MCI	HC
Number of subjects	51	99	52
Age	75.2 ± 7.4	75.3 ± 7.0	75.3 ± 5.2
Education	14.7 ± 3.6	15.9 ± 2.9	15.8 ± 3.2
MMSE	23.8 ± 1.9	27.1 ± 1.7	29.0 ± 1.2
ADAS-Cog	18.3 ± 6.0	11.4 ± 4.4	7.4 ± 3.2

AD Alzheimer's disease, *HC* healthy control, *MCI* mild cognitive impairment, *MMSE* mini-mental state examination, *ADAS-Cog* Alzheimer's disease assessment scale-cognitive subscale

included, thus leading to a total of 202 subjects (including 51 AD patients, 99 MCI patients, and 52 HC). Table 1.8 lists the demographics of these subjects. Image pre-processing is same as literature [41].

To evaluate the performance of regression methods, we use both a square RMSE and correlation coefficient (CORR) as performance measures. We use a tenfold cross-validation strategy to compute the average RMSE and CORR measures. The RVM regression learning machine is implemented using Sparse Bayesian toolbox,[1] with Gauss kernel and default kernel-width. Iterations $\boldsymbol{T}$ $(1 \leq \boldsymbol{T} \leq 99)$ and the number of nearest neighbor $\boldsymbol{k}$ $(1 \leq \boldsymbol{k} \leq 20)$ are learned based on the training samples by leave-10-out cross validation. The weights in the MRVR are learned based on the training samples, through a grid search using the range from 0 to 1 at a step size of 0.1. For each feature f_i in the training samples, a common feature normalization scheme was adopted, i.e., $f_i = \left(f_i - \overline{f_i}\right)/\sigma_i$, where $\overline{f_i}$ and σ_i are, respectively, the mean and standard deviation of the i-th feature across all training samples. The estimated $\overline{f_i}$ and σ_i will be used to normalize the corresponding feature of each test sample.

Table 1.9 shows the performance measures (including RMSE and CORR) of our SMRVR method, using different combinations of MRI, PET, and CSF modalities. As we can see from Table 1.9, the combination of MRI, PET, and CSF can consistently achieve better results than any other methods. Specifically, SM-RVR using all three modalities can achieve an RMSE of 1.919 and a CORR of 0.801 for MMSE scores, and an RMSE of 4.448 and a CORR of 0.782 for ADAS-Cog scores, as shown in Fig. 1.6 which give the scatterplots of actual clinical scores vs. predicted scores. On the other hand, Table 1.9 also indicates that the use of two modalities can improve the regression performance, although they are inferior to the use of all three modalities together. These results validate the advantage of multi-modal regression over the conventional single-modal regression in estimation of clinical scores.

Table 1.10 shows the comparison of SMRVR with supervised multi-modal relevance vector regression (MRVR). It is worth noting that, for fair comparison, we implement two versions of MRVR, i.e., one using only AD and HC subjects as

[1] http://www.miketipping.com/index.php?page=rvm

Table 1.9 Regression performance of SMRVR with respect to different combination of MRI, PET and CSF modalities

	MMSE		ADAS-Cog	
Modality	RMSE	CORR	RMSE	CORR
MRI	2.171	0.731	5.157	0.700
PET	2.461	0.618	5.041	0.706
CSF	2.449	0.600	5.617	0.641
MRI + PET	2.095	0.755	4.732	0.762
MRI + CSF	2.032	0.771	4.982	0.738
PET + CSF	2.383	0.663	4.891	0.734
MRI + PET + CSF	1.919	0.801	4.448	0.782

MMSE mini-mental state examination, *ADAS-Cog* Alzheimer's disease assessment scale-cognitive subscale, *RMSE* root mean square error, *CORR* correlation coefficient

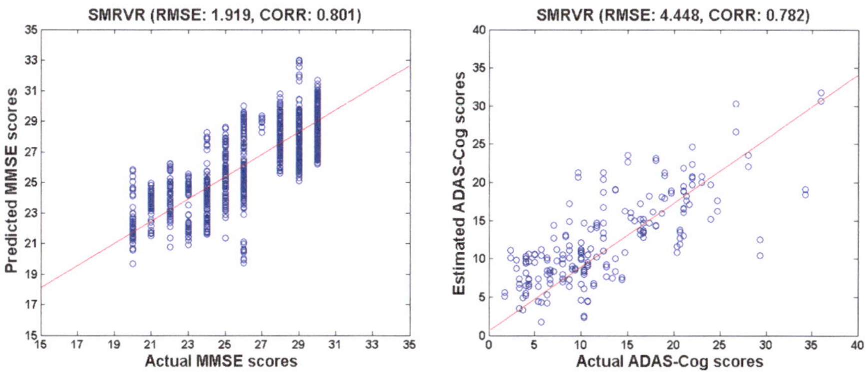

Fig. 1.6 Scatterplots of actual clinical scores vs. predicted scores for MMSE (*left*) and ADAS-Cog (*right*) (*MMSE* mini-mental state examination, *ADAS-Cog* Alzheimer's disease assessment scale-cognitive subscale, *RMSE* root mean square error, *CORR* correlation coefficient)

Table 1.10 Comparison of regression performance of SMRVR and MRVR

	MMSE		ADAS-Cog	
Methods	RMSE	CORR	RMSE	CORR
MRVR (51 AD + 52HC)	2.216	0.729	4.917	0.733
MRVR (51 AD + 52HC + 99MCI)	2.170	0.526	4.691	0.640
SMRVR(51 AD + 52HC + 99MCI)	1.919	0.801	4.448	0.782

MMSE mini-mental state examination, *ADAS-Cog* Alzheimer's disease assessment scale-cognitive subscale, *RMSE* root mean square error, *CORR* correlation coefficient

training sample and another using all (AD, HC and MCI) subjects as training samples. As can be seen from Table 1.10, SMRVR consistently outperforms MRVR (including both versions) on each performance measure, which validates the efficacy of our SMRVR method that uses MCI subjects only as unlabeled samples in a semi-supervised regression framework. Also, from Table 1.10, it is interesting to note that MRVR using all subjects achieves slightly better performance in terms of RMSE, but much worse performance in terms of CORR, compared with MRVR using only AD and HC subjects. This implies that the clinical scores of MCI subjects may contain more noise than those of AD or HC subjects.

Summary

In the past two decades, machine learning techniques have been proven to be important for effective neurodegenerative disorders diagnosis and progression, particularly for AD and MCI. Essentially, machine learning techniques that have been applied for AD and MCI diagnosis and prognosis can be categorized into classification and regression-based approaches. Some recent developments in this area have been discussed in this chapter. Specifically, in pattern classification approaches, we first extracted the ROI-based features (i.e., GM and WM volumes, and regional mean cortical thickness) from the subject's MR volumes and then constructed the correlative features from the regional mean cortical thickness. These ROI-based features and correlative morphological features are finally integrated via a multi-kernel SVM for AD and MCI prediction. Then, a random patch-based subspace ensemble classification method is proposed for AD and MCI prediction. For pattern regression approaches, M3T learning can effectively estimate the MMSE and ADAS-Cog scores and also the classification label in both AD vs. HC and MCI vs. HC classifications, and it can further predict the 2-year MMSE and ADAS-Cog changes and the classification label in MCI-C vs. MCI-NC classification. On the other hand, SMRVR is used to predict clinical scores of subjects (including AD, HC or MCI) from both imaging and biological biomarkers, i.e., MRI, PET, and CSF. The experimental results on the ADNI dataset show the efficacy of all these proposed methods.

References

1. Brookmeyer R, Johnson E, Ziegler-Graham K, Arrighi HM (2007) Forecasting the global burden of Alzheimer's disease. Alzheimers Dement 3:186–191
2. Johnson SC, Schmitz TW, Moritz CH, Meyerand ME, Rowley HA, Alexander AL, Hansen KW, Gleason CE, Carlsson CM, Ries ML, Asthana S, Chen K, Reiman EM, Alexander GE (2006) Activation of brain regions vulnerable to Alzheimer's disease: the effect of mild cognitive impairment. Neurobiol Aging 27:1604–1612
3. Thompson PM, Apostolova LG (2007) Computational anatomical methods as applied to ageing and dementia. Br J Radiol 80:S78–S91
4. Whitwell JL, Przybelski SA, Weigand SD, Knopman DS, Boeve BF, Petersen RC, Jack CR Jr (2007) 3D maps from multiple MRI illustrate changing atrophy patterns as subjects progress from mild cognitive impairment to Alzheimer's disease. Brain 130:1777–1786

5. Grundman M, Petersen RC, Ferris SH, Thomas RG, Aisen PS, Bennett DA (2004) Mild cognitive impairment can be distinguished from Alzheimer's disease and normal aging for clinical trials. Arch Neurol 61:59–66
6. Bischkopf J, Busse A, Angermeyer MC (2002) Mild cognitive impairment - a review of prevalence, incidence and outcome according to current approaches. Acta Psychiatr Scand 106:403–414
7. de Leon MJ, Mosconi L, Li J, De Santi S, Yao Y, Tsui WH, Pirraglia E, Rich K, Javier E, Brys M, Glodzik L, Switalski R, Saint Louis LA, Pratico D (2007) Longitudinal CSF isoprostane and MRI atrophy in the progression to AD. J Neurol 254:1666–1675
8. Fjell AM, Walhovd KB, Fennema-Notestine C, McEvoy LK, Hagler DJ, Holland D, Brewer JB, Dale AM (2010) CSF biomarkers in prediction of cerebral and clinical change in mild cognitive impairment and Alzheimer's disease. Neurobiol Dis 30:2088–2101
9. Du AT, Schuff N, Kramer JH, Rosen HJ, Gorno-Tempini ML, Rankin K, Miller BL, Weiner MW (2007) Different regional patterns of cortical thinning in Alzheimer's disease and frontotemporal dementia. Brain 130:1159–1166
10. McEvoy LK, Fennema-Notestine C, Roddey JC, Hagler DJ Jr, Holland D, Karow DS, Pung CJ, Brewer JB, Dale AM (2009) Alzheimer disease: quantitative structural neuroimaging for detection and prediction of clinical and structural changes in mild cognitive impairment. Radiology 251:195–205
11. De Santi S, de Leon MJ, Rusinek H, Convit A, Tarshish CY, Roche A, Tsui WH, Kandil E, Boppana M, Daisley K, Wang GJ, Schlyer D, Fowler J (2001) Hippocampal formation glucose metabolism and volume losses in MCI and AD. Neurobiol Aging 22:529–539
12. Morris JC, Storandt M, Miller JP, McKeel DW, Price JL, Rubin EH, Berg L (2001) Mild cognitive impairment represents early-stage Alzheimer disease. Arch Neurol 58:397–405
13. Shaw LM, Vanderstichele H, Knapik-Czajka M, Clark CM, Aisen PS, Petersen RC, Blennow K, Soares H, Simon A, Lewczuk P, Dean R, Siemers E, Potter W, Lee VM, Trojanowski JQ (2009) Cerebrospinal fluid biomarker signature in Alzheimer's disease neuroimaging initiative subjects. Ann Neurol 65:403–413
14. Mattsson N, Zetterberg H, Hansson O, Andreasen N, Parnetti L, Jonsson M, Herukka SK, van der Flier WM, Blankenstein MA, Ewers M, Rich K, Kaiser E, Verbeek M, Tsolaki M, Mulugeta E, Rosen E, Aarsland D, Visser PJ, Schroder J, Marcusson J, de Leon M, Hampel H, Scheltens P, Pirttila T, Wallin A, Jonhagen ME, Minthon L, Winblad B, Blennow K (2009) CSF biomarkers and incipient Alzheimer disease in patients with mild cognitive impairment. JAMA 302:385–393
15. Bouwman FH, van der Flier WM, Schoonenboom NS, van Elk EJ, Kok A, Rijmen F, Blankenstein MA, Scheltens P (2007) Longitudinal changes of CSF biomarkers in memory clinic patients. Neurology 69:1006–1011
16. Westman E, Simmons A, Zhang Y, Muehlboeck J-S, Tunnard C, Liu Y, Collins L, Evans A, Mecocci P, Vellas B, Tsolaki M, Kloszewska I, Soininen H, Lovestone S, Spenger C, Wahlund L-O (2010) AddNeuroMed consortium: multivariate analysis of MRI data for Alzheimer's disease, mild cognitive impairment and healthy controls. Neuroimage 54:1178–1187
17. Fan Y, Batmanghelich N, Clark CM, Davatzikos C (2008) The Alzheimer's disease neuroimaging initiative: spatial patterns of brain atrophy in MCI patients, identified via high-dimensional pattern classification, predict subsequent cognitive decline. Neuroimage 39:1731–1743
18. Lao Z, Shen D, Xue Z, Karacali B, Resnick SM, Davatzikos C (2004) Morphological classification of brains via high-dimensional shape transformations and machine learning methods. Neuroimage 21:46–57
19. Chetelat G, Baron JC (2003) Early diagnosis of Alzheimer's disease: contribution of structural neuroimaging. Neuroimage 18:525–541
20. Jack CR Jr, Petersen RC, Xu YC, O'Brien PC, Smith GE, Ivnik RJ, Tangalos EG, Kokmen E (1998) Rate of medial temporal lobe atrophy in typical aging and Alzheimer's disease. Neurology 51:993–999

21. Thompson PM, Hayashi KM, Sowell ER, Gogtay N, Giedd JN, Rapoport JL, de Zubicaray GI, Janke AL, Rose SE, Semple J, Doddrell DM, Wang Y, van Erp TG, Cannon TD, Toga AW (2004) Mapping cortical change in Alzheimer's disease, brain development, and schizophrenia. Neurobiol Dis 23:S2–S18
22. Dickerson BC, Bakkour A, Salat DH, Feczko E, Pacheco J, Greve DN, Grodstein F, Wright CI, Blacker D, Rosas HD, Sperling RA, Atri A, Growdon JH, Hyman BT, Morris JC, Fischl B, Buckner RL (2009) The cortical signature of Alzheimer's disease: regionally specific cortical thinning relates to symptom severity in very mild to mild AD dementia and is detectable in asymptomatic amyloid-positive individuals. Cereb Cortex 19:497–510
23. Thompson PM, Mega MS, Woods RP, Zoumalan CI, Lindshield CJ, Blanton RE, Moussai J, Holmes CJ, Cummings JL, Toga AW (2001) Cortical changes in Alzheimer's disease detected with a disease-specific population-based brain atlas. Cereb Cortex 11:1–16
24. Chupin M, Gerardin E, Cuingnet R, Boutet C, Lemieux L, Lehericy S, Benali H, Garnero L, Colliot O (2009) Alzheimer's disease neuroimaging initiative: fully automatic hippocampus segmentation and classification in Alzheimer's disease and mild cognitive impairment applied on data from ADNI. Hippocampus 19:579–587
25. Colliot O, Chetelat G, Chupin M, Desgranges B, Magnin B, Benali H, Dubois B, Garnero L, Eustache F, Lehericy S (2008) Discrimination between Alzheimer disease, mild cognitive impairment, and normal aging by using automated segmentation of the hippocampus. Radiology 248:194–201
26. Diehl J, Grimmer T, Drzezga A, Riemenschneider M, Forstla H, Kurz A (2004) Cerebral metabolic patterns at early stages of frontotemporal dementia and semantic dementia. A PET study. Neurobiol Aging 25:1051–1056
27. Wang Y, Fan Y, Bhatt P, Davatzikos C (2010) High-dimensional pattern regression using machine learning: from medical images to continuous clinical variables. Neuroimage 50:1519–1535
28. Duchesne S, Caroli A, Geroldi C, Frisoni G, Collins D (2005) Predicting clinical variable from MRI features: application to MMSE in MCI. Medical Image Computing and Computer-Assisted Intervention (MICCAI 2005) Lecture notes in computer science, Volume 3749: 392–399
29. Duchesne S, Caroli A, Geroldi C, Collins DL, Frisoni GB (2009) Relating one-year cognitive change in mild cognitive impairment to baseline MRI features. Neuroimage 47:1363–1370
30. Stonnington CM, Chu C, Kloppel S, Jack CR Jr, Ashburner J, Frackowiak RS (2010) Predicting clinical scores from magnetic resonance scans in Alzheimer's disease. Neuroimage 51:1405–1413
31. Fan Y, Kaufer D, Shen D (2010) Joint estimation of multiple clinical variables of neurological diseases from imaging patterns. In Proceedings of 2010 IEEE international symposium on biomedical imaging: from nano to macro (ISBI 2010), 852–855
32. Davatzikos C, Bhatt P, Shaw LM, Batmanghelich KN, Trojanowski JQ (2011) Prediction of MCI to AD conversion, via MRI, CSF biomarkers, and pattern classification. Neurobiol Aging 32:2322.e19–27
33. Davatzikos C, Fan Y, Wu X, Shen D, Resnick SM (2008) Detection of prodromal Alzheimer's disease via pattern classification of magnetic resonance imaging. Neurobiol Aging 29:514–523
34. Vemuri P, Wiste HJ, Weigand SD, Shaw LM, Trojanowski JQ, Weiner MW, Knopman DS, Petersen RC, Jack JCR (2009) On behalf of the Alzheimer's disease neuroimaging initiative: MRI and CSF biomarkers in normal, MCI, and AD subjects: predicting future clinical change. Neurology 73:294–301
35. Kloppel S, Stonnington CM, Chu C, Draganski B, Scahill RI, Rohrer JD, Fox NC, Jack CR Jr, Ashburner J, Frackowiak RSJ (2008) Automatic classification of MR scans in Alzheimer's disease. Brain 131:681–689
36. Fan Y, Gur RE, Gur RC, Wu X, Shen D, Calkins ME, Davatzikos C (2008) Unaffected family members and Schizophrenia patients share brain structure patterns: a high-dimensional pattern classification study. Biol Psychiatry 63:118–124

37. Fan Y, Resnick SM, Wu X, Davatzikos C (2008) Structural and functional biomarkers of prodromal Alzheimer's disease: a high-dimensional pattern classification study. Neuroimage 41:277–285
38. Vemuri P, Gunter JL, Senjem ML, Whitwell JL, Kantarci K, Knopman DS, Boeve BF, Petersen RC, Jack CR Jr (2008) Alzheimer's disease diagnosis in individual subjects using structural MR images: validation studies. Neuroimage 39:1186–1197
39. Fan Y, Shen D, Gur RC, Gur RE, Davatzikos C (2007) COMPARE: classification of morphological patterns using adaptive regional elements. IEEE Trans Med Imaging 26:93–105
40. Davatzikos C, Resnick SM, Wu X, Parmpi P, Clark CM (2008) Individual patient diagnosis of AD and FTD via high-dimensional pattern classification of MRI. Neuroimage 41:1220–1227
41. Zhang D, Wang Y, Zhou L, Yuan H, Shen D (2011) The Alzheimer's Disease Neuroimaging Initiative: Multimodal classification of Alzheimer's disease and mild cognitive impairment. Neuroimage 55:856–867
42. Magnin B, Mesrob L, Kinkingnehun S, Pelegrini-Issac M, Colliot O, Sarazin M, Dubois B, Lehericy S, Benali H (2009) Support vector machine-based classification of Alzheimer's disease from whole-brain anatomical MRI. Neuroradiology 51:73–83
43. Wright J, Yang AY, Ganesh A, Sastry SS, Ma Y (2009) Robust face recognition via sparse representation. IEEE Trans Pattern Anal Mach Intell 31:210–227
44. Majumdar A, Ward RK (2009) Fast group sparse classification. Can J Electr Comput Eng 34:136–144
45. Huang K, Aviyente S (2007) Sparse representation for signal classification. Adv Neural Inf Process Syst 19:609–612
46. Chu C, Kloppel SS, Draganski CSB, Jack C Jr, Ashburner J, Frackowiak RSJ (2007) Regression analysis for clinical scores of Alzheimer's disease using multivariate machine learning method. Hum Brain Mapp Poster, Chicago, IL, USA
47. Fan Y, Kaufer D, Shen D (2009) Estimating clinical variables from brain images using Bayesian regression. Alzheimer & Dementia 5:372
48. Franke K, Ziegler G, Kloppel S, Gaser C (2010) Estimating the age of healthy subjects from T1-weighted MRI scans using kernel methods: exploring the influence of various parameters. Neuroimage 50:883–892
49. Ashburner J (2007) A fast diffeomorphic image registration algorithm. Neuroimage 38:95–113
50. Folstein MF, Folstein SE, McHugh PR (1975) Mini-mental state. A practical method for grading the cognitive state of patients for the clinician. J Psychiatr Res 12:189–198
51. Rosen WG, Mohs RC, Davis KL (1984) A new rating scale for Alzheimer's disease. Am J Psychiatr 141:1356–1364
52. Desikan RS, Segonne F, Fischl B, Quinn BT, Dickerson BC, Blacker D, Buckner RL, Dale AM, Maguire RP, Hyman BT, Albert MS, Killiany RJ (2006) An automated labeling system for subdividing the human cerebral cortex on MRI scans into gyral based regions of interest. Neuroimage 31:968–980
53. He Y, Chen ZJ, Evans AC (2008) Structural insights into aberrant topological patterns of large-scale cortical networks in Alzheimer's disease. Neurobiol Dis 28:4756–4766
54. Stam CJ, Jones BF, Nolte G, Breakspear M, Scheltens P (2007) Small-world networks and functional connectivity in Alzheimer's disease. Cereb Cortex 17:92–99
55. Ding C, Peng H (2005) Minimum redundancy feature selection from microarray gene expression data. J Bioinform Comput Biol 3:185–205
56. Peng H, Long F, Ding C (2005) Feature selection based on mutual information: criteria of max-dependency, max-relevance, and min-redundancy. IEEE Trans Pattern Anal Mach Intell 27:1226–1285
57. Guyon I, Weston J, Barnhill S, Vapnik V (2004) Gene selection for cancer classification using support vector machines. Mach Learn 46:389–422
58. Rakotomamonjy A (2003) Variable selection using SVM based criteria. J Mach Learn Res 3:1357–1370

59. Elad M, Aharon M (2006) Image denoising via sparse and redundant representations over learned dictionaries. IEEE Trans Image Process 15:3736–3745
60. Fadili M, Starck JL, Murtagh F (2009) Inpainting and zooming using sparse representations. Comput J 52:64–79
61. Hazan T, Polak S, Shashua A (2005) Sparse image coding using a 3D non-negative tensor factorization. In Proceedings of the Tenth IEEE international conference on computer vision (ICCV 2005), Volume 1:50–57
62. Liu M, Zhang D, Shen D (2012) Ensemble sparse classification of Alzheimer's disease. Neuroimage 60:1106–1116
63. Sled JG, Zijdenbos AP, Evans AC (1998) A nonparametric method for automatic correction of intensity nonuniformity in MRI data. IEEE Trans Med Imaging 17:87–97
64. Shen D, Davatzikos C (2003) Very high resolution morphometry using mass-preserving deformations and HAMMER elastic registration. Neuroimage 18:28–41
65. Chen SS, Donoho DL, Saunders MA (2001) Atomic decomposition by basis pursuit. SIAM Rev 43:129–159
66. Candes E, Romberg J (2005) l1-magic: recovery of sparse signals via convex programming. http://www.acm.caltech.edu/l1magic/downloads/l1magic.pdf
67. Boyd SP, Vandenberghe L (2004) Convex optimization. Cambridge University Press, Cambridge
68. Kim SJ, Koh K, Lustig M, Boyd S, Gorinevsky D (2007) An interior-point method for large-scale l1-regularized least squares. IEEE J Sel Top Signal Process 1:606–617
69. Zhang D, Shen D (2012) Multi-modal multi-task learning for joint prediction of multiple regression and classification variables in Alzheimer's disease. Neuroimage 59:895–907
70. Obozinski G, Taskar B, Jordan MI (2006) Multi-task feature selection. Statistics Department, UC, Berkeley
71. Tibshirani R (1996) Regression shrinkage and selection via the lasso. J R Stat Soc 58:267–288
72. Liu J, Ji S, Ye J (2009) SLEP: sparse learning with efficient projections. Arizona State University. http://www.public.asu.edu/~jye02/Software/SLEP
73. Tipping ME (2001) Sparse Bayesian learning and the relevance vector machine. J Mach Learn Res 1:211–244
74. Jack CR Jr, Bernstein MA, Fox NC, Thompson P, Alexander G, Harvey D, Borowski B, Britson PJ, L Whitwell J, Ward C, Dale AM, Felmlee JP, Gunter JL, Hill DL, Killiany R, Schuff N, Fox-Bosetti S, Lin C, Studholme C, DeCarli CS, Krueger G, Ward HA, Metzger GJ, Scott KT, Mallozzi R, Blezek D, Levy J, Debbins JP, Fleisher AS, Albert M, Green R, Bartzokis G, Glover G, Mugler J, Weiner MW (2008) The Alzheimer's disease neuroimaging initiative (ADNI): MRI methods. J Magn Reson Imaging 27:685–691
75. Chang CC, Lin CJ (2001) LIBSVM: a library for support vector machines. http://www.csie.ntu.edu.tw/~cjlin/libsvm/
76. Wee CY, Yap PT, Shen D (2013) The Alzheimer's disease neuroimaging initiative: prediction of Alzheimer's disease and mild cognitive impairment using cortical morphological patterns. Hum Brain Mapp

Chapter 2
The Role of Content-Based Image Retrieval in Mammography CAD

Issam El Naqa and Yongyi Yang

Abstract There has been a tremendous increase in the amount of stored medical images, making manual search infeasible for a busy radiology clinic. Content-based image retrieval (CBIR) offers a computerized solution that aims to query images for diagnostic information based on the content or extracted features of the images rather than their textual annotation. Potentially, this approach would provide the radiologist with archived examples that are relevant to the case being evaluated. In this chapter, we review recent advances in CBIR technology and discuss its expanding role in medical imaging and its particular application to mammography. We provide two examples based on our experience using CBIR in mammography; one example is to model perceptual similarity in CBIR and the other example is to apply CBIR to achieve case-adaptive classification in computer-aided diagnosis (CAD). We also highlight the potential opportunities in this field for CAD research and clinical decision-making.

Introduction

Breast cancer is the most frequently diagnosed cancer in women after skin cancer. According to the American Cancer Society, an estimated 226,870 new cases of invasive breast cancer are expected to occur among women in the USA during 2012; about 2,190 new cases are expected in men. Approximately 39,510 women

---

I. El Naqa
Montreal General Hospital, Room #L5-112, 1650 Cedar Avenue,
Montreal, QC, Canada H3G 1A4
e-mail: issam.elnaqa@mcgill.ca

Y. Yang (✉)
Department of Electrical and Computer Engineering, Illinois Institute of Technology,
3301 S. Dearborn Street, Chicago, IL 60616, USA
e-mail: yangyo@iit.edu

K. Suzuki (ed.), *Computational Intelligence in Biomedical Imaging*,
DOI 10.1007/978-1-4614-7245-2_2,

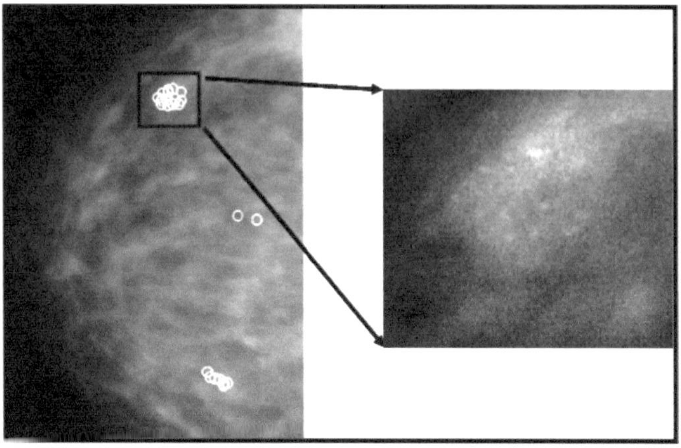

Fig. 2.1 A mammogram image with suspected areas highlighted, and a magnified view of a region with clustered microcalcifications

and 410 men are anticipated to die from breast cancer in the same year [1]. Research has shown that the key to successfully treating breast cancer is early detection. The combination of early detection and improvements in treatment options has led to 2–3.3 % decline in the mortality rate among women in recent years [1].

Breast lesions can manifest as masses or clustered microcalcifications (MCs). As an example, Fig. 2.1 shows a mammogram image with clustered MCs.

Mammography currently provides the most effective strategy for early detection of breast cancer. The sensitivity of mammography could be up to approximately 90 % for patients without symptoms [2]. However, this sensitivity is highly dependent on the patient's age, the size and conspicuity of the lesion, the hormonal status of the tumor, the density of a woman's breasts, the overall image quality, and the interpretative skills of the radiologist [3]. Therefore, the overall sensitivity of mammography could range between from 90 to 70 % only [4]. Furthermore, it is very difficult to distinguish mammographically benign lesions from malignant ones. It has been estimated that one third of regularly screened women experience at least one false-positive (benign lesions being biopsied) screening mammogram over a period of 10 years [5]. A population-based study that included about 27,394 screening mammograms, which were interpreted by 1,067 radiologists showed that the radiologists had substantial variations in the false-positive rates ranging from 1.5 to 24.1 % [6]. Unnecessary biopsy is often cited as one of the risks of screening mammography. Surgical, needle-core, and fine-needle aspiration biopsies are expensive, invasive, and traumatic for the patient.

The last two decades have witnessed a great deal of research for developing computer-aided detection (CADe)/diagnosis (CADx) tools for detection and diagnosis of breast cancer [7–10]. This intensive research has resulted in several FDA approved commercial systems since the late 1990s, which aim to play the role of a virtual "second reader" by highlighting suspicious areas for further review by the radiologist in association with their own reading. Improvement in cancer detection and diagnosis has been reported in retrospective and prospective studies [11–13]. However, this was not without controversies [14]. A multi-institutional study of 43 facilities showed that the current CAD systems were associated with reduced accuracy of interpretation for screening mammograms [14]. In any case, these negative results may strongly urge the need for utilizing more improved techniques for analyzing mammogram images.

Content-based image retrieval (CBIR) may potentially provide new and exciting opportunities for the analysis and the interpretation of mammogram images. The underlying principle in CBIR is analogous to textual search engines (e.g., Google), in which a search engine aims to retrieve information that is relevant (or similar) to the user's query. Instead of textual description, however, in CBIR the information is embedded in the form of an image or its extracted features. CBIR could serve as a diagnostic tool for aiding radiologists by comparing current cases with previously diagnosed ones in a medical archive.

In this chapter, we provide an overview of CBIR in recent years in the medical imaging literature and specifically for mammography. We discuss its expanding role and provide examples based on our experience using CBIR in mammography and highlight its strong potential as a valuable tool for computerized detection and diagnosis in mammography.

Background

Content-Based Image Retrieval

Image retrieval has been one of the most exciting and fastest growing research areas in image processing over the past decade [15]. There have been several general-purpose image retrieval systems developed. For instance, Guo et al. [16] developed a supervised approach for learning similarity measures for natural images, while Chen et al. [17] investigated unsupervised clustering-based image retrieval. Interested readers are referred to [15] for further examples on general-purpose CBIR systems. However, an evolving application of CBIR in recent years has been in the area of medical imaging [18]. CBIR has been developed as a visual-based approach to overcome some of the difficulties and problems associated with human perception subjectivity and annotation impreciseness in text-based retrieval systems. However, despite the significant developments over the past decade with respect to similarity measures, objective image interpretations, feature extraction, and semantic descriptors [18, 19], some fundamental difficulties still remain pertaining to CBIR applications. First, it is understood that similarity measures can vary with the different aspects of perceptual similarity between images; the selection of an appropriate similarity measure thus becomes problem-dependent. Second, the relation between the low-level visual features and the high-level human interpretation of similarity is not well defined when comparing two images; it is thus not

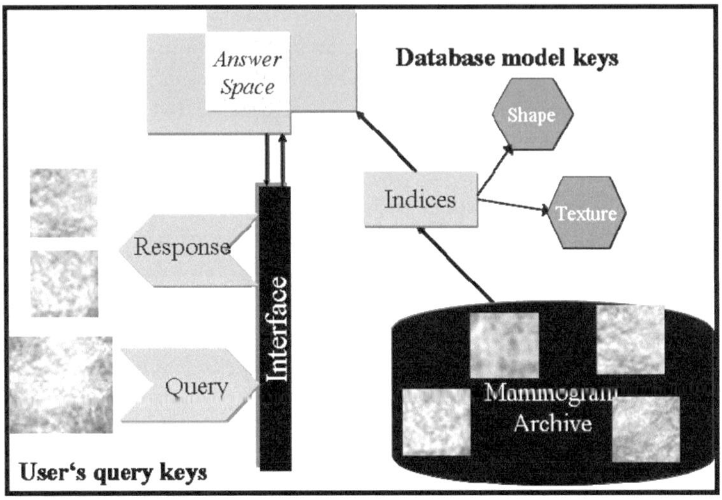

Fig. 2.2 Image retrieval framework for mammography [73]. Reprinted by permission of the publisher

exactly clear what features or combination of them are relevant for such judgment [20, 21]. Finally, while the user may understand more about the query, the database system can only guess (possibly through interactive learning) what the user is looking for during the retrieval process. This is an indispensable challenge in information retrieval, where the correct answer may not always be clearly identified. In Fig. 2.2, we show a diagram to illustrate a typical scenario of image retrieval from mammography databases, where an archive is organized into mammogram images, which in turn is organized into indices (i.e., a data structure of selected image features) for rapid lookup. The user formulates his/her retrieval problem as an expression in the query language (e.g., by presenting the images of the current case as query). The query is then translated into the language of indices and matched against those in the database, and those images with matching indices are retrieved.

CBIR as a CAD Tool

Historically, the concept of image retrieval in medical images was first introduced by Swett et al. [22], who developed a rudimentary, rule-based expert system to display radiographs from a library of images as illustrative examples for helping radiologists' diagnosis. However, application of CBIR for medical images is a quite challenging task due to the complexity of image content in relation to the disease conditions. As a consequence, many of the useful image features in traditional CBIR are no longer adequate in medical imaging. For example, global image features (such as grayscale histogram) would not be salient for describing the characteristics of pathological regions or lesions which are typically localized in the images [18]. In such a case, it is important to derive quantitative features that correlate well with the anatomical or functional information perceived as important for diagnostic purposes by the physicians. Therefore, present medical CBIR systems mostly focus on a specific topic, thus offering support only for a restricted variety of image types and feature sets, such as high-resolution computed tomography (HRCT) scans of the lung [23]. This system was referred to as the ASSERT system, where a rich set of texture features was derived from the disease bearing regions. In [24], a new hierarchical approach to CBIR called "customized-queries" approach is applied to lung images. In [25], a system called CBIR2 was developed for retrieval of spine X-ray images. Three-dimensional MR image retrieval was studied in [26] based on anatomical structure matching. An online pathological neuroimage retrieval system was investigated in [27] under the framework of classification-driven feature selection. Cai et al. [28] presented a prototype design for content-based functional image retrieval for dynamic PET images. Tobin et al. [29] developed a CBIR system for retrieving diabetic retinopathy cases using a k-nearest neighbors (KNN)-based approach. Application to different medical databases such as dermatological images [30], cervicographic images [31], and microscopic pathology databases [32] was explored in the literature. More recently, there has also been growing interest in retrieving reference images from PACS, and CBIR has now become an important research direction in radiological sciences [18, 33, 34].

Despite the extensive research efforts in CBIR, current imaging standards such as DICOM v3.0 still rely on textual attributes of images (e.g., study, patient, and other parameters), which are still to date the only information used to select relevant images within PACS [35]. However, in recent years several research-oriented image retrieval projects and prototypes have been developed for management of medical images for research and teaching purposes. Examples of such systems include: the ASSERT mentioned above; CasImage [36], which retrieves a variety of images ranging from CT, MR, and radiographs to color photos based on color and textural features; IRMA (image retrieval in medical applications) [37], a development platform of components intended for CBIR in medical applications; NHANES II (the second national health and nutrition examination survey) [38] for retrieval of cervical and lumbar spine X-ray images based on the shape of the vertebra. In the rest of this chapter, we will focus on CBIR application to mammography due to its important role in breast cancer management.

Mammography

Mammograms are low-energy X-ray images of the breast of patients. Typically, they are in the order of 0.7 mSv. A mammogram can detect a cancerous or precancerous tumor in the breast even before the tumor is large enough to be palpable. The results are interpreted according to an American College of Radiology (ACR) score known as the Breast Imaging Reporting and Data System (BI-RADS™) with values ranging from 0 (incomplete) to 6 (known biopsy—proven malignancy) [39]. To date mammography remains the modality of choice for early screening of breast cancer. As mentioned earlier, there has been intensive development of CAD systems for computerized lesion detection; however, this was not without controversies about the value of such systems compared to human readers [14]. It is expected that human decision-making is much more complex than what a detection algorithm can provide. *We share the belief that the potential value for application of CAD systems to mammography could be facilitated through the development of information systems based on CBIR.*

CBIR for Mammography

Review of Existing Methods

Since the pioneering work by Swett et al. [22], there have been extensive efforts to apply CBIR to medical imaging in general and mammography in particular. Sklansky et al. [40] developed a technique that produces a two-dimensional (2D) map based on the decision space of a neural network classifier, in which images that are close to each other are selected for purposes of visualization; the neural network was trained for separating "biopsy recommended" and "biopsy not recommended" classes. Qi and Snyder [41] demonstrated the potential use of CBIR in PACS using a digital mammogram database based on the shape and size information of mass lesions. At about the same time, we started developing our perceptual similarity approach for retrieval of MC lesions in mammograms [42–44]. Giger et al. [45] developed an intelligent workstation interface that displays known malignant and benign cases similar to lesions in question (based on one or more selected features or computer estimated likelihood of malignancy), and demonstrated that radiologists' performance, especially specificity, increases with the use of such aid tool. Tourassi et al. [46–48] developed an approach for retrieval and detection of masses in mammograms based on the use of information-theoretic measures (such as mutual information), where a decision index is calculated based on the query's best matches. Zheng et al. [49] applied a KNN algorithm and further used observer-rated spiculation levels to improve the similarity of breast masses and subsequently investigated the use of mutual information [50] to improve the similarity measure. An unsupervised learning approach based on Kohonen self-organizing map (SOM) was proposed in [51]. The SOM was trained using a set of 88 features for each mammogram, which included common shape factors, texture, and moment features as well as angular projections and morphological features derived from segmented fibroglandular tissues.

As noted above, CBIR has been studied recently by researchers as a useful tool for exploring known cases from a reference library that can assist radiologists in diagnosis. The idea is to provide evidence for case-based reasoning with information from the retrieved cases [52]. As an indication of the predictive value of retrieved cases, the correlation in disease condition between the query and the retrieved cases was examined in previous work [21, 53]. The ratio of malignant cases among all retrieved cases was used as a useful predictor for the query [54, 55]; conceptually, this can be viewed as a KNN classifier using only the retrieved cases. The similarity level between a retrieved case and the query was used by Zheng et al. [49] as a weighting factor in the prediction. A genetic algorithm was used by Mazurowski et al. [56] to adjust the weighting factors of the retrieved cases. An observer study was used by Nakayama et al. [57] to investigate the potential diagnostic value of similar cases. These studies provide evidence on the positive predictive value of similar cases in CADx.

Evaluation Metrics

Retrieval systems are typically evaluated using the so-called precision-recall curves [58]. The retrieval precision is defined as the proportion of the images among all the retrieved that are truly relevant to a given query; the term recall is measured by the proportion of the images that are actually retrieved among all the relevant images to a query. Mathematically, they are given by:

$$\begin{aligned} \text{Precision} &= \frac{\text{The number of relevant images that are retrieved}}{\text{The total number of retrieved images}} \\ \text{Recall} &= \frac{\text{The number of relevant images that are retrieved}}{\text{The total number of relevant images}}. \end{aligned} \tag{2.1}$$

The precision-recall curve is a plot of the retrieval precision versus the recall over a continuum of the operating threshold. An example of precision-recall curves is given later in Fig. 2.4 in section "Case-Study Example."

Other metrics to quantify the accuracy of a retrieval system could be defined on the similarity measure used, such as the mean-squared error (MSE) of the model score compared to the observer score. In addition, to evaluate the merit of the similarity measure for cancer diagnosis, criteria such as cumulative neighbor matching rate could be used [59]. In this case, for each query image, the ratio of top k images that actually match the disease condition of the query is computed and averaged over all the queries.

For statistical validation of the retrieval performance, resampling techniques such as cross-validation and bootstrap are typically used. In cross-validation, the data samples are divided into a number of subsets which are permuted for training and testing in a round-robin fashion, whereas in bootstrap, the data samples are randomly selected for training and testing for many times. Bootstrap could be regarded as a smoothed version of cross-validation. It is thought to be more realistic in modeling real life scenarios [60].

Finally, we add that besides these rather generic measures used in information retrieval, it is also necessary to evaluate the retrieval efficiency based on specific clinical tasks.

Example 1: Similarity Learning for CBIR

In this section, we present a CBIR application to mimic radiologists' perceptual similarity using machine learning methods. As an example, we will consider in particular lesions with clustered MCs, which can be an important early sign of breast cancer in women. Their clustering patterns play an important role in determining malignancy risk following the BI-RADS criteria as mentioned in section "Mammography."

Similarity as Nonlinear Regression Functional

In this approach, the notion of similarity is modeled as a nonlinear function of the image features in a pair of mammogram images containing lesions of interest, e.g., microcalcification clusters (MCCs). If we let vectors **u** and **v** denote the features of two MCCs at issue, the following regression model could be used to determine their similarity coefficient (SC):

$$SC(\mathbf{u},\mathbf{v}) = f(\mathbf{u},\mathbf{v}) + \zeta, \tag{2.2}$$

where $f(\mathbf{u},\mathbf{v})$ is a function determined using a machine learning approach, which we choose to be support vector machine (SVM) learning [61], and ζ is the modeling error. The similarity function $f(\mathbf{u},\mathbf{v})$ in Eq. (2.2) is trained using data samples collected in an observer study. For convenience, we denote $f(\mathbf{u},\mathbf{v})$ by $f(\mathbf{x})$ with $\mathbf{x} = [\mathbf{u}^T, \mathbf{v}^T]^T$.

Assume that we have a set of N training samples, denoted by $Z = \{(\mathbf{x}_i, y_i)\}_{i=1}^N$, where y_i denotes the user similarity score for the MCC pair denoted by $\mathbf{x}_i$, $i = 1, 2, \ldots, N$. The regression function $f(\mathbf{x})$ is written in the following form:

$$f(\mathbf{x}) = \mathbf{w}^T \mathbf{\Phi}(\mathbf{x}) + b, \tag{2.3}$$

where $\mathbf{\Phi}(\mathbf{x})$ is a mapping implicitly defined by a so-called kernel function which we introduce below. The parameters **w** and b in Eq. (2.3) are determined through minimization of the following structured risk:

$$R(\mathbf{w}, b) = \frac{1}{2}\mathbf{w}^T\mathbf{w} + C\sum_{i=1}^{N} L_\varepsilon(\mathbf{x}_i), \tag{2.4}$$

where $L_\varepsilon(\bullet)$ is the so-called ε-insensitive loss function, which has the property that it does not penalize errors below the parameter ε. The constant C in Eq. (2.4) determines the trade-off between the model complexity and the training error. In this study the Gaussian radial basis function is used for the SVM kernel function $K(\cdot,\cdot)$, where $K(\cdot,\cdot) = \mathbf{\Phi}^T(\mathbf{x})\mathbf{\Phi}(\mathbf{x})$. The regression function $f(\mathbf{x})$ in Eq. (2.2) is characterized by a set of so-called support vectors:

$$f(\mathbf{x}) = \sum_{j=1}^{Ns} \gamma_j K(\mathbf{x}_j, \mathbf{x}) + b, \tag{2.5}$$

where $\mathbf{x}_j$ are the support vectors and N_s is the number of the support vectors.

To model the similarity between two feature vectors, we want to learn a symmetric function satisfying $f(\mathbf{u},\mathbf{v}) = f(\mathbf{v},\mathbf{u})$, i.e., the notion of similarity is commutative. This can be achieved by duplicating the training image pairs, i.e., first with $(\mathbf{u}, \mathbf{v})$ and then with $(\mathbf{v}, \mathbf{u})$. We can explicitly enforce this property in the SVM cost function as:

$$R(\mathbf{w}, b) = \frac{1}{2}\mathbf{w}^T\mathbf{w} + C\sum_{i=1}^{N} L_\varepsilon(\mathbf{x}_i) + C\sum_{i=1}^{N} L_\varepsilon(\mathbf{x}_i^s). \tag{2.6}$$

Here $y(\mathbf{x}_i) = y(\mathbf{x}_i^s)$, $\mathbf{x}_i = (\mathbf{u}_i^T, \mathbf{v}_i^T)^T$, $\mathbf{x}_i^s = (\mathbf{v}_i^T, \mathbf{u}_i^T)^T$.

With this formulation the SVM training algorithm yields the global optimum of a symmetric Lagrangian. The resulting regression function can be written as:

$$f(\mathbf{x}) = \sum_{j=1}^{Ns} \gamma_j \left[K(\mathbf{x}_j, \mathbf{x}) + K\left(\mathbf{x}_j^s, \mathbf{x}\right)\right] + b. \tag{2.7}$$

That is, if a training sample $\mathbf{x}_j$ is a support vector, i.e., $|y_j - f(\mathbf{x}_j)| \geq \varepsilon$, then its symmetric sample $\mathbf{x}_j^s$ is also a support vector and $\gamma_j = \gamma_j^s$. This will ensure that the solution is symmetric: $f(\mathbf{x}) = f(\mathbf{x}^s)$. A detailed proof of this is given in [59].

Case-Study Example

A database of mammogram images provided by the Department of Radiology at the University of Chicago is used for demonstration purposes. The database consists of a total of 200 different mammogram images of dimension 1,024 × 1,024 (a few are 512 × 512) from 104 patients with known pathology (46 malignant, 58 benign), digitized with a spatial resolution of 0.1 mm/pixel and 10-bit grayscale. All these images contain MCCs. The MCCs in each image had been identified by expert radiologists and a total of 600 image pairs were scored by a group of six mammogram readers. Following intraobserver and interobserver consistency analyses, scores from four observers with the highest consistency were selected and their scores were averaged for each of the 600 image pairs.

To characterize the similarity data by the experts, we considered image features derived from MCCs which were demonstrated to have high discriminating power for cancer diagnosis [62, 63]. We applied a sequential feature selection procedure to obtain 12 features for characterizing an MC cluster, namely: (1) compactness of the cluster; (2) eccentricity of the smallest ellipse fitting the region; (3) the number of MCs per unit area; (4) the average of the inter-distances between neighboring MCs; (5) the standard deviation of the inter-distances between neighboring MCs; (6) solidity of the cluster region defined as the ratio between cross-sectional area and the area of the convex hull formed by the MCs; (7) the moment signature of the cluster region computed based on the distance deviation of a boundary point from the center of the region; (8) the number of MCs in the cluster; (9) the mean effective volume (area times effective thickness) of individual MCs; (10) the relative standard deviation of the effective thickness; (11) the relative standard deviation of the effective volume; and (12) the second highest MC-shape-irregularity measure. In our experiments, all the feature components were normalized to have the same dynamic range (0, 1).

The SVM similarity model was trained using the observer data. Besides the human scores for the 600 image pairs, we also added the following pairs for training:

1. $SC(\mathbf{u}, \mathbf{u}) = 10$, and
2. $SC(\mathbf{u}, \mathbf{v}) = 10$ if $\mathbf{u}$ and $\mathbf{v}$ are different views from the same case.

With a leave-one-out procedure, the SVM model achieved an MSE of 0.0334 per image pair compared to the observer scores. The trained SVM similarity model was tested with the 200 images in the database, where each of the 200 images in the dataset was used in turn as a query image. A retrieval example is shown in Fig. 2.3. The average matching rate between SVM prediction and disease pathology reached 72 % for the top retrieved images. The precision-recall analysis achieved by the SVM model is shown in Fig. 2.4. Note that the performance can be further refined by incorporating user's response through an adaptive process called relevance feedback (RFB) [64, 65]. Figure 2.4 also shows the resulting precision-recall curves obtained by RFB with different number of feedback samples.

Example 2: Adaptive CADx with CBIR

In recent years, we have been investigating a case-adaptive approach to boost the performance of a CADx classifier based on retrieval of cases with similar image features from a reference library. In traditional CADx, a classifier $f(\mathbf{x})$ is first optimized on a set of training samples, which is often limited in size; subsequently, this classifier is applied to classify a new case $\mathbf{x}$ under consideration (called query). In our approach, we will first obtain from a reference database (e.g., a PACS system) a set of known cases with similar features to the query case $\mathbf{x}$, and use these retrieved cases to adapt the classifier $f(\mathbf{x})$ so as to improve its classification accuracy on the query case.

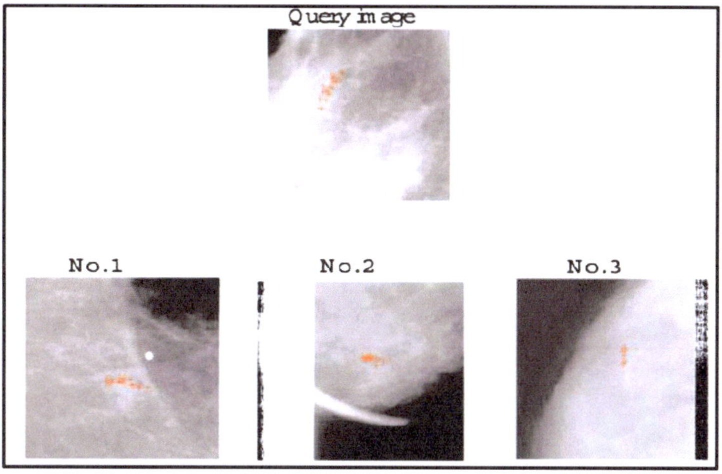

Fig. 2.3 A retrieval example of similar cases using SVM similarity learning [73]. Reprinted by permission of the publisher

Fig. 2.4 Precision-recall curve of MC retrieval using SVM machine learning methods and refinement of precision-recall accuracy using relevance feedback (RFB) with different number of image samples [65]. Reprinted by permission of the publisher

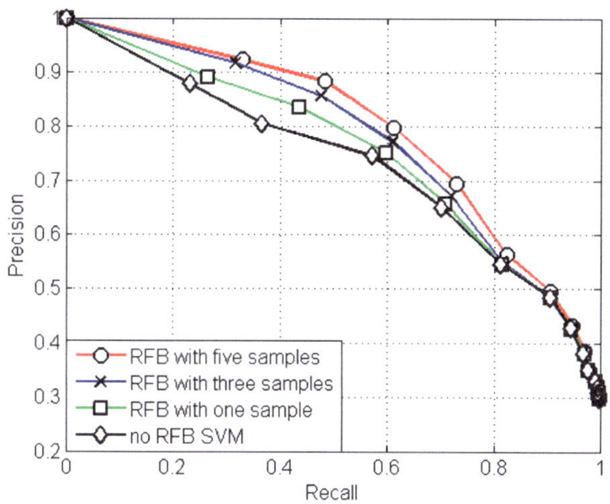

The problem of classifying clustered MCs into malignant or benign is treated as a two-class classification problem. Let $f(\cdot)$ denote a classifier that has been trained on a set of training samples $\{(\mathbf{x}_i, y_i), i = 1, \ldots, N\}$, where $\mathbf{x}_i \in R^n$ denotes the feature vector of each sample and $y_i \in \{-1, +1\}$ denotes its corresponding class label. Now, consider a new lesion with feature vector $\mathbf{x}$. Our goal is to make use of a set of retrieved cases to improve the accuracy of the classifier $f(\cdot)$ on $\mathbf{x}$. Below we first describe our approach using a linear classifier, based on logistic regression, which is attractive in practice owing to its numerical simplicity. This approach can be readily extended to a nonlinear classifier using the technique of kernel principal component analysis (KPCA) [66].

Case-Adaptive Linear Classifier

Mathematically, a linear classifier is of the form

$$f(\mathbf{x}) = \mathbf{w}^T\mathbf{x} + b, \tag{2.8}$$

where $\mathbf{x}$ is a vector denoting an input pattern (i.e., lesion), and $f(\mathbf{x})$ is the classifier output, which is typically compared against an operating threshold for decision on $\mathbf{x}$. In practice, the discriminant vector $\mathbf{w}$ and bias parameter b are both determined from training.

We consider the approach of logistic regression for determining the unknown $\mathbf{w}$ and b from the training set $\{(\mathbf{x}_i, y_i),\ i = 1, \ldots, N\}$ [67], which is to maximize the following log-likelihood function:

$$L(\mathbf{w}, b) = \sum_{i=1}^{N} \log p(y_i|\mathbf{x}_i; \mathbf{w}, b), \tag{2.9}$$

where each probability term is given by

$$p(y_i = 1|\mathbf{x}_i; \mathbf{w}, b) = \frac{1}{1 + \exp(-\mathbf{w}^T\mathbf{x}_i - b)}, \tag{2.10}$$

and $p(y_i = -1|\mathbf{x}_i; \mathbf{w}, b) = 1 - p(y_i = 1|\mathbf{x}_i; \mathbf{w}, b)$.

Now consider a query lesion $\mathbf{x}$ to be classified. Let $\{(\mathbf{x}_i^{(r)}, y_i^{(r)}),\ i = 1, \ldots, N_r\}$ be a set of N_r cases obtained from a reference library, which are similar to $\mathbf{x}$. In our case-adaptive approach, we modify the objective function in Eq. (2.9) by these retrieved cases as

$$\widetilde{L}(\mathbf{w}, b) = \sum_{i=1}^{N} \log p(y_i|\mathbf{x}_i; \mathbf{w}, b) + \sum_{i=1}^{N_r} \beta_i \log p\left(y_i^{(r)} \middle| \mathbf{x}_i^{(r)}; \mathbf{w}, b\right), \tag{2.11}$$

where the weighting coefficients $\beta_i > 1$ are used to put more emphasis on the retrieved samples, particularly those more similar to the query, the goal being to refine the decision boundary of the classifier in the neighborhood of the query $\mathbf{x}$. Indeed, the first term in Eq. (2.11) simply corresponds to the log-likelihood function in Eq. (2.9), while the second term can be viewed as a weighted likelihood of those retrieved similar samples. Intuitively, the retrieved samples are used to steer the pre-trained classifier from Eq. (2.9) to achieve more emphasis in the neighborhood of the query $\mathbf{x}$.

Note that the objective function in Eq. (2.11) has the same mathematical form as that in the original optimization problem in Eq. (2.9), which can be solved efficiently by the method of iteratively reweighted least square (IRLS).

Database of MC Cases for CBIR

To demonstrate the proposed CBIR approach, we used a dataset of digitized, standard-view, screen-film mammographic images collected from two sources: one is from the Department of Radiology, The University of Chicago (UC), and the other from the DDSM dataset maintained at The University of South Florida [68]. The DDSM dataset consists of images collected from three different institutions: The Massachusetts General Hospital (MGH), Wake Forest University School of Medicine, and Sacred Heart Hospital and ISMD, Incorporated. It has 14 benign volumes, 15 cancer volumes, 12 normal volumes and 2 benign without callback volumes. The normal and benign without callback volumes are not used in this work since they contain no lesions with verified pathology. To maximize the yield, we extracted all those cases with only MC lesions from all the benign and cancer volumes in DDSM.

The mammogram images from the different institutions were digitized with five different scanners with different resolutions. To reduce their differences, the mammogram images were first converted to a common resolution (100 μm) using cubic interpolation and calibrated such that their gray levels correspond to the same optical density. Altogether, there were a total of 1,006 cases (646 benign, 360 malignant) collected in the dataset.

To characterize clustered MCs in these images, we applied a sequential forward procedure [69] with a linear classifier using logistic regression on a set of training images. In the end, a total of nine features were selected for characterizing MC lesions. These features are: (1) number of MCs in the cluster; (2) density of the cluster, measured by the number of MCs in a unit area; (3) mean of the MC size in the cluster; (4) eccentricity of the cluster; (5) standard deviation of the distance from individual MCs to the geometric center of the cluster; (6) maximum of the mean intensity of MCs; (7) mean of the average intensity in each MC window; (8) standard deviation of the contrast of MCs; and (9) standard deviation of the fourth order central moment of MCs.

With all the cases in the library characterized by their feature vectors, for a given query case $\mathbf{x}$, the similar cases to $\mathbf{x}$ can then be obtained by comparing its feature vector against that of library cases according to a similarity measure. These retrieved cases are then incorporated into the case-adaptive classifier in Eq. (2.11) via the weighting coefficients β_i. In this study, we implemented the following strategy for adjusting β_i according to the similarity level of a retrieved sample $\mathbf{x}_i^{(r)}$ to the query $\mathbf{x}$:

$$\beta_i = 1 + k\frac{\alpha_i}{\max\limits_{j=1,\ldots,N_r}\{\alpha_j\}},\quad i = 1,\ldots,N_r, \tag{2.12}$$

where α_i denotes the similarity measure between $\mathbf{x}_i^{(r)}$ and $\mathbf{x}$, and $k > 0$ is used to control the degree of emphasis on the retrieved samples relative to other training samples. The choice of the form in Eq. (2.12) is such that the weighting factor increases linearly with the similarity level of a retrieved case to **x**, with the most similar case among the retrieved receiving maximum weight $1 + k$, which corresponds to k times more influence than the existing training samples in the objective function in Eq. (2.11).

As a similarity measure for retrieved cases, we used the Gaussian RBF kernel function

$$\alpha_i = \exp\left(-\left\|\mathbf{x}_i^{(r)} - \mathbf{x}\right\|^2/\gamma^2\right), \quad i = 1, \ldots, N_r, \tag{2.13}$$

where γ is a scaling factor controlling the sensitivity of α_i with respect to the distance between the query and a retrieved case. In our experiments, the parameter γ was set to the tenth percentile of the distance between every possible image pairs in the training set. Such a choice is out of the consideration that most of the cases in a database are typically not similar to each other. Those cases with a large distance away from query **x** will receive a low similarity measure consequently.

Performance Evaluation

To demonstrate the case-adaptive classification approach, we used the following setting in this study. We first partitioned the dataset of all 1,006 cases randomly into two subsets, denoted by A and B, respectively, such that subset A consisted of 175 cases (100 benign, 75 malignant), and subset B had the remaining 831 cases (546 benign, 285 malignant). The cases in A were used to train and optimize a baseline CADx classifier, while the cases in B were set aside as a library of known cases for retrieval, which was used to boost the baseline CADx classifier (trained on subset A).

For efficient use of subset B, the cases in B were also used to test the CADx classifier. To remove the effect of case distributions, we applied a bootstrapping methodology for testing the performance of the classifiers [70, 71]. A total of 10,000 bootstrap sample sets were used, of which each was obtained by sampling with replacement from the cases in B; subset A was fixed during this process. The classifier performance was subsequently obtained over each bootstrap sample set.

To avoid any potential bias, we applied a leave-one-out (LOO) procedure when testing the adaptive classifier as follows: for each case used for testing, we excluded this case from B and retrieved known cases only from the rest of the data set to boost the CADx classifier. The resulting classifier was then applied to classify the test case. This was to ensure that the test case itself would not be used in any way for boosting the adaptive classifier.

To evaluate the classification performance, we conducted a receiver operating characteristic (ROC) analysis, which is now routinely used for performance evaluation in classification tasks. As a summary measure of overall diagnostic performance, the area under an ROC curve (denoted by AUC) is often used. A larger AUC means better classification performance. In our experiments the ROCKIT program [72] was used to calculate the AUC values for the different classifiers.

Fig. 2.5 Classification performance (AUC) achieved by the case-adaptive linear classifier (ada-LR). The number of retrieved cases N_r was varied from 6 to 200. For comparison, results are also shown for the baseline classifier (LR)

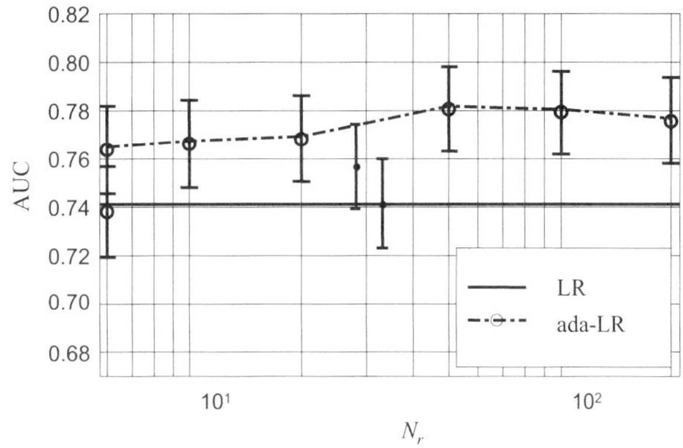

We summarize in Fig. 2.5 the performance results achieved by the case-adaptive linear classifier (ada-LR). To demonstrate the impact of retrieved cases, in the experiments we also varied the number of retrieved cases N_r for a query case. In Fig. 2.5, the area under the ROC curve, AUC, is shown for different values of N_r; for comparison, the performance result by the baseline classifier (LR) (i.e., prior to boosting) is also shown.

From Fig. 2.5 it can be seen that the AUC value of the adaptive classifier is notably higher than that of the baseline classifier. In particular, with $N_r = 10$ the adaptive classifier achieved AUC = 0.7663; with $N_r = 50$, the AUC value of the adaptive classifier was further increased to 0.7807 compared to AUC = 0.7415 for the baseline classifier (p-value = 0.0001). No additional improvement was observed when N_r was further increased. We believe that this is because the number of similar cases for a given query case is limited in the reference library and the benefit of retrieving additional cases diminishes.

Current Challenges and Recommendations

Despite the increasing number of research systems developed in recent years, the application of CBIR for medical applications is very much still at its infancy [73]. For content-based mammogram retrieval, there remain several technical issues that would require further investigation, which may include the following seven different aspects:

1. How to incrementally improve the retrieval performance through accumulating experts' query log remains a challenge. Our proposed approach of using perceptual similarity could be used to improve precision in image retrieval. This concept has been studied by other researchers [74–76]. For instance, the results in [75] demonstrate good concordance consistency even among three different types of

readers (13 breast radiologists, 10 general radiologists, and 10 non-radiologists), which indicates the reliability of the similarity ratings obtained from observer studies.

2. Inclusion of semantics-based similarity features such as patient history, age, and view besides the low-level image features to improve retrieval accuracy.
3. Investigation of advanced RFB techniques to refine the retrieval process. Adaptive learning algorithms can be incorporated into the learning approach as in our previous study [64].
4. System integration into PACS or other medical image databases. This is an essential step for the clinical use of retrieval systems [18]. PACS systems are now widely used in the hospitals to manage the storage and distribution of images. Thus, CBIR is expected to have a great impact on PACS and health database management [77]. An important issue in medical practice is to keep patient's private information from any unauthorized access in accordance with the Health Insurance Portability and Accountability Act (HIPAA). Security requirements need to be embedded into the design of a database system, so that users would have access to data that they only have privilege over. This may add additional burdens to achieve high efficiency for CBIR within the mandated security constraints. Experiences from textual relational database management systems (RDBMS) could be helpful in this regard.
5. Human–computer interaction and usability. This would involve the development of efficient search methods in a high-dimensional feature space. Search in the presence of user-dependent similarity measures is largely unsolved [15]. Possible solutions may involve the need to develop faster methods for extracting relevant features from the given query image and to pre-store the image features using efficient data structures (e.g., linked-list tree structures) for rapid retrieval. To further speed up the retrieval process for an online environment, one can also employ a two-stage approach in which a computationally efficient linear-classifier is used to quickly discard any non-similar entries from further consideration [21, 42, 44, 59, 62, 63, 78].
6. Performance evaluation framework and standard. The problem of how to evaluate the retrieval quality is an important topic as well. Retrieval systems need to be compared in order to sort out the different techniques [18]. Due to the complexity of medical images, how to construct a common test bed for medical CBIR is an interesting research issue [79]. To construct a test bed for medical CBIR, a number of factors such as imaging modalities, regions of interest, and orientations of images should be taken into account.
7. Validation of many of the proposed methods for clinical use on large databases. To fully evaluate the benefit of a retrieval system, it is desirable to establish a benchmark database, which is large enough so that it would maximize the yield of truly relevant images. In practice, this can be an expensive process. It is noted that there exist several public domain mammogram databases such as DDSM (Digital Database for Screening Mammography) maintained by the University of South Florida and MIAS (Mammographic Image Analysis Society maintained by the University of Manchester). These databases are mainly used for comparing

different CAD systems. It would be beneficial to augment these databases with additional image similarity information so that they could be used as a benchmark for comparing different CBIR systems.

Conclusions

CBIR for mammography is a promising field for improving automated detection and diagnosis of breast cancer lesions. In this chapter, we provided an overview of recent advances in CBIR technology and its application to mammographic databases. In addition, we presented examples from our experience in building CBIR systems for mammography. In our approach, we investigated the use of a supervised learning methodology in content-based mammogram retrieval based on perceptual similarity from expert observers. This approach was demonstrated using a set of clinical mammograms to achieve significant improvement in retrieval performance over competing unsupervised learning methods. Moreover, we also demonstrated that the use of CBIR could further improve the performance in a CADx classifier. We also discussed some of the current problems in the field and highlighted the potential opportunities for future research and clinical implementation. These areas could benefit from existing expertise in the computer vision community. If successful, CBIR approaches could realize their potential to improve current clinical decision-making processes for patients with breast cancer.

Acknowledgments This work was supported in part by NIH/NIBIB Grant R01EB009905 and the Natural Sciences and Engineering Research Council of Canada under grant NSERC-RGPIN 397711-11.

References

1. American Cancer Society (2012) Cancer facts and figures. American Cancer Society, Atlanta
2. Mushlin AI, Kouides RW, Shapiro DE (1998) Estimating the accuracy of screening mammography: a meta-analysis. Am J Prev Med 14:143–153
3. Urbain JL (2005) Breast cancer screening, diagnostic accuracy and health care policies. CMAJ 172:210–211
4. Kolb TM, Lichy J, Newhouse JH (2002) Comparison of the performance of screening mammography, physical examination, and breast US and evaluation of factors that influence them: an analysis of 27,825 patient evaluations. Radiology 225:165–175
5. Elmore JG, Barton MB, Moceri VM, Polk S, Arena PJ, Fletcher SW (1998) Ten-year risk of false positive screening mammograms and clinical breast examinations. N Engl J Med 338:1089–1096
6. Tan A, Freeman DH Jr, Goodwin JS, Freeman JL (2006) Variation in false-positive rates of mammography reading among 1067 radiologists: a population-based assessment. Breast Cancer Res Treat 100:309–318
7. Bazzocchi M, Mazzarella F, Del Frate C, Girometti F, Zuiani C (2007) CAD systems for mammography: a real opportunity? A review of the literature. Radiol Med 112:329–353

8. Collins MJ, Hoffmeister J, Worrell SW (2006) Computer-aided detection and diagnosis of breast cancer. Semin Ultrasound CT MR 27:351–355
9. Hadjiiski L, Sahiner B, Helvie MA, Chan HP, Roubidoux MA, Paramagul C, Blane C, Petrick N, Bailey J, Klein K, Foster M, Patterson SK, Adler D, Nees AV, Shen J (2006) Breast masses: computer-aided diagnosis with serial mammograms. Radiology 240:343–356
10. Malich A, Fischer DR, Bottcher J (2006) CAD for mammography: the technique, results, current role and further developments. Eur Radiol 16:1449–1460
11. Dean JC, Ilvento CC (2006) Improved cancer detection using computer-aided detection with diagnostic and screening mammography: prospective study of 104 cancers. AJR Am J Roentgenol 187:20–28
12. Georgian-Smith D, Moore RH, Halpern E, Yeh ED, Rafferty EA, D'Alessandro HA, Staffa M, Hall DA, McCarthy KA, Kopans DB (2007) Blinded comparison of computer-aided detection with human second reading in screening mammography. AJR Am J Roentgenol 189:1135–1141
13. Yang SK, Moon WK, Cho N, Park JS, Cha JH, Kim SM, Kim SJ, Im JG (2007) Screening mammography-detected cancers: sensitivity of a computer-aided detection system applied to full-field digital mammograms. Radiology 244:104–111
14. Fenton JJ, Taplin SH, Carney PA, Abraham L, Sickles EA, D'Orsi C, Berns EA, Cutter G, Hendrick RE, Barlow WE, Elmore JG (2007) Influence of computer-aided detection on performance of screening mammography. N Engl J Med 356:1399–1409
15. Smeulders AWM, Worring M (2000) Content-based image retrieval at the end of the early years. IEEE Trans Pattern Anal Mach Intell 22:32 p
16. Guo GD, Jain AK, Ma WY, Zhang HJ (2002) Learning similarity measure for natural image retrieval with relevance feedback. IEEE Trans Neural Netw 13:811–820
17. Chen Y, Wang JZ, Krovetz R (2005) CLUE: cluster-based retrieval of images by unsupervised learning. IEEE Trans Image Process 14:1187–1201
18. Müller H, Michoux N, Bandon D, Geissbuhler A (2004) A review of content-based image retrieval systems in medical applications – clinical benefits and future directions. Int J Med Inform 73:1–23
19. Bustos B, Keim D, Saupe D, Schreck T (2007) Content-based 3D object retrieval. IEEE Comput Graph Appl 27:22–27
20. Bhanu B, Peng J, Qing S (1998) Learning feature relevance and similarity metrics in image database. In: IEEE workshop proceedings on content-based access of image and video libraries. IEEE Computer Society, Washington, DC, USA, pp 14–18
21. El Naqa I, Yang Y, Galatsanos NP, Nishikawa RM, Wernick MN (2004) A similarity learning approach to content-based image retrieval: application to digital mammography. IEEE Trans Med Imaging 23:1233–1244
22. Swett HA, Mutalik PG, Neklesa VP, Horvath L, Lee C, Richter J, Tocino I, Fisher PR (1998) Voice-activated retrieval of mammography reference images. J Digit Imaging 11:65–73
23. Shyu CR, Brodley CE, Kak AC, Kosaka A, Aisen A, Broderick LS (1999) ASSERT: a physician-in-the-loop content-based retrieval system for HRCT image database. Comput Vis Image Underst 75(1–2):111–132
24. Dy JG, Brodley CE, Kak A, Broderick LS, Aisen AM (2003) Unsupervised feature selection applied to content-based retrieval of lung images. IEEE Trans Pattern Anal Mach Intell 25:373–378
25. Antani S, Long LR, Thoma GR (2004) Content-based image retrieval for large biomedical image archives. Stud Health Technol Inform 107:829–833
26. Guimond A, Subsol G (1997) Automatic MRI database exploration and applications. Pattern Recognit Artif Intell 11:1345–1365
27. Liu Y, Lazar N, Rothfus W (2002) Semantic-based biomedical image indexing and retrieval. In: Proceedings of the international conference on diagnostic imaging and analysis, pp 18–20
28. Cai W, Feng DD, Fulton R (2000) Content-based retrieval of dynamic PET functional images. IEEE Trans Inf Technol Biomed 4:152–158

29. Tobin KW, Abramoff MD, Chaum E, Giancardo L, Govindasamy VP, Karnowski TP, Tennant MTS, Swainson S (2008) Using a patient image archive to diagnose retinopathy. In: 30th annual international conference of the IEEE. Engineering in Medicine and Biology Society (EMBS), Vancouver, Canada, pp 5441–5444
30. Dorileo EAG, Frade MAC, Roselino AMF, Rangayyan RM, Azevedo-Marques PM (2008) Color image processing and content-based image retrieval techniques for the analysis of dermatological lesions. In: 30th annual international conference of the IEEE. Engineering in Medicine and Biology Society (EMBS), Vancouver, Canada, pp 1230–1233
31. Xue Z, Antani S, Long LR, Jeronimo J, Thoma GR (2007) Investigating CBIR techniques for cervicographic images. In: Proceedings of the 2007 annual symposium of the American Medical Information Association (AMIA), Chicago, pp 826–830
32. Zheng L, Wetzel AW, Gilbertson J, Becich MJ (2003) Design and analysis of a content-based pathology image retrieval system. IEEE Trans Inf Technol Biomed 7:249–255
33. Muller H, Rosset A, Garcia A, Vallee JP, Geissbuhler A (2005) Informatics in radiology (infoRAD): benefits of content-based visual data access in radiology. Radiographics 25:849–858
34. Vannier MW, Summers RM (2003) Sharing images. Radiology 228:23–25
35. Lehmann TM, Gould MO, Thies C, Fischer B, Keysers M, Kohnen D, Schubert H, Wein BB (2003) Content-based image retrieval in medical applications for picture archiving and communication systems. In: Proceedings SPIE medical imaging, vol 5033, San Diego, pp109–117
36. Muller H, Rosset A, Vallee J, Geissbuhler A (2004) Comparing features sets for content-based image retrieval in a medical-case database. In: PACS and Imaging Informatics IS&T/SPIE Medical Imaging, San Diego, CA, pp 99–109
37. Lehmann T, Guld M, Thies C, Plodowski B, Keysers D, Ott B (2004) IRMA – content-based image retrieval in medical applications. In: 14th world congress on medical informatics. IOS, Amsterdam, pp 842–848
38. Antani S, Lee DJ, Long LR, Thoma GR (2004) Evaluation of shape similarity measurement methods for spine X-ray images. J Vis Commun Image Represent 15:285–302
39. American College of Radiology (2003) American College of Radiology (ACR) Breast Imaging Reporting and Data System Atlas (BI-RADS® Atlas). American College of Radiology, Reston
40. Sklansky J, Tao EY, Bazargan M, Ornes CJ, Murchison RC, Teklehaimanot S (2000) Computer-aided, case-based diagnosis of mammographic regions of interest containing microcalcifications. Acad Radiol 7:395–405
41. Qi H, Snyder WE (1999) Content-based image retrieval in picture archiving and communications systems. J Digit Imaging 12:81–83
42. El Naqa I (2002) Content-based image retrieval by similarity learning for digital mammography in electrical engineering. Illinois Institute of Technology, Chicago
43. El Naqa I, Wernick M, Yang Y, Galatsanos N (2000) Image retrieval based on similarity learning. In: IEEE international conference on image processing, Vancouver, pp 722–725
44. El Naqa I, Wernick M, Yang Y, Galatsanos N (2002) Content-based image retrieval for digital mammography. In: IEEE international conference on image processing, Rochester, pp 141–144
45. Giger M, Huo Z, Vyborny C, Lan L, Bonta I, Horsch K (2002) Intelligent CAD workstation for breast imaging using similarity to known lesions and multiple visual prompt aids. In: Proceedings of the SPIE, vol 4684, San Diego, pp 768–773
46. Tourassi GD, Harrawood B, Singh S, Lo JY, Floyd CE (2007) Evaluation of information-theoretic similarity measures for content-based retrieval and detection of masses in mammograms. Med Phys 34:140–150
47. Tourassi GD, Ike R 3rd, Singh S, Harrawood B (2008) Evaluating the effect of image preprocessing on an information-theoretic CAD system in mammography. Acad Radiol 15:626–634

48. Tourassi GD, Vargas-Voracek R, Catarious DM Jr, Floyd CE Jr (2003) Computer-assisted detection of mammographic masses: a template matching scheme based on mutual information. Med Phys 30:2123–2130
49. Zheng B, Lu A, Hardesty LA, Sumkin JH, Hakim CM, Ganott MA, Gur D (2006) A method to improve visual similarity of breast masses for an interactive computer-aided diagnosis environment. Med Phys 33:111–117
50. Zheng B, Mello-Thoms C, Wang X, Gur D (2007) Improvement of visual similarity of similar breast masses selected by computer-aided diagnosis schemes. In: 4th IEEE international symposium on biomedical imaging: from nano to macro, Washington, DC, pp 516–519
51. Kinoshita SK, de Azevedo-Marques PM, Pereira RR Jr, Rodrigues JA, Rangayyan RM (2007) Content-based retrieval of mammograms using visual features related to breast density patterns. J Digit Imaging 20:172–190
52. Holt A, Bichindaritz I, Schmidt R, Perner P (2005) Medical applications in case-based reasoning. Knowl Eng Rev 20:289–292
53. Wei L, Yang Y, Nishikawa R, Wernick M (2006b) Learning of perceptual similarity from expert readers for mammogram retrieval. In: IEEE international symposium medical imaging: macro to nano, Arlington, pp 1356–1359
54. Bilska-Wolak AO, Floyd CE Jr (2002) Development and evaluation of a case-based reasoning classifier for prediction of breast biopsy outcome with BI-RADS lexicon. Med Phys 29:2090–2100
55. Floyd CE, Lo JY, Tourassi GD (2000) Case-based reasoning computer algorithm that uses mammographic findings for breast biopsy decisions. Am J Roentgenol 175:1347–1352
56. Mazurowski MA, Habas PA, Zurada JM, Tourassi GD (2008) Decision optimization of case-based computer-aided decision systems using genetic algorithms with application to mammography. Phys Med Biol 53:895–908
57. Nakayama R, Abe H, Shiraishi J, Doi K (2009) Potential usefulness of similar images in the differential diagnosis of clustered microcalcifications on mammograms. Radiology 253:625–631
58. Del Bimbo A (1999) Visual information retrieval. Morgan Kaufmann Publishers, San Francisco
59. Wei L, Yang Y, Wernick MN, Nishikawa RM (2009) Learning of perceptual similarity from expert readers for mammogram retrieval. IEEE J Sel Top Signal Process 3:53–61
60. Efron B, Tibshirani R (1993) An introduction to the bootstrap. Chapman & Hall, New York
61. Vapnik V (1998) Statistical learning theory. Wiley, New York
62. Wei L, Yang Y, Nishikawa RM, Jiang Y (2005) A study on several machine-learning methods for classification of malignant and benign clustered microcalcifications. IEEE Trans Med Imaging 24:371–380
63. El Naqa I, Yang Y, Galatsanos NP, Wernick MN (2004b) Mammogram retrieval based on incremental learning. In: IEEE international symposium on biomedical imaging: nano to macro, vol 2, Arlington, pp 1163–1166
64. Oh JH, Yang Y, El Naqa I (2010) Adaptive learning for relevance feedback: application to digital mammography. Med Phys 37:4432–4444
65. El Naqa I, Oh J, Yang Y (2012) Machine learning in computer-aided diagnosis. In: Suzuki K (ed) Medical imaging intelligence and analysis. IGI Global, Hershey
66. Scholkopf B, Smola A, Muller KR (1998) Nonlinear component analysis as a kernel eigenvalue problem. Neural Comput 10:1299–1319
67. Bishop CM (2006) Pattern recognition and machine learning. Springer, New York
68. Heath M, Bowyer K, Kopans D, Moore R, Kegelmeyer P (2001) The digital database for screening mammography. In: 5th international workshop on digital mammography (IWDM). Medical Physics Publishing Corp, Madison, pp 212–218
69. Guyon I, Elissee A (2003) An introduction to variable and feature selection. J Mach Learn Res 3:1157–1182
70. Samuelson FW, Petrick N (2006) Comparing image detection algorithms using resampling. In: International symposium on biomedical imaging, Arlington, pp 1312–1315

71. Bandos AI, Rockette HE, Gur D (2005) A permutation test sensitive to differences in areas for comparing ROC curves from a paired design. Stat Med 24:2873–2893
72. Metz CE, Herman BA, Shen JH (1998) Maximum likelihood estimation of receiver operating characteristic (ROC) curves from continuously-distributed data. Stat Med 17:1033–1053
73. El Naqa I, Wei L, Yang Y (2010) Ubiquitous health and medical informatics. In: Mohammed S, Fiaidhi J (eds) The ubiquity 2.0 trend and beyond. IGI Global, Hershey
74. Li Q, Li F, Shiraishi J, Katsuragawa S, Sone S, Doi K (2003) Investigation of new psychophysical measures for evaluation of similar images on thoracic CT for distinction between benign and malignant nodules. Med Phys 30:2584–2593
75. Muramatsu C, Li Q, Schmidt R, Suzuki K, Shiraishi J, Newstead G, Doi K (2006) Experimental determination of subjective similarity for pairs of clustered microcalcifications on mammograms: observer study results. Med Phys 33:3460–3468
76. Muramatsu C, Li Q, Suzuki K, Schmidt RA, Shiraishi J, Newstead GM, Doi K (2005) Investigation of psychophysical measure for evaluation of similar images for mammographic masses: preliminary results. Med Phys 32:2295–2304
77. Aggarwal P, Sardana HK, Jindal G (2009) Content based medical image retrieval: theory gaps and future directions. ICGST-GVIP J 9:27–37
78. Wei L, Yang Y, Nishikawa RM, Wernick MN, Edwards A (2005) Relevance vector machine for automatic detection of clustered microcalcifications. IEEE Trans Med Imaging 24:1278–1285
79. Wei C, Li C, Wilson R (2006) Database modeling for industrial data management: emerging technologies and applications. Idea Group Publishing, Hershey, pp 258–291

Chapter 3
A Novel Image-Based Approach for Early Detection of Prostate Cancer Using DCE-MRI

Ahmad Firjani, Fahmi Khalifa, Ahmad Elnakib, Georgy Gimel'farb, Mohammed Abou El-Ghar, Adel Elmaghraby, and Ayman El-Baz

Abstract A novel noninvasive approach for early diagnosis of prostate cancer from dynamic contrast-enhanced magnetic resonance imaging (DCE-MRI) is proposed. The proposed approach consists of four main steps. The first step is to isolate the prostate from the surrounding anatomical structures based on a maximum a posteriori (MAP) estimate of a log-likelihood function that accounts for the shape priori, the spatial interaction, and the current appearance of the prostate tissues and its background (surrounding anatomical structures). In the second step, a nonrigid registration algorithm is employed to account for any local deformation that could occur in the prostate during the scanning process due to patient breathing and local motion. In the third step, the perfusion curves that show propagation of the contrast agent into the tissue are obtained from the segmented prostate of the whole image sequence of the patient. In the final step, we collect two features from these curves

---

A. Firjani
BioImaging Laboratory, Department of Bioengineering, University of Louisville,
304 Lutz Building, Louisville, KY 40292, USA

Department of Computer Engineering and Computer Science, University of Louisville,
Louisville, KY 40292, USA

F. Khalifa • A. Elnakib • A. El-Baz (✉)
BioImaging Laboratory, Department of Bioengineering, University of Louisville,
304 Lutz Building, Louisville, KY 40292, USA
e-mail: aselba01@louisville.edu

G. Gimel'farb
Department of Computer Science, University of Auckland, Auckland, New Zealand

M. Abou El-Ghar
Radiology Department, Urology and Nephrology Center, Mansoura University,
Mansoura 35516, Egypt

A. Elmaghraby
Department of Computer Engineering and Computer Science, University of Louisville,
Louisville, KY 40292, USA

K. Suzuki (ed.), *Computational Intelligence in Biomedical Imaging*,
DOI 10.1007/978-1-4614-7245-2_3,

and use a k-nearest neighbor (KNN) classifier to distinguish between malignant and benign detected tumors. Moreover, in this chapter we introduce a new approach to generate color maps that illustrate the propagation of the contrast agent in the prostate tissues based on the analysis of the 3D spatial interaction of the change of the gray-level values of prostate voxel using a generalized Gauss–Markov random field (GGMRF) image model. Finally, the tumor boundaries are determined using a level set deformable model controlled by the perfusion information and the spatial interactions between the prostate voxels. Experimental results on 30 clinical DCE-MRI data sets yield promising results.

Introduction

Prostate cancer is the most frequently diagnosed malignancy in the American male population and the second leading cause of cancer death. Recent prostate cancer studies reported an estimated 217,730 new cases and a mortality rate of close to 32,000 in 2010 [1]. The growth of the population is a major cause of the high number of prostate cancer cases and will contribute to an increase in the global burden. Fortunately, the survival rate is very high for patients with an early diagnosis.

The techniques currently used for diagnosing prostate cancer are unsatisfactory. For example, prostate specific antigen (PSA) screening doesn't offer accurate information about the location and extent of the lesion(s). In addition, PSA is associated with a high-risk of over diagnosis of prostate cancer [2–5].

Medical imaging tools [e.g., transrectal ultrasound (TRUS), MR spectroscopy (MRS), dynamic contrast-enhanced MRI (DCE-MRI)], are favorable since they provide reliable information about the size and shape of prostate gland and can localize the cancer foci, which would improve the accuracy of diagnosis and enable more efficient treatment. One of the most common modalities is the TRUS imaging [6–9]. It is widely used for guided needle biopsy due to the real time nature of the imaging system, ease of use, and portability. However, TRUS images have low signal-to-noise ratio (SNR) and detection of malignant tissues is difficult. Another traditional imaging modality is computed tomography (CT). It is widely used for diagnosis and follow-up of prostate cancer, but it has poor soft-tissue contrast resolution which does not allow precise distinction of the internal or external anatomy of the prostate. Magnetic resonance (MR) imaging has recently been suggested for improved visualization and localization of the prostate. It provides valuable pathological and anatomical information [10]. Recently, new MR modalities, such as MRS, DCE-MRI, and diffusion MRI, have gained considerable attention as important tools for the early detection of prostate cancer.

In this chapter, we will focus on DCE-MRI based computer-aided diagnostic (CAD) systems since they have shown more capabilities in determining the size and the shape of the prostate gland and localizing the cancer foci. The principles of DCE-MRI lie in the analysis of signal-time or kinetic curves at a specific location in MR images. A sequential set of MR images is acquired before and during an intravenous bolus injection of paramagnetic gadolinium chelate, preferably by using a power injector. The contrast agent will induce an increased signal intensity on an MR image at vessel lumen and interstitial space. Such intensity curves obtained from the prostate are called wash-in and wash-out perfusion curves and can be used to distinguish between malignant and benign detected tumors [11]. Generally, any early diagnosis of prostate cancer using DCE-MRI requires intermediate image processing steps, such as prostate segmentation and classification. Therefore, in the following sections we will introduce the related work on both prostate segmentation and CAD systems.

Related Work in Prostate Segmentation

The prostate segmentation is an essential step in developing any noninvasive CAD system for detecting prostate cancer and calculating the prostate gland volume during biopsy. However, the segmentation of the prostate in MR images is a challenge due to large variations of prostate shape within a specific time series as well as across subjects, lack of strong edges and diffused prostate boundaries, and the similar intensity profile of the prostate and surrounding tissues. Although manual outlining of the prostate border enables the prostate volume to be determined, it is time consuming. Moreover, traditional edge detection methods (e.g., [10]) are unable to extract the correct boundaries of the prostate since the gray-level distributions of the prostate and the surrounding organs are hardly distinguishable.

The most successful known approaches (e.g., [8–12]) have addressed the segmentation challenges of the prostate by modeling object appearance and shape. In particular, Zhu et al. [12] used a combination of an active shape model (ASM) and 3D statistical shape modeling to segment the prostate. Toth et al. [13] presented an algorithm for the automatic segmentation of the prostate in multi-modal MRI. Their algorithm starts by isolating the region of interest (ROI) from MRS data. Then, an ASM within the ROI is used to obtain the final segmentation. Klein et al. [14] presented an atlas-based segmentation approach to extract the prostate from MR images. The segmentation of the prostate is obtained as the average of the best-matched registered atlas set to the test image (image to be segmented). Recently, Vikal et al. [15] used a priori knowledge of prostate shape to detect the contour in each slice and then refined them to form a 3D prostate surface. Martin et al. [16] developed an atlas-based approach for segmenting the prostate from 3D MR images by mapping probabilistic anatomical atlas to the test image. The resulting map is used to constrain a deformable model-based segmentation framework.

However, in most of these methods the segmentation reliability is not very high due to many reasons. First, parametric shape models fail in the presence of large gray-level variability across subjects and time. Second, edge detection methods are not suitable for discontinued objects. Moreover, deformable models tend to fail in the case of excessive noise, poor image resolution, diffused boundaries or occluded objects if they do not incorporate a priori models (e.g., shape and appearance).

To overcome the aforementioned limitations, in this chapter we present a general prostate segmentation framework, based on a maximum a posteriori (MAP) estimate of a new likelihood function. To handle the object inhomogeneities and variability and overcome image noise, the proposed likelihood function accounts for the visual appearances of the prostate and background, 3D spatial interaction between the prostate voxels, and a 3D prior prostate shape. The prostate shape is adaptively learned from the co-aligned segmented 3D prostate DCE-MRI. The visual appearances of the object and background are described with marginal gray-level distributions of the prostate and its background. The spatial interactions between the prostate voxels is modeled by a second-order rotation-variant Markov–Gibbs random field (MGRF) of object/background labels with analytically estimated potentials.

Related Work in Computer-Aided Detection and Diagnosis Systems for Prostate Cancer

When prostate cancer is suspected, a systematic biopsy guided by TRUS is usually used to confirm the diagnosis [17]. Twenty-three percent of all prostate cancers detected by TRUS-guided biopsy are missed in the first screening [18]. Even when biopsy results are true negatives some patients have to repeat biopsy before their cancers are detected. In 66–71 % of patients undergoing TRUS-biopsy for the first time, the results are negative [18, 19].

Initial results suggest that T2-weighted MRI and DCE-MRI holds promise for improving cancer detection, thereby reducing the need for prostate biopsy [20–30]. To the best of our knowledge, the first computerized prostate image analysis using MRI was developed by Chan et al. [20]. In this study, they present an in vivo computer-aided diagnosis system that uses multi-modal MRI to estimate malignancy likelihood in the peripheral zone. They constructed summary statistical maps from T2-weighted MRI images, diffusion-weighted images, PD maps, and T2 maps. Then they combined the statistic maps with textural and anatomical features in prostate cancer areas. However, this study doesn't include benign regions. A similar procedure with some extensions was used by Madabhushi et al. [21]. This study is based on T2-weighted MRI and showed the additional value of combining numerous features. Unfortunately, no discrimination performance was calculated and the method is limited to 2D ex vivo MRI.

Ocak et al. [22] developed a predictor by using a generalized estimating equation and logistic regression model, which comprehensively analyzed the T2-weighted MRI scans. Futterer et al. [23] developed a system to compare the accuracies of T2-weighted MRI and DCE-MRI imaging for prostate cancer localization in 14 ROIs. The results showed higher accuracy in DCE-MRI than they achieved with T2-weighted MRI.

Rouvière et al. [24] compared T2-weighted MRI and DCE-MRI in the detection of post-radiotherapy recurrence in 22 patients, using biopsy results as the reference standard. The results showed higher accuracy in DCE-MRI than they achieved with T2-weighted MRI.

Kim et al. [25] demonstrated that parametric imaging of the wash-in rate was more accurate for the detection of prostate cancer in the peripheral zone than was T2-weighted imaging alone. However, they also observed significant overlap between the wash-in rate for cancer and that for normal tissue in the transitional zone.

Puech et al. [26] developed a CAD system for prostate cancer detection using perfusion DCE-MRI data. The operator draws a polygon around the lesion within an enhanced image of the prostate. Semiautomatic lesion segmentation is initiated by a user-selected seed point. Region growing occurs from the seed point and the growing process stops when a different tissue (based on the contrast-enhanced time sequence) is encountered. Lesions are classified as benign, malignant, or indeterminate based on the analysis of the median wash-in and wash-out values. Although the results looked promising, manual interaction was still required.

Engelbrecht et al. [27] showed the usefulness of measurements of relative peak enhancement and wash-out rates for prostate cancer detection and localization. From their analysis of receiver operating characteristic curves, they concluded that the relative peak enhancement was the most accurate perfusion parameter for cancer detection in the peripheral zone and central region of the gland.

Vos et al. [28] developed a semiautomatic CAD system for prostate lesion classification using quantitative pharmacokinetic (PK) maps and T1 estimates. Pharmacokinetic features are extracted from a user defined ROI around the prostate and a support vector machine is used to estimate the likelihood of malignancy. Results show that the system has an accuracy of 92 % in classification of all ROIs from within the peripheral region and an accuracy of 83 % in classification of the ROIs with abnormal enhancement patterns. However, this study focused on the peripheral zone of the prostate gland and excluded central and transitional zones in which up to 35 % of prostate cancers can occur. Viswanath et al. [29] proposed a CAD system for DCE-MRI data. In this system, the authors rely on a nonrigid (elastic) registration scheme and unsupervised classification (k-means) procedure. The CAD system improves the objective annotation of prostate cancer, but the corresponding slices still need to be selected.

Most prostate CAD researchers have focused on the initial voxel classification stage. They obtained likelihood maps by combining information from MR images using mathematical descriptors. These studies showed on a voxel basis that the discrimination between benign and malignant tissue is feasible with good performances. However, these studies require user interaction to select an ROI around the prostate. In addition to the localization of the ROI of the tumor, the final diagnosis and patient management is left to the radiologist.

However, the majority of these studies were performed by radiologists who selected an ROI (a small window) around the prostate and followed signal change within this ROI. Unfortunately, such approaches not only require manual interaction of the operators, but also ROI selection biases the final decision and brings up the same issue of over or underestimating the problem in the entire graft, just as with biopsy. Moreover, manual window selection and generating a function curve from this window over a time-sequence of images assumes that the prostates (prostate contours) remain exactly the same from scan to scan. However, prostate contours may not always exactly match due to patient movement or breathing effects; therefore, image registration schemes should be applied first before ROI selection. Also, to automate the algorithm and to cancel ROI dependency, segmentation algorithms that can separate the prostate from the surrounding structures are needed. To overcome these limitations, we propose an automatic framework for the early diagnosis of prostate cancer using DCE-MRI. The proposed framework segments the prostate from the surrounding anatomical structures based on a learned shape model and an identifiable joint MGRF model of DCE-MRI and "object–background" region maps. Following segmentation, a nonrigid registration algorithm is employed to account for any local deformation that could occur in the prostate during the scanning process. Once all the images are aligned, the perfusion curves that show propagation of the contrast agent into the tissue are obtained, and then used to collect two features to distinguish between malignant and benign detected tumors.

The rest of this chapter is organized as follows. Section "Methods" discusses in detail the steps of the proposed framework, the experimental results are presented in section "Experimental Results," and the study is concluded in section "Conclusion" with speculation about future work.

Methods

In this chapter we introduce a new, automated, and noninvasive framework for early diagnosis of prostate cancer from DCE-MRI. Figure 3.1 demonstrates the steps of the proposed CAD system.

Segmentation of the Prostate Using a Joint MGRF Model

The segmentation of the prostate is a challenge, since the gray-level distribution of the prostate and surrounding organs is not highly distinguishable and because of the anatomical complexity of prostate. This stage proposes a powerful framework for prostate segmentation based on a learned shape model and an identifiable joint MGRF model of DCE-MRI and "object–background" region maps.

The joint-MGRF model is fundamentally a model that relates the joint probability of an image and its object–background region map to geometric structure and to the energy of repeated patterns within the image [31]. The basic theory behind such models is that they assume that the signals associated with each pixel depend on the signals of the neighboring pixels, and thus explicitly take into account their spatial interactions, and other features, such as shape.

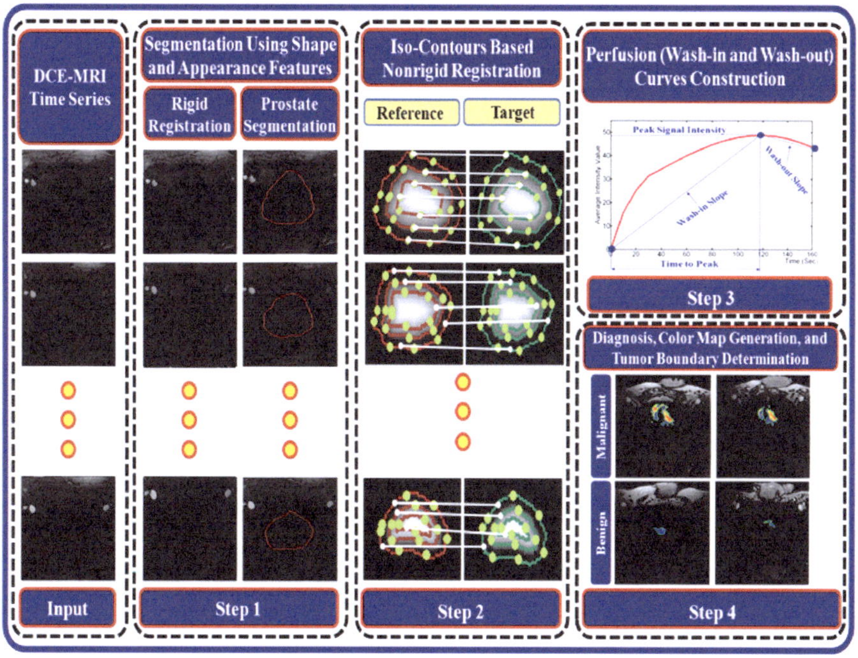

Fig. 3.1 The proposed CAD system for automatic detection of cancer

Let $\mathbf{Q} = \{0, 1, \ldots, Q - 1\}$, $\mathbf{L} = \{\mathbf{ob}, \mathbf{bg}\}$, and $\mathbf{U} = [\mathbf{0}, \mathbf{1}]$ be a set of Q integer gray-level, a set of object ("ob") and background ("bg") labels, and a unit interval, respectively. Let a 3D arithmetic grid $\mathrm{R} = \{(x,y,z) : x = 0, 1, \ldots, X - 1; y = 0, 1, \ldots, Y - 1; z = 0, 1, \ldots Z - 1\}$ support a grayscale DCE-MRI $\mathbf{g} : \mathbf{R} \rightarrow \mathbf{Q}$ and their binary region maps $\mathbf{m} : \mathbf{R} \rightarrow \mathbf{L}$, and probabilistic shape model $\mathbf{s} : \mathbf{R} \rightarrow \mathbf{U}$. The shape model allows for registering (aligning) 3D prostate DCE-MRI. The DCE-MR data $\mathbf{g}$ and their region maps $\mathbf{m}$ are described with a joint probability model:

$$P(\mathbf{g}, \mathbf{m}) = P(\mathbf{g}|\mathbf{m}) P_h(\mathbf{m}) \tag{3.1}$$

where $P_h(\mathbf{m})$ is a second-order MGRF of region maps and $P(\mathbf{g}|\mathbf{m})$ is a conditionally independent random field of image intensities given the map. The map model $P_h(\mathbf{m}) = P_s(\mathbf{m})\ P(\mathbf{m})$ has two parts: a shape prior probability being a spatially variant independent random field of region labels $P_s(\mathbf{m})$, for a set of co-aligned training DCE-MR data, and a second-order MGRF model $P(\mathbf{m})$ of a spatially homogeneous evolving map.

The Bayesian MAP estimate of the map, given the DCE-MR data g, $\mathrm{m}^* = \arg \max_{\mathbf{m}} L(\mathbf{g}, \mathbf{m})$ maximize the log-likelihood function:

$$L(\mathbf{g}, \mathbf{m}) = \log(P(\mathbf{g}|\mathbf{m})) + \log(P_h(\mathbf{m}))$$

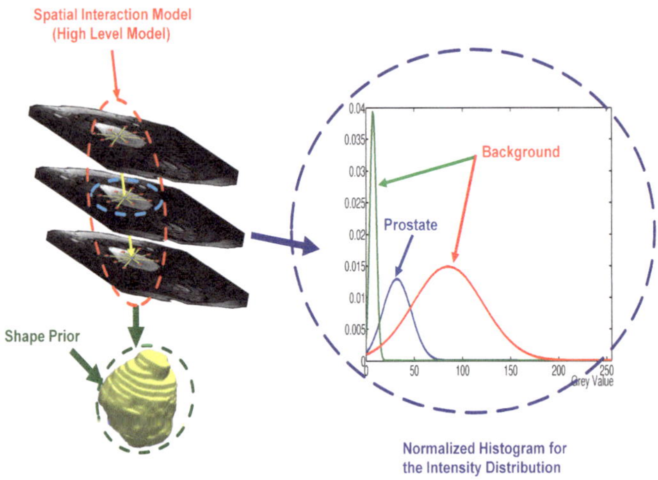

Fig. 3.2 Joint Markov–Gibbs random field model of DCE-MRI

In this work we focus on accurate identification of the spatial interaction between the prostate voxels $P(\mathbf{m})$, and the intensity distribution for the prostate tissues, $P(\mathbf{g}|\mathbf{m})$, and the prior distribution $P_s(\mathbf{m})$ of the prostate shape, as shown in Fig. 3.2.

To perform the initial prostate segmentation, a given 3D DCE-MRI is aligned to one of the training 3D DCE-MRI. The shape model provides the voxel-wise object and background probabilities being used, together with the conditional image intensity model $P(\mathbf{g}|\mathbf{m})$, to build an initial region map. The final Bayesian segmentation is performed using the identified joint MGRF model of the DCE-MRI and region maps.

Conditional Intensity Model

The specific visual appearance of the prostate in each data set to be segmented is taken into account by modeling a marginal gray-level distribution with a linear combination of discrete Gaussians (LCDG) [32, 33]. Close approximation with LCDG separates each factor of the joint empirical gray-level distribution, $P(\mathbf{g}) = \prod_{(x,y)\in\mathbf{R}} p_{mix}(g_{x,y})$, into two (object and background) components, $(p(q|\lambda);$ $q \in \mathbf{Q}, \textit{and}\ \lambda \in \mathbf{L})$. The LCDG modeling restores transitions between these components more accurately than conventional mixtures of only positive Gaussians, thus yielding a better initial region map formed by voxel-wise classification of the image gray values. The similar intensity profile of the prostate and surrounding tissues.

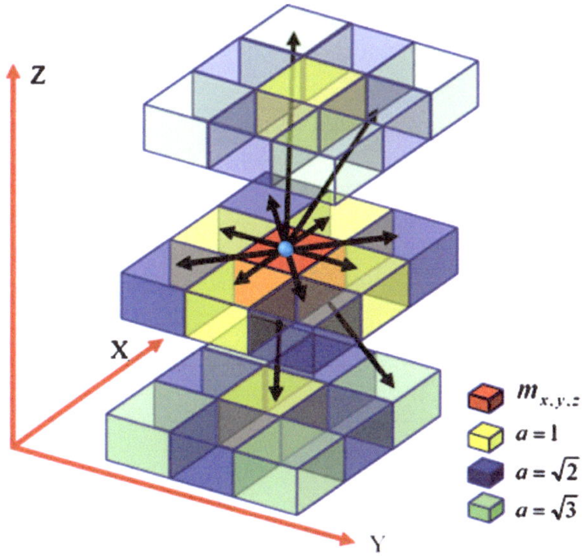

Fig. 3.3 Three-dimensional second-order MRF neighborhood system. The reference voxel is shown in *red*

Spatial Voxel Interaction Model

To overcome noise effect and to ensure the homogeneity of the segmentation, spatially voxel interactions between the region labels are also taken into account.

A generic MGRF of region maps [34] accounts only for pairwise interaction between each region label and its characteristic neighbors. Generally, the interaction structure and the Gibbs potentials can be arbitrary and are identified from the training data. For simplicity, we restrict the interaction structure to the nearest voxel 26-neighborhood only as shown in Fig. 3.3. By symmetry considerations, we assume that the potentials are independent of relative orientation of each voxel pair and depend only on intra- or inter-region position (i.e., whether the labels are equal or not). Under these restrictions, it is the 3D extension of the conventional auto-binomial, or Potts model differing only in that the potentials are estimated analytically.

The 26-neighborhood has three types of symmetric pairwise interactions specified by the absolute distance a between two voxels in the same and adjacent MRI slices ($a = 1$, $\sqrt{2}$, and $\sqrt{3}$, respectively): (1) the closest pairs with the inter-voxel $\mathbf{N}_1 = \{(1,0,0),(0,1,0),(0,0,1)\}$ coordinate offsets; (2) the diagonal pairs with the offsets $\mathbf{N}_{\sqrt{2}} = \{(0,1,\pm 1),(1,0,\pm 1),(1,\pm 1,0)\}$; and (3) the farthest diagonal pairs with the offsets $\mathbf{N}_{\sqrt{3}} = \{(1,\pm 1,\pm 1)\}$. The Gibbs potentials of each type are bi-valued because only label coincidence is accounted for: $\mathbf{V}_a = \{V_{a,eq}; V_{a,ne}\}$

where $V_{a,eq} \equiv V_a(l,l')$ if $l = l'$ and $V_{a,ne} \equiv V_a(l,l')$ if $l \neq l'$; $a \in \mathbf{A} = \{1, \sqrt{2}, \sqrt{3}\}$. Then the MGRF model of region maps is as follows:

$$P(\mathbf{m}) = \frac{1}{Z} \exp \sum_{(x,y,z) \in \mathbf{R}} \sum_{a \in \mathbf{A}} \sum_{(\xi,\eta,\kappa) \in \mathbf{N}_a} V_a\left(m_{x,y,z}, m_{x+\xi,y+\eta,z+\kappa}\right) \tag{3.2}$$

where Z is the normalizing factor (partition function).

To identify the MGRF in Eq. (3.1), approximate analytical maximum likelihood estimate of the 3D Gibbs potentials, $V_{a,eq}$ and $V_{a,ne}$ are derived in line with [34]:

$$V_{a,eq} = -V_{a,ne} = 2\left(f_{a,eq}(m) - \frac{1}{2}\right) \tag{3.3}$$

where $f_{a,eq}(m)$ denotes the relative frequency of the equal labels in the equivalent voxel pairs $\{((x,y,z),(x+\xi, y+\eta, z+\kappa)) : (x,y,z) \in \mathbf{R}; (x+\xi, y+\eta, z+\kappa) \in \mathbf{R}; (\xi,\eta,\kappa) \in \mathbf{N}_a\}$ of a region map m of a given DCE-MRI aligned in accord with the prior shape model.

Probabilistic Shape Model

To enhance the segmentation accuracy, additional constraints based on the expected shape of the prostate are introduced by co-aligning each given DCE-MR data to a training database and using a soft probabilistic 3D prostate shape model $P_s(m) = \prod_{(x,y,z) \in \mathbf{R}} S_{mx,y,z}$; where $S_{mx,y,z}$ is the empirical probability that the voxel (x,y,z) belongs to the prostate ($L = $ 'ob') or the background ($L = $ 'bg') given the map (see Figs. 3.4 and 3.5).

Prostate Shape Model Algorithm

Initialization:

- Co-align the 3D DCE-MRI training sets collected from different subjects using a rigid 3D registration maximizing their mutual information (MI) [35].
- Manually segment the prostate from the aligned sets.
- Estimate the voxel-wise probabilities by counting how many times each voxel (x,y,z) was segmented as the prostate.

Updating Prior Shape Model:

- To enhance the segmentation of the current prostate volume, the prior probabilistic shape model is updated by adding the previous segmented 3D prostate data to the prior calculated shape model.

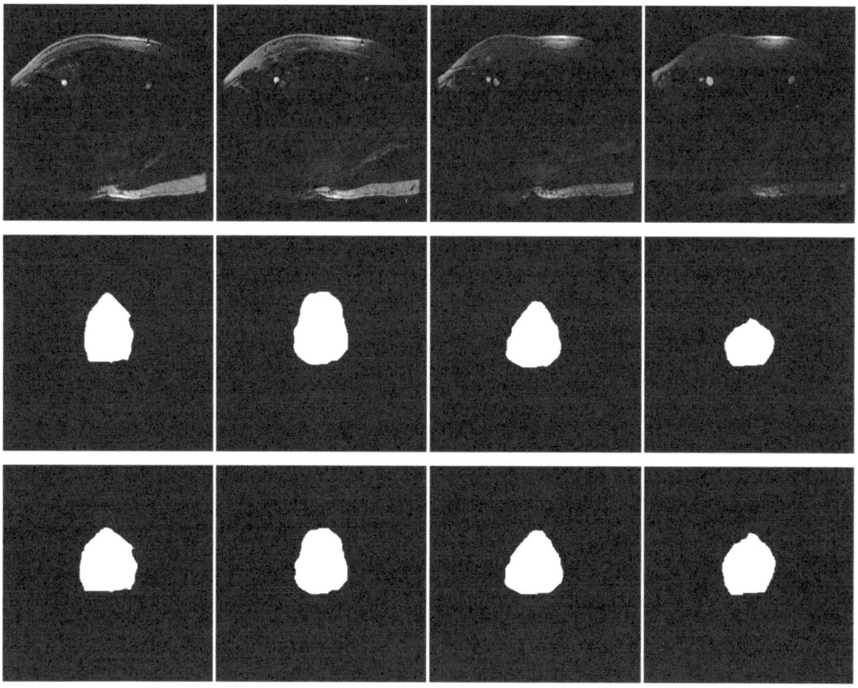

Fig. 3.4 Forming prostate shape prior projected onto 2D:0020 *top row*-training samples; *middle row*—manually segmented prostate regions, and *bottom row*—their affine MI-based alignment

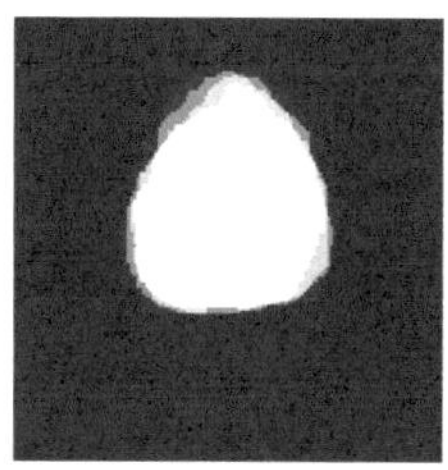

Fig. 3.5 Two-dimensional axial projection of gray-coded prostate region shape prior

Segmentation Algorithm

In total, the proposed prostate segmentation process involves the following steps:

1. Perform an affine alignment of a given 3D MRI to an arbitrary prototype prostate from the training set using mutual information [35] as a similarity measure to obtain the learned probabilistic shape model $P(\mathbf{s}|\mathbf{m})$.
2. Estimate the conditional intensity model $P(\mathbf{g}|\mathbf{m})$ by identifying the bimodal LCDG.
3. Use the intensity model found and the learned probabilistic shape model to perform an initial segmentation of the prostate, i.e., to form an initial region map.
4. Use the initial region map to estimate the potential for the Potts model using (3) and to identify the MGRF model $P(\mathbf{m})$ of region maps.

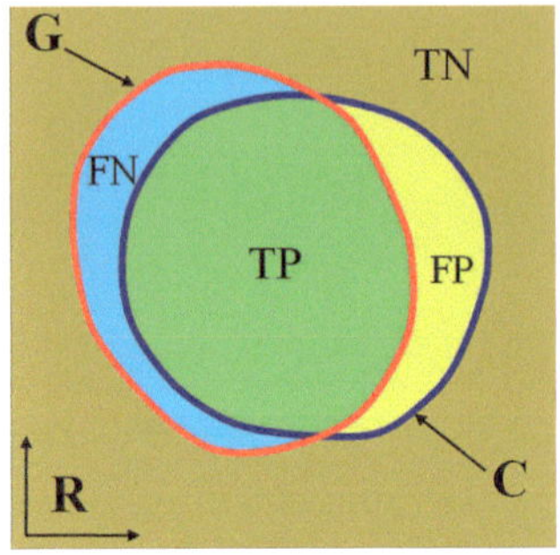

Fig. 3.6 Two-dimensional schematic illustration of measuring segmentation errors

5. Improve the region map using voxel-wise stochastic relaxation (iterative conditional mode—ICM [36]) through successive iterations to maximize the log-likelihood function of Eq. (3.1) until the log-likelihood remains almost the same for two successive iterations.
6. Output: The 3D prostate segmentation is the final estimate region map, **m**.

Performance Evaluation of the Proposed Segmentation Algorithm

To evaluate the performance of the proposed segmentation algorithm, we measured true positive (TP), true negative (TN), false positive (FP), and false negative (FN) segmentation (Fig. 3.6) Let C and G denote the segmented region, its "ground truth" counterpart, and the whole image lattice, respectively. Let $|z|$ denote the volume (in the number of voxels) of a region z. Then $TP = |C \cap G|$ is the overlap between C and G the false positive $FP = |C - C \cap G|$ is the difference between the segmented object and the TP; the false negative $FN = |G - C \cap G|$ is the difference between the ground truth and the TP; and $TN = |R - C \cup G|$ The positive predictive value (PPV), Sensitivity (Sens), and dice similarity coefficient (DSC) are defined as:

$$PPV = \frac{TP}{TP + FP} \tag{3.4}$$

$$Sens = \frac{TP}{TP + FN} \tag{3.5}$$

$$DSC = \frac{2 \times TP}{2 \times TP + FP + FN} \tag{3.6}$$

Nonrigid Registration

Due to patient breathing and local movement, accurate registration is a main issue in DCE-MRI sequences. A tremendous number of nonrigid image registration techniques have been developed, e.g., [37, 38]. However, more robust, efficient,

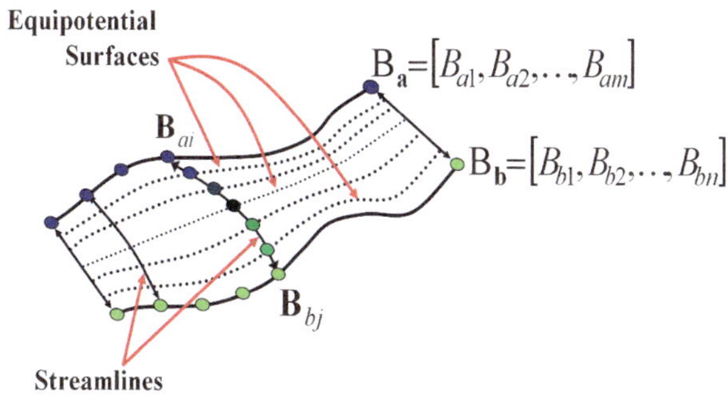

Fig. 3.7 Two-dimensional schematic illustration of correspondences by a potential field

and sophisticated registration techniques are required. In this chapter, the nonrigid registration of the DCE-MR data is performed by solving the second-order linear partial differential Laplace equation:

$$\nabla^2 \gamma = \frac{\partial^2 \gamma}{\partial x^2} + \frac{\partial^2 \gamma}{\partial y^2} = 0 \tag{3.7}$$

for a scalar function $\gamma(x,y)$ between the target and the reference prostate objects. This PDE arises in various scientific and engineering applications including fluid mechanics, electromagnetic theory, potential theory, solid mechanics, heat conduction, geometry, probability theory, etc. The solution of a planar Laplace equation between two boundaries results in intermediate equipotential surfaces (dashed lines in Fig. 3.7) and streamlines that connect both boundaries and are everywhere orthogonal to all the equipotential surfaces (see, e.g., the line connecting the points B_{ai} and B_{bj} in Fig. 3.7).

The streamlines establish natural point-to-point correspondences between the boundaries. Based on solving the Laplace equation, we perform the nonrigid registration as follows:

1. Generate the distance maps inside the prostate regions as shown in Fig. 3.8a, b.
2. Use these distance maps to generate equispaced iso-contours (Fig. 3.8c, d).
3. Solve the Laplace equation between respective reference and target iso-contours to find the point-to-point correspondence.

Wash-In and Wash-Out Perfusion Curves

After the nonrigid alignment, the wash-in and wash-out curves are constructed by calculating the average intensities of prostate regions for each time sequence. These curves show the response of the prostate tissues as the contrast agent perfuses for each image section (see Fig. 3.9).

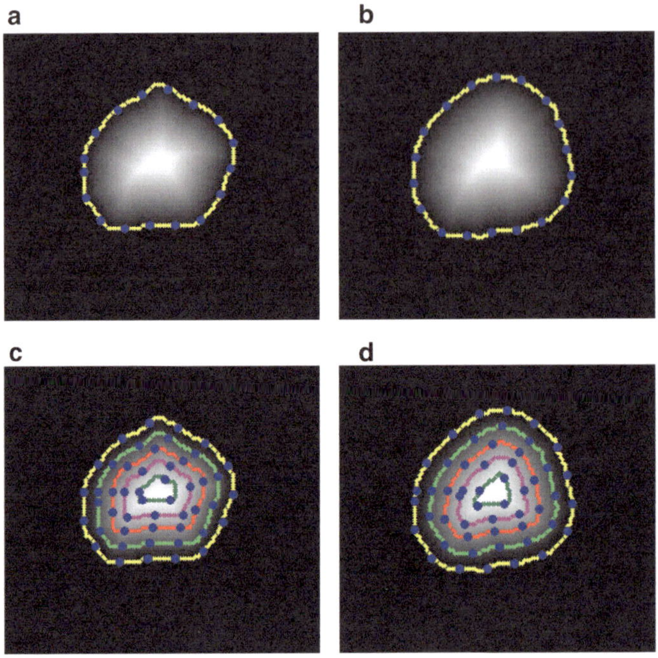

Fig. 3.8 The distance maps (**a**, **b**) and the iso-contours (**c**, **d**) of the two prostates

Color Map Generation and Tumor Boundary Determination

To characterize the physiological data, color-coded maps that illustrate the propagation of the contrast agent in the prostate tissues are constructed. To construct the initial color maps, we have to estimate the changes in image signals $\delta_{x,y,z}$ due to the contrast agent. These changes are estimated from the constructed perfusion curves as the difference between the signals of image sequences at t_p and t_0 (see Fig. 3.9). To preserve continuity (remove inconsistencies), the initial estimated $\delta_{x,y,z}$ values are considered as samples from a generalized Gauss–Markov random field (GGMRF) image model [39] of measurements with the 26-voxel neighborhood (Fig. 3.3). Continuity of the constructed 3-D volume (Fig. 3.10) is amplified by using their MAP estimates as shown in [28]:

$$\hat{\delta}_{x,y,z} = \arg\min_{\tilde{\delta}_{x,y,z}} \left\{ \left|\delta_{x,y,z} - \tilde{\delta}_{x,y,z}\right|^{\alpha} + \rho^{\alpha}\lambda^{\beta} \sum_{(x',y',z') \in \nu_{(x,y,z)}} \eta_{(x,y,z),(x',y',z')} \left|\tilde{\delta}_{x,y,z} - \delta_{x',y',z'}\right|^{\beta} \right\}$$

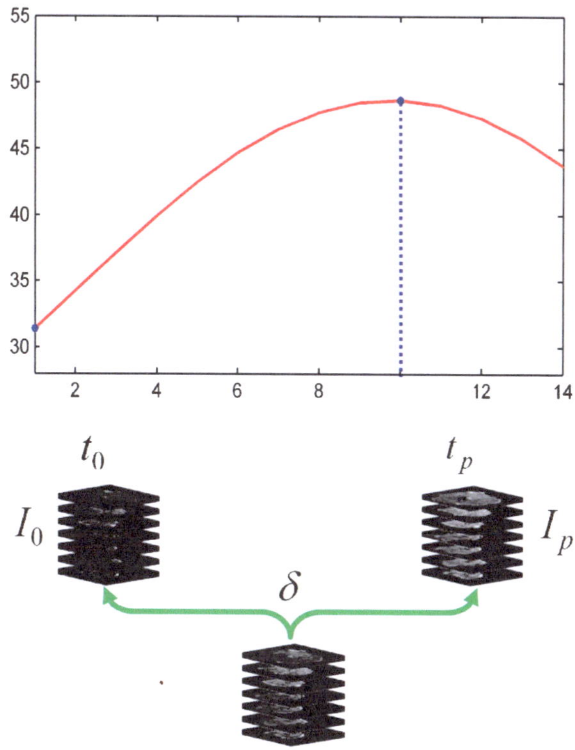

Fig. 3.9 Estimating δ from the perfusion curve as the difference between the peak and initial signal of image sequences

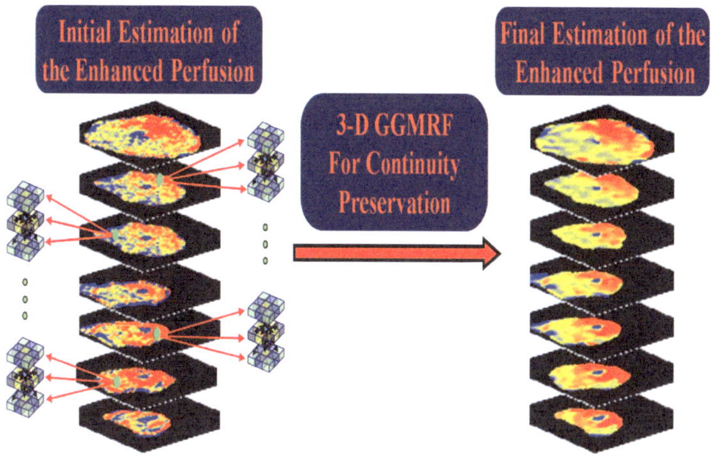

Fig. 3.10 Enhanced perfusion estimation and continuity analysis using the 3-D GGMRF image model

where $\delta_{x,y,z}$ and $\widetilde{\delta}_{x,y,z}$ denote the original values and their expected estimates, $\nu_{(x,y,z)}$ is the 26-neighborhood voxel set (Fig. 3.3), $\eta_{(x,y,z),(x',y',z')}$ is the GGMRF potential, and ρ and λ are scaling factors. The parameter $\beta \in [1.01, 2.0]$ controls the level of smoothing (e.g., smooth, $\beta = 2$, vs. relatively abrupt edges, $\beta = 1.01$). The parameter $\alpha \in \{1; 2\}$ determines the Gaussian, $\alpha = 2$, or Laplace, $\alpha = 1$, prior distribution of the estimator. Then, the color maps are generated based on the final estimated $\widetilde{\delta}$ (see Fig. 3.10).

Finally, to allocate the boundary of the detected tumors, which is important to determine the cancer stage in case of malignancy, we used a level set-based deformable model controlled by a stochastic speed function [40]. The latter accounts for the perfusion information and spatial interactions between the prostate voxels.

Experimental Results

Data Acquisition

During development of this study, we observed that good selection of a DCE-MR imaging protocol is as important as the image analysis, if not more important. The key point in the protocol is to take the images as quickly as possible while trying to conserve the quality. A compromise on image quality results in too much noise and partial volume effects; on the other hand, a compromise on speed results in fewer data points, which prevents us from being able to classify signals. Therefore, with collaborative efforts, the protocol was modified a number of times to acquire standard and better quality imaging. The protocol described below has been found to be optimal with the current MRI hardware (Signa Horizon GE 1.5 tesla MR scanner using an additional pelvic coil).

In our protocol, gradient-echo T2 imaging was employed by a Signa Horizon GE 1.5 tesla MR scanner using an additional pelvic coil. Images were taken at a 7 mm thickness with an interslice gap of 0.5 mm. The repetition time (TR) was 50 ms, the TE was minimum with flip angle at 60°, the band width was 31.25 kHz, the field of view (FOV) was 28 cm, and the number of slices was seven. The DCE-MRI process started with a series of MRI scans which were used to establish a baseline in image intensity. These scans were performed without the administration of contrast enhancing agents so that the tissue's nonenhanced image intensity could be established. In the next stage, 10 cc of gadoteric acid (Dotarem 0.5 mmol/mL; Guerbet, France) was administered intravenously at a rate of 3 mL/s. At this point, a series of MRI scans was performed every 10 s for 3 min, and every series contained seven slices. Note all the subjects were diagnosed using a biopsy (ground truth). A sample of what a DCE-MRI looks like with this protocol is shown in Fig. 3.11.

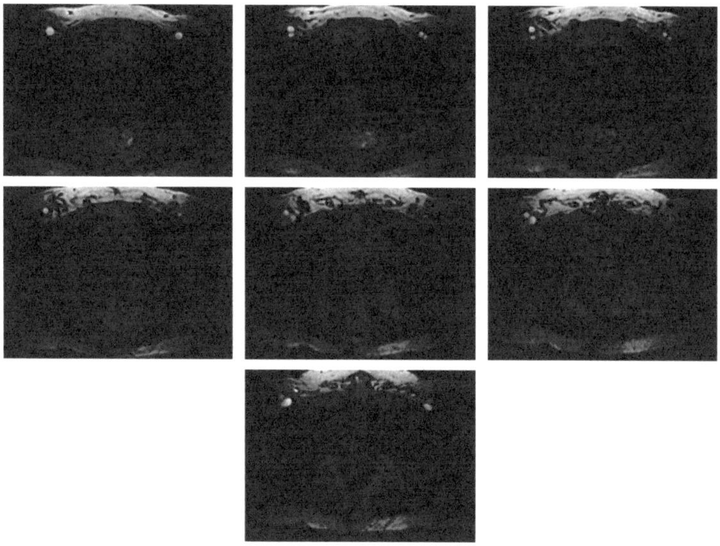

Fig. 3.11 Example of a DCE-MRI slices images from one patient. For each patient, 128 images are taken

Segmentation Results

The proposed segmentation approach has been tested on DCE-MRI sequences for 30 independent subjects. Figure 3.12 demonstrates some segmentation results of the prostate region at selected image sections for different subjects and their associated false positive (FP) and false negative (FN) errors. For comparison, our segmentation results are compared to the radiologist's tracing based on the PPV, Sensitivity (Sens), and DSC [41]. Table 3.1 represents the PPV, Sens, and DSC statistics obtained for the test subjects involved in this study.

For comparison, all time series images have been segmented using the shape-based approach proposed in Tsai et al. [42]. The comparative results for a few of them are shown in Fig. 3.13. Table 3.2 compares the segmentation results over all test data sets with the known ground truth (manual tracing by an imaging expert) and the differences are shown to be statistically significant by the unpaired t-test (the two-tailed value P is less than 0.0001).

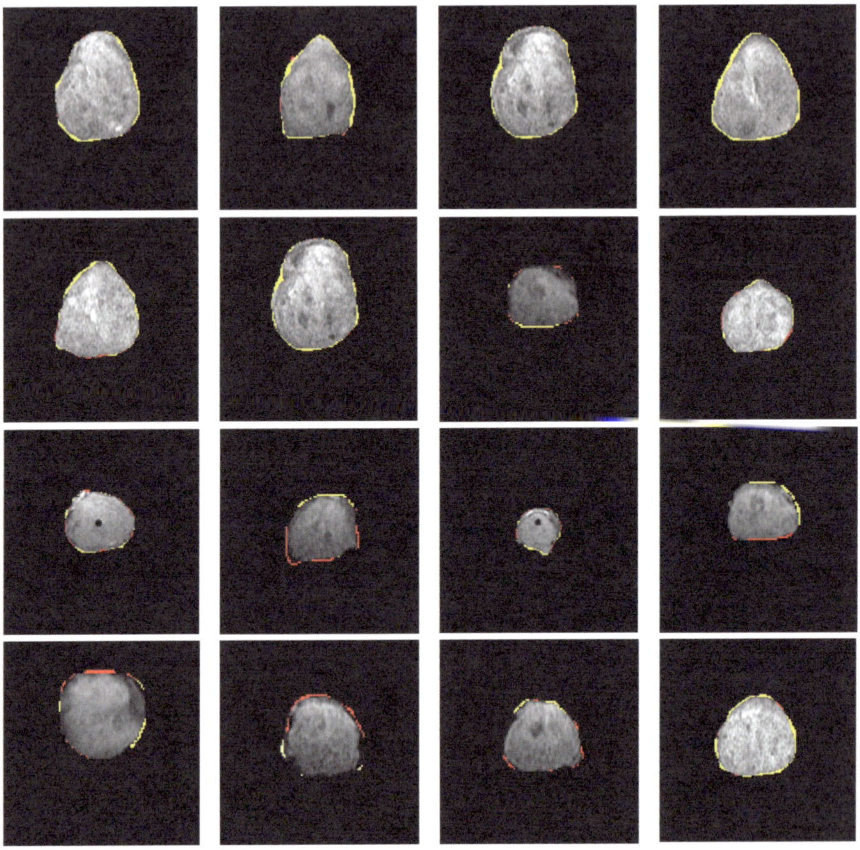

Fig. 3.12 Segmentation results: the segmentation results with error referenced to the ground truth G is outlined in *yellow* [false negative (FN): pixels segmented as the prostate in G but not segmented as the prostate with our approach] and *red* [false positive (FP): pixels segmented as the prostate with our approach but not segmented as the prostate in the G]

Table 3.1 Error statistics over all test data sets

Performance measures			
	PPV	Sens	DSC
Minimum	0.972	0.837	0.909
Maximum	0.989	0.851	0.930
Mean	0.982	0.846	0.923
Standard deviation	0.004	0.004	0.004

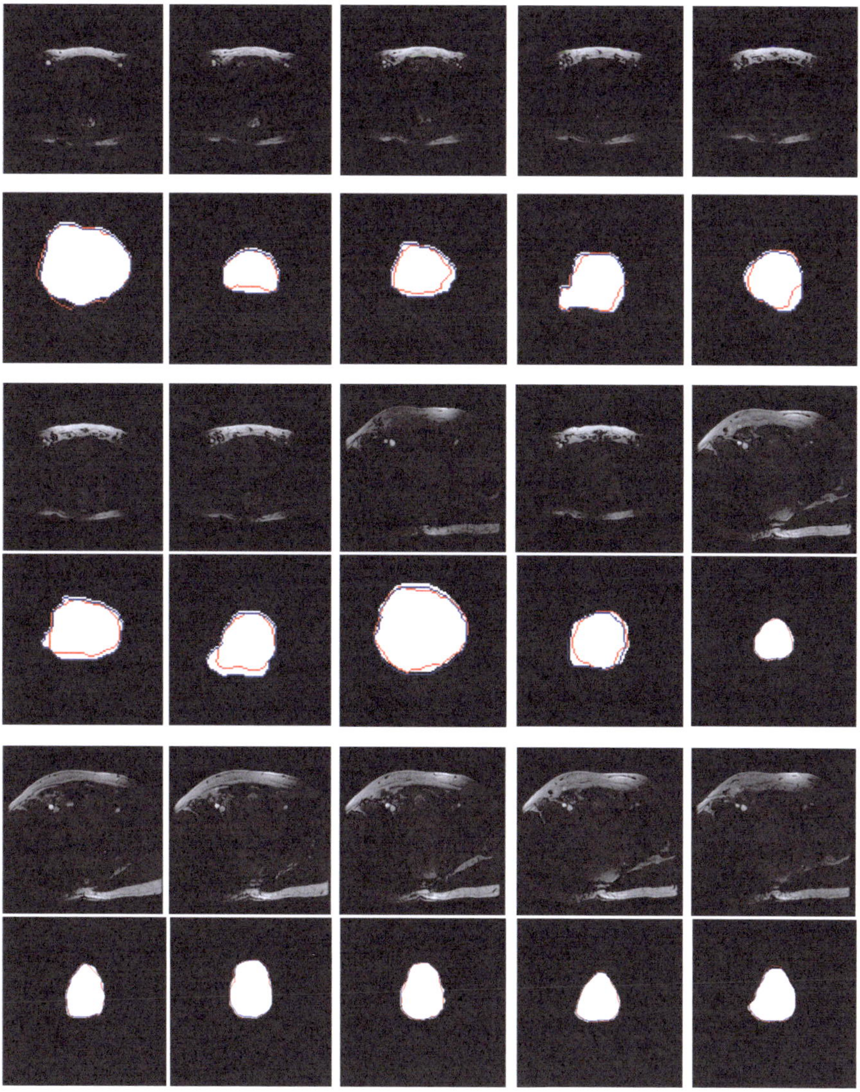

Fig. 3.13 Accuracy of our segmentation in comparison with [42]. Our segmentation is outlined in *blue* and [42] in *red* with reference to the ground truth G in *white*

Table 3.2 Comparative segmentation accuracies over all test data sets

	Algorithm	
	Our	[42]
Minimum error (%)	0	2.51
Maximum error (%)	1.50	11.92
Average error (%)	0.53	5.91
Standard deviation (%)	0.33	4.44
Two-tailed P-value		0.0001

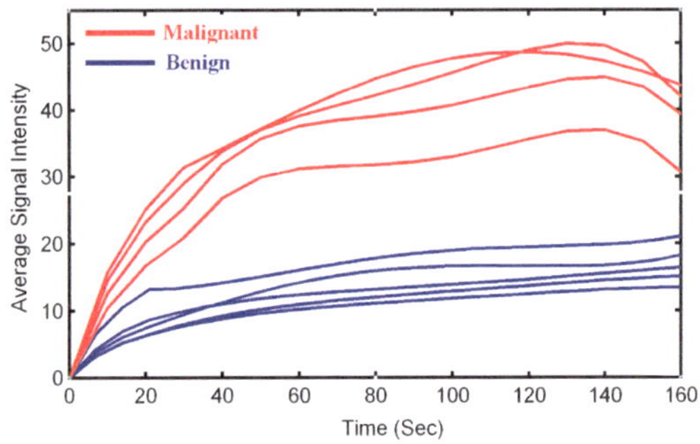

Fig. 3.14 Perfusion curves from nine subjects with respect to scan number. Subjects in *red* are malignant, and subjects in *blue* are benign

Diagnostic Results

The ultimate goal of the proposed framework is to successfully distinguish between malignant and benign detected tumors by constructing the perfusion curves from the DCE-MRI sequences. The curves show the response of the prostate tissues as the contrast agent perfuses. The malignant subjects show an abrupt increase to the higher perfusion values and the benign subjects show a delay in reaching their peak perfusion (see Fig. 3.14). From these curves, we have been able to conclude that the peak perfusion value and the wash-in slope are the two major extracted features for classification. To distinguish between benign and malignant cases, we used a *k*-nearest neighbor (KNN) classifier to learn the statistical characteristics of both benign and malignant subjects from the perfusion curves of the training sets. In our approach, we used nine data sets for the training (see Fig. 3.14) and the other 21 for testing. The KNN-based classification classifies both training and testing data correctly, so the overall accuracy of the proposed approach is 100 %. Following the classification, a visual assessment is made. Figure 3.15 presents the color-coded maps over all image sections before and after applying the 3-D GGMRF smoothing for three subjects involved in our study. Figures 3.16 and 3.17 show two examples of the tumor contours determination for benign subjects, and Figs. 3.18 and 3.19 show two examples of the tumor contours determination for malignant subjects.

Conclusion

In this chapter, we present a framework for detecting prostate cancer using DCE-MRI. The framework includes prostate segmentation, nonrigid registration, and KNN-based classification. For prostate segmentation, we introduced a new 3D

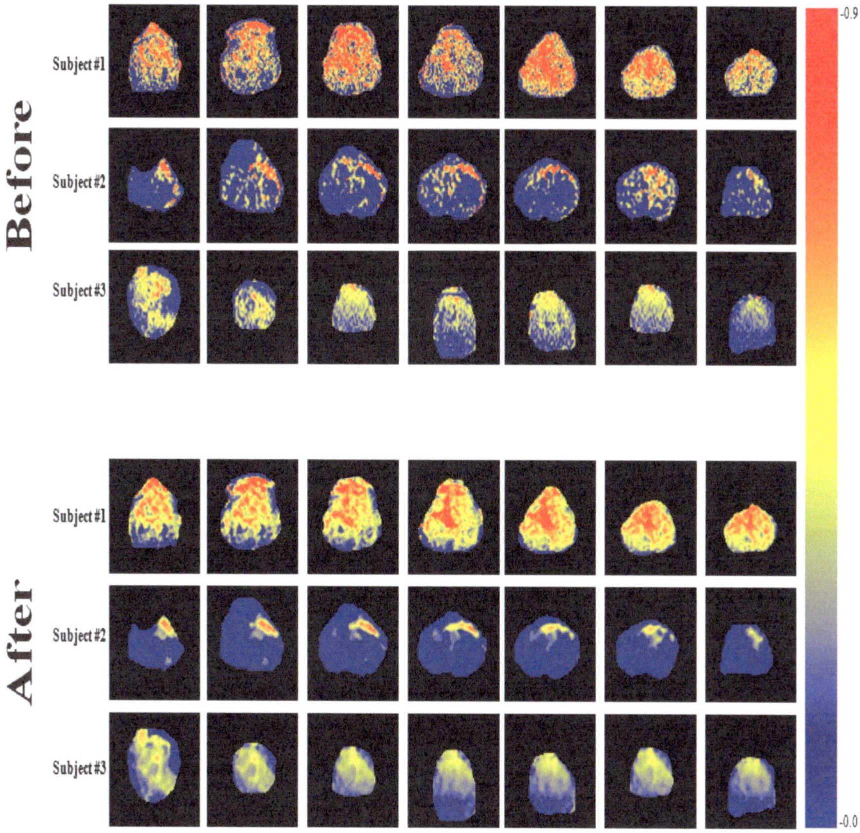

Fig. 3.15 Color-coded maps for three of the test subjects before and after the 3-D GGMRF smoothing with $\rho = 1$, $\lambda = 5$, $\beta = 1{:}01$, $\alpha = 2$, and $\eta_{(x,y,z),(x',y',z')} = \sqrt{2}$ and their respective color-coded maps. The *red* and *blue* ends of the color scale relate to the maximum and minimum changes, respectively

approach that is based on a MAP estimate of a new log-likelihood function that accounts for the shape priori, the spatial interaction, and the current appearance of the prostate tissues and its background. Following segmentation, we introduced a nonrigid registration approach that deforms the prostate object on iso-contours instead of a square lattice, which provides more degrees of freedom to obtain accurate deformation. The perfusion curves of the segmented prostate region are calculated and the features extracted from these curves undergo KNN-based

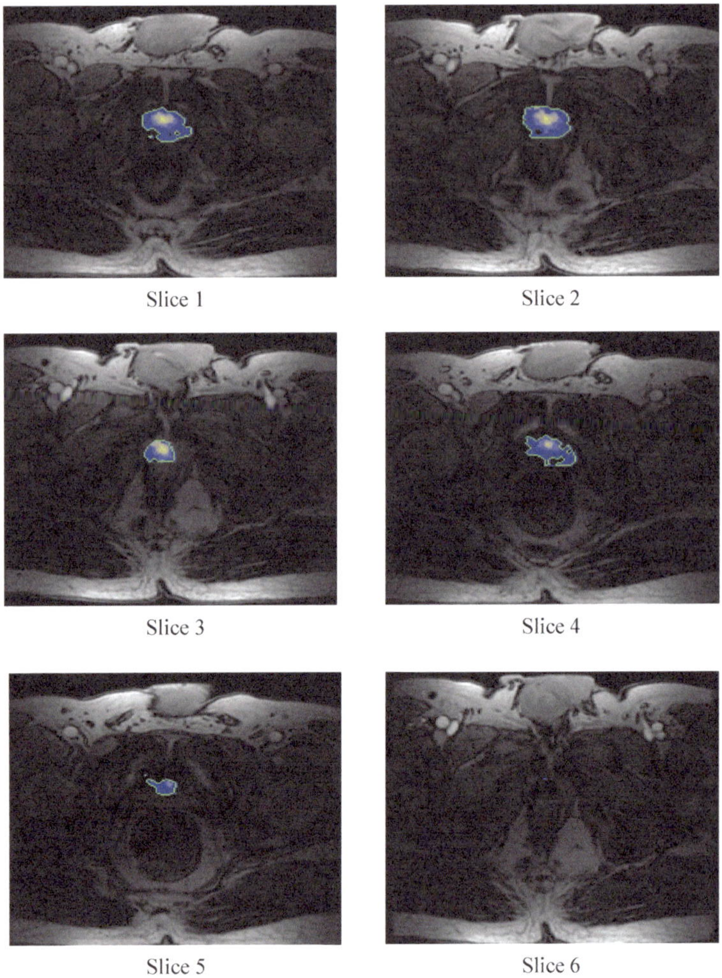

Fig. 3.16 Dynamic contrast-enhanced MRI images of the pelvis with local tumor progression of the first benign subject. Tumor's contour determination (*green*)

classification. Applications of the proposed approach yield promising results that would, in the near future, replace the use of current technologies to determine the type of prostate cancer.

Our future work will include testing more patients. In addition, we will try to implement a fusion between DCE-MRI and Diffusion MRI to get better diagnosis results.

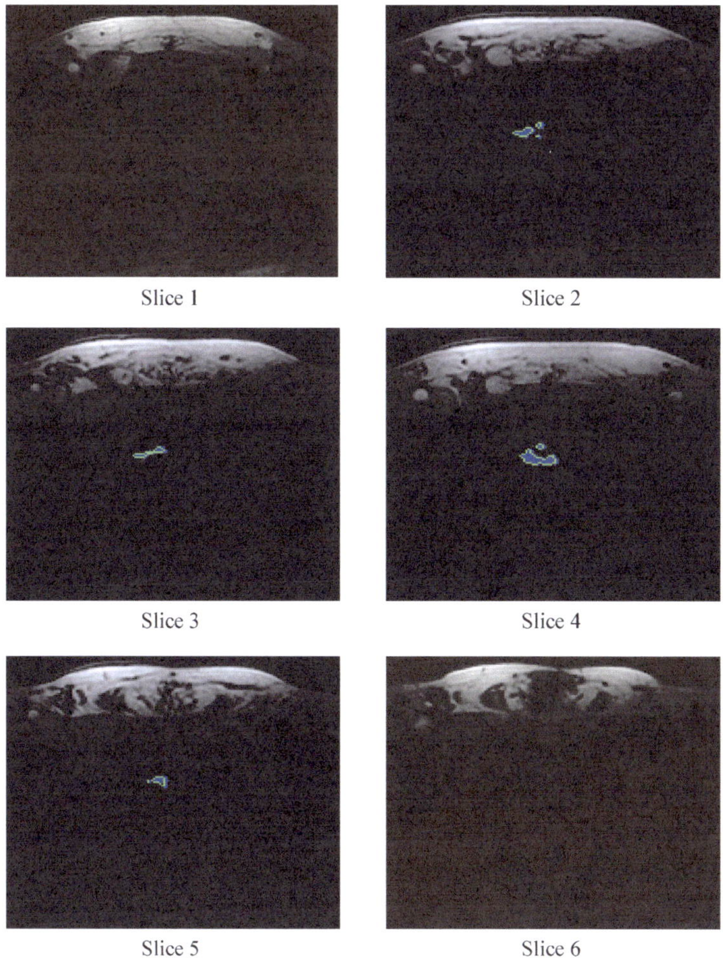

Fig. 3.17 Dynamic contrast-enhanced MRI images of the pelvis with local tumor progression of second benign subject. Tumor's contour determination (*green*)

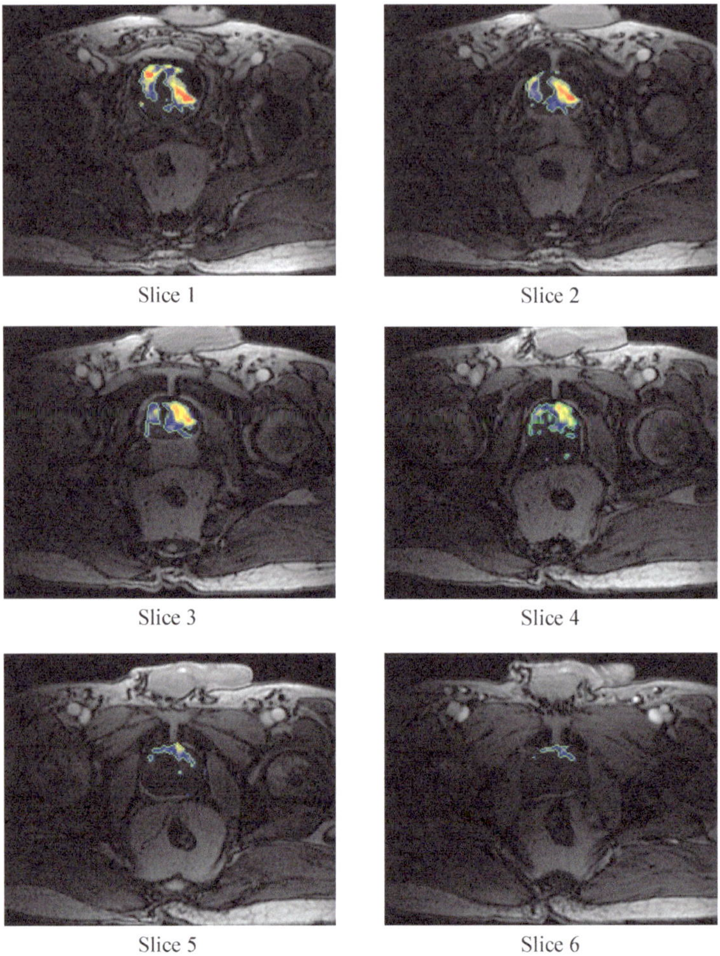

Fig. 3.18 Dynamic contrast-enhanced MRI images of the pelvis with local tumor progression of the first malignant subject. Tumor's contour determination (*green*)

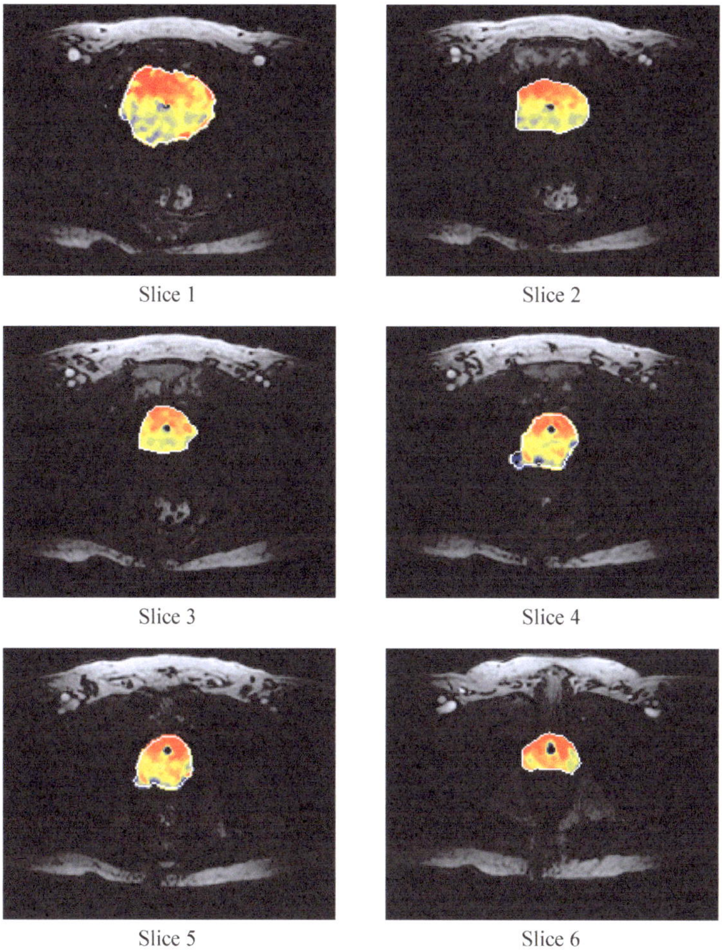

Fig. 3.19 Dynamic contrast-enhanced MRI images of the pelvis with local tumor progression of first malignant subject

References

1. Jemal A, Siegel R, Xu J, Ward E (2010) Cancer statistics 2010. CA Cancer J Clin 60:277–300
2. Crawford ED (2003) Epidemiology of prostate cancer. Urology 62(6 Suppl 1):3–12
3. Lin K, Lipsitz R, Miller T, Janakiraman S, Force UPST (2008) Benefits and harms of prostate-specific antigen screening for prostate cancer: an evidence update for the U.S. preventive services task force. Ann Intern Med 149(3):192–199
4. Schroder FH (2010) Prostate cancer around the world. An overview. Urol Oncol 28 (6):663–667
5. Hugosson J, Carlsson S, Aus G, Bergdahl S, Khatami A, Lodding P, Pihl C, Stranne J, Holmberg E, Lilja H (2010) Mortality results from the Goteborg randomised population-based prostate-cancer screening trial. Lancet Oncol 11(8):725–732
6. Shen D, Zhan Y, Davatzikos C (2003) Segmentation of prostate boundaries from ultrasound images using statistical shape model. IEEE Trans Med Imaging 22(4):539–551
7. Ladak HM, Mao F, Wang Y, Downey DB, Steinman DA, Fenster A (2000) Prostate boundary segmentation from 2D ultrasound images. Med Phys 27:1777–1788
8. Zhan Y, Shen D (2003) Automated segmentation of 3D US prostate images using statistical texture-based matching method. In: Medical image computing and computer-assisted intervention (MICCAI), vol 2878, Montreal, 16–18 Nov 2003, pp 688–696
9. Gong L, Pathak SD, Haynor DR, Cho PS, Kim Y (2004) A parametric shape modeling using deformable super ellipses for prostate segmentation. IEEE Trans Med Imaging 23:340–349
10. Zwiggelaar R, Zhu Y, Williams S (2003) Semi-automatic segmentation of the prostate. In: Proceedings of first Iberian Conference on Pattern Recognition and Image (ibPRIA'03), Puerto de Andratx, Mallorca, Spain, 4–6 June 2003, pp 1108–1116
11. Trkbey B, Thomasson D, Pang Y, Bernardo M, Choyke P (2010) The role of dynamic contrast-enhanced MRI in cancer diagnosis and treatment. Turk Soc Radiol 16:186–192
12. Zhu Y, Williams S, Zwiggelaar R (2004) Segmentation of volumetric prostate MRI data using hybrid 2D+3D shape modeling. In: Proceeding Medical Image Understanding and Analysis, London, UK, pp 61–64
13. Toth R, Tiwari P, Rosen M, Kalyanpur A, Pungavkar S, Madabhushi A (2008) A multimodal prostate segmentation scheme by combining spectral clustering and active shape models. In: Proceedings of SPIE Medical Imaging: Image Processing, vol 6914, San Diego, CA, 16 February 2008
14. Klein S, van der Heidi UA, Raaymakers BW, Kotte A, Staring M, Pluim J (2007) Segmentation of the prostate in MRI images by atlas matching. In: Proceedings of IEEE international symposium on biomedical imaging: From nano to macro, Washington, DC, USA, 12–16 April 2007, pp 1300–1303
15. Vikal S, Haker S, Tempany C, Fichtinger G (2009) Prostate contouring in MRI guided biopsy. In: Proceedings of SPIE Medical Imaging: Image Processing, vol 7259, Lake Buena Vista, FL, USA, February 2009, pp 1–11
16. Martin S, Daanenc V, Troccaz J (2010) Automated segmentation of the prostate in 3D MRI images using a probabilistic atlas and a spatially constrained deformable model. Med Phys 37:1579–1590
17. Thompson I, Thrasher JB, Aus G, Burnett AL, Canby-Hagino ED, Cookson MS, D'Amico AV, Dmochowski RR, Eton DT, Forman JD, Goldenberg SL, Hernandez J, Higano CS, Kraus SR, Moul JW, Tangen CM (2007) AUA Prostate Cancer Clinical Guideline Update Panel Guideline for the management of clinically localized prostate cancer: 2007 update. J Urol 177:2106–2131
18. Roehl K, Antenor J, Catalona W (2002) Serial biopsy results in prostate cancer screening study. J Am Urol Assoc 167:2435–2439
19. Keetch D, Catalona W, Smith D (1994) Serial prostatic biopsies in men with persistently elevated serum prostate specific antigen values. J Am Urol Assoc 151:1571–1574

20. Chan I, Wells W, Mulkern RV, Haker S, Zhang J, Zou KH, Maier SE, Tempany CMC (2003) Detection of prostate cancer by integration of line-scan diffusion, T2-mapping and T2-weighted magnetic resonance imaging; a multichannel statistical classifier. Med Phys 30 (9):2390–2398
21. Madabhushi A, Feldman M, Metaxas D, Tomaszeweski J, Chute D (2005) Automated detection of prostatic adenocarcinoma from high-resolution ex-vivo MRI. IEEE Trans Med Imaging 24(12):1611–1625
22. Ocak I, Bernardo M, Metzger G, Barrett T, Pinto P, Albert PS, Choyke PL (2007) Dynamic contrast-enhanced MRI of prostate cancer at 3 T: a study of pharmacokinetic parameters. Am J Roentgenol 189:849–853
23. Fütterer JJ, Heijmink SW, Scheenen TW, Veltman J, Huisman HJ, Vos P, Hulsbergen Van de Kaa CA, Witjes JA, Krabbe PF, Heerschap A, Barentsz JO (2006) Prostate cancer localization with dynamic contrast-enhanced MR imaging and proton MR spectroscopic imaging. Radiology 241:449–458
24. Rouvière O, Valette O, Grivolat S, Colin-Pangaud C, Bouvier R, Chapelon J, Gelet A, Lyonnet D (2004) Recurrent prostate cancer after external beam radiotherapy: value of contrast-enhanced dynamic MRI in localizing intraprostatic tumor correlation with biopsy findings. Urology 63:922–927
25. Kim J, Hong S, Choi Y et al (2005) Wash-in rate on the basis of dynamic contrast-enhanced MRI: usefulness for prostate cancer detection and localization. J Magn Reson Imaging 22:639–646
26. Puech P, Betrouni N, Makni N, Dewalle AS, Villers A, Lemaitre L (2009) Computer-assisted diagnosis of prostate cancer using DCE-MRI data: design, implementation and preliminary results. Int J Comput Assist Radiol Surg 4:1–10
27. Engelbrecht M, Huisman H, Laheij R et al (2003) Discrimination of prostate cancer from normal peripheral zone and central gland tissue by using dynamic contrast-enhanced MR imaging. Radiology 229:248–254
28. Vos PC, Hambrock T, Hulsbergen-van de Kaa CA, Futterer JJ, Barentsz JO, Huisman HJ (2008) Computerized analysis of prostate lesions in the peripheral zone using dynamic contrast enhanced MRI. Med Phys 35:888–899
29. Viswanath S, Bloch BN, Genega E, Rofsky N, Lenkinski R, Chappelow J, Toth R, Madabhushi A (2008) A comprehensive segmentation, registration, and cancer detection scheme on 3 tesla in vivo prostate DCE-MRI. In: Proceedings of International Conference on Image Computing and Computer Assisted Intervention (MICCAI'08), New York, NY, USA, September 6–10, 2008, pp 662–671
30. Reinsberg SA, Payne GS, Riches SF, Ashley S, Brewster JM, Morgan VA, deSouza NM (2007) Combined use of diffusion-weighted MRI and 1h MR spectroscopy to increase accuracy in prostate cancer detection. Am J Roentgenol 188:91–98
31. Gímel'farb G (1999) Image textures and Gibbs random fields. Kluwer, Dordrecht
32. El-Baz A, Gimel'farb G (2007) EM based approximation of empirical distributions with linear combinations of discrete Gaussians. In: Proceedings of IEEE international conference on image processing, vol 4. San Antonio, 16–19 Sept 2007, pp 373–376
33. El-Baz A, Elnakib A, Khalifa F, Abou El-Ghar M, McClure P, Soliman A, Gimel'farb GL (2012) Precise segmentation of 3-D magnetic resonance angiography. IEEE Trans Biomed Eng 59(7):2019–2029
34. Farag A, El-Baz A, Gimelfarb G (2006) Precise segmentation of multimodal images. IEEE Trans Image Process 15(4):952–968
35. Viola P, Wells WM III (1995) Alignment by maximization of mutual information. Int J Comput Vis 24:137–154
36. Besag J (1986) On the statistical analysis of dirty pictures. J R Stat Soc B 48(3):259–302
37. Studholme C, Constable RT, Duncan J (2000) Accurate alignment of functional EPI data to anatomical MRI using a physics-based distortion model. IEEE Trans Med Imaging 19 (11):1115–1127

38. Avants BB, Gee JC (2004) Geodesic estimation for large deformation anatomical shape averaging and interpolation. Neuroimage 23(1):139–150
39. Bouman CA, Sauer K (1993) A generalized Gaussian image model for edge-preserving MAP estimation. IEEE Trans Image Process 2(3):296–310
40. Khalifa F, Beache GM, Gimel'farb G, Giridharan GA, El-Baz A (2012) Accurate automatic analysis of cardiac cine images. IEEE Trans Biomed Eng 59(2):445–455
41. Dice R (1945) Measures of the amount of ecologic association between species. Ecol Soc Am 26(3):297–302
42. Tsai A, Yezzi A, Wells W, Tempany C, Tucker D, Fan A, Grimson E, Willsky A (2003) A shape-based approach to curve evolution for segmentation of medical imagery. IEEE Trans Med Imaging 22(2):137–154

Chapter 4
Computational Intelligent Image Analysis for Assisting Radiation Oncologists' Decision Making in Radiation Treatment Planning

Hidetaka Arimura, Taiki Magome, Genyu Kakiuchi, Jumpei Kuwazuru, and Asumi Mizoguchi

Abstract This chapter describes the computational image analysis for assisting radiation oncologists' decision making in radiation treatment planning for high precision radiation therapy. The radiation therapy consists of five steps, i.e., diagnosis, treatment planning, patient setup, treatment, and follow-up, in which computational intelligent image analysis and pattern recognition methods play important roles in improving the accuracy of radiation therapy and assisting radiation oncologists' or medical physicists' decision making. In particular, the treatment planning step is substantially important and indispensable, because the subsequent steps must be performed according to the treatment plan. This chapter introduces a number of studies on computational intelligent image analysis used for the computer-aided decision making in radiation treatment planning. Moreover, the authors also explore computer-aided treatment planning methods including automated beam arrangement based on similar cases, computerized contouring of lung tumor regions using a support vector machine (SVM) classifier, and a computerized method for determination of robust beam directions against patient setup errors in particle therapy.

Introduction

Malignant neoplasms, cardiac disease, and cerebrovascular disease are the top three major causes of death in Japan. Malignant neoplasms have been the top cause of death since 1981, and their mortality rate has consistently increased in Japan. The mortality due to malignant neoplasm was 30 % of all-cause mortality in 2009 [1].

H. Arimura (✉) • T. Magome • G. Kakiuchi • J. Kuwazuru • A. Mizoguchi
Division of Medical Quantum Sciences, Department of Health Sciences, Faculty of Medical Sciences, Kyushu University, 3-1-1, Maidashi, Higashi-ku, Fukuoka 812-8582, Japan
e-mail: arimurah@med.kyushu-u.ac.jp

K. Suzuki (ed.), *Computational Intelligence in Biomedical Imaging*,
DOI 10.1007/978-1-4614-7245-2_4,

The three major treatment strategies for malignant neoplasms are surgical intervention, chemotherapy, and radiation therapy, but usually patients are treated using the combination of two or more modalities instead of a single approach, which is called combined modality therapy.

Radiation therapy, which of course does not require physical incision of the patient's body like surgical intervention, has attracted considerable attention, because it can preserve organ function and reduce the physical burden of patients, particularly elderly patients. This treatment modality is especially important for developed countries such as the USA and Japan, which have been moving toward an aging society. In Japan, the percentage of elderly people is currently estimated to be more than 20 %, and the average lifespan was 86 years for females and 79 for males in 2008. Therefore, radiotherapy would provide great benefits for many patients, including elderly patients, and thereby enhance their quality of life.

The primary aim of radiation therapy is to deliver as high a dose as possible to the tumor, while causing as little damage as possible to normal tissues and organs at risks (OARs) and thus avoiding adverse effects [2, 3]. The OARs are the normal tissues whose radiation sensitivity may significantly influence radiation treatment planning (RTP) and/or the prescribed dose [4]. In order to protect these tissues, several techniques using high precision radiation therapy have been developed, such as stereotactic body radiation therapy (SBRT), intensity modulated radiation therapy (IMRT), adaptive radiotherapy (ART), real-time tracking radiotherapy (RTRT), and image-guided radiation therapy (IGRT), and these advances have led to impressive progress in radiation precision in recent years. As a result, high precision radiation therapy has been reported to provide outcomes comparable to surgery for some cancers [5]. In these high precision radiation therapies, computational intelligent image analysis and pattern recognition methods play important roles in improving the accuracy of radiation therapy and assisting radiation oncologists' or medical physicists' decision making.

The radiation therapy consists of four steps, i.e., diagnosis, treatment planning, treatment, and follow-up. The computational intelligent image processing and pattern recognition techniques are employed to assist radiation oncology staff members in the decision making at each step of the radiation therapy. Figure 4.1 shows the five steps of radiation therapy and examples of image processing techniques at each step.

The first step is the diagnosis of the patient. In this step, a radiation oncologist determines the treatment policy, e.g., curative treatment or palliative treatment, but computer-aided diagnosis techniques may also be useful if the oncologist decides to use multiple modalities.

The second step is the treatment planning. In this step, the treatment planner should extract the gross tumor volume (GTV) and the OAR, and should formulate an "optimum" plan by arranging beams to maximize the tumor dose and minimize the OAR dose. Various automated segmentation methods have been developed and are still being researched for the extraction of tumor and OAR regions. Image registration techniques are very useful for segmenting tumors using fused images that combine morphological and functional images such as planning CT images and positron emission tomography (PET) images. In particle therapy, treatment

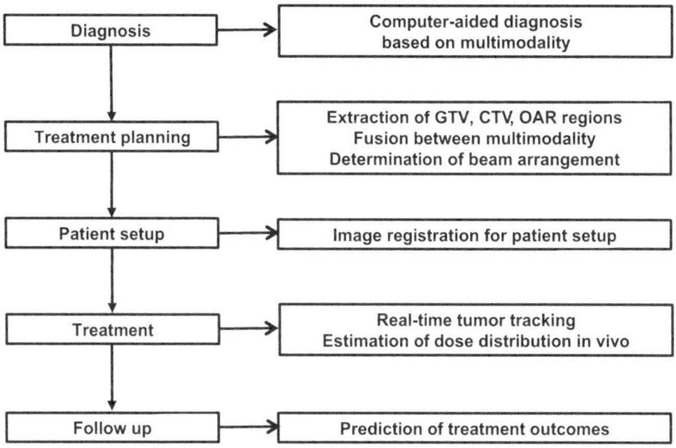

Fig. 4.1 Five steps of radiation therapy and examples of image processing techniques in each step

planners should take into account patient setup error when the beam directions are determined; otherwise, the actual dose distribution in the patient during treatment may be strongly degraded compared with the planned dose distribution.

The third step is the patient setup. In this step, the radiation therapists position a patient on the treatment couch. Image registration techniques, which register a moving image to a reference image using corresponding feature points between the two images, are employed for correction of a patient's setup errors. Previous studies have demonstrated that these techniques are indeed effective for reducing the setup errors [6, 7]. In general, digitally reconstructed radiograph (DRR) images and planning CT images are used as the reference images, and electronic portal imaging device (EPID) and cone-beam CT (CBCT) images produced using kilovoltage or megavoltage X-rays at the treatment time are employed as the moving images.

The fourth step is the treatment itself. An X-ray or particle beam is delivered to the patient according to the treatment plan. One of the major issues is the radiation delivery for moving tumors such as lung or liver cancers. Pattern recognition techniques, such as the detection of tumors and fiducial markers (e.g., gold marker), are essential for minimizing the treatment time in these cases. For instance, a real-time tumor tracking radiography (RTRT) system has been developed, which employs pattern recognition techniques by following a gold marker within the tumor in order to track the tumor and switch the X-ray beam on and off [8].

Finally, the fifth step is the follow-up. In this step, the radiation oncologist evaluates the treatment outcomes using multimodality imaging devices. Pattern recognition techniques have also been applied during the follow-up to predict the radiation therapy outcomes and normal tissue complications [9–13].

In this chapter, we will consider computational and intelligent approaches in the radiation treatment planning, because the treatment planning step is indispensable, and largely dictates the subsequent steps. Therefore, a number of studies on computational intelligent image analysis used for computer-aided decision making in the radiation treatment planning have been introduced, including automated beam arrangement based on similar cases, computerized contouring of lung tumor regions using a support vector machine (SVM) classifier, and a computerized method for determination of robust beam directions against patient setup errors in hadron particle therapy.

Computer-Aided Decision Making for the Determination of Beam Arrangements

Background

Stereotactic body radiotherapy (SBRT) has been widely used for the treatment of early stage lung cancers in recent decades [14]. The survival rate for SBRT has been encouraging and potentially comparable to that for surgery [5]. Daily doses in conventional external beam radiotherapy are typically delivered in the range of 1.8–2.0 Gy (total doses: 60–70 Gy), whereas stereotactic body radiotherapy (SBRT) is generally administered at five or fewer fractions of high doses of 10–20 Gy per fraction. The shortened treatment time with fewer fractions would result in significant benefits to both patients and hospitals, which have limited inpatient capabilities. However, high doses per treatment have been considered dangerous in the past due to limitations in the treatment delivery technology, such as incomplete immobilization, that raised concerns about potential toxicity if large volumes of normal tissues or OAR were exposed to high dose radiation during each treatment. With the recent advances in treatment techniques, it has become possible to concentrate very large doses of radiation to tumors and to minimize the doses to surrounding normal tissues by using multiple beams directed in coplanar and non-coplanar directions [15]. However, the determination of beam arrangement is a substantially demanding task for inexperienced treatment planners and affects the critical dose distribution with steep dose gradients.

Treatment planning skills are developed by repeated planning in clinical practice, often under the guidance of experienced planners or appropriate textbooks. In this way, treatment planners should memorize many planning patterns and construct an evolving "database" in their memory, which can then be searched for previous cases similar to the case under consideration. However, although a number of automated methods for determination of beam arrangements have been developed [16, 17], there are currently no such methods for determining beam arrangements based on similar previous cases. On the other hand, in the field of diagnostic radiology, the presentation of similar cases as a diagnostic assist has been suggested for diagnosis of chest images [18], lung computed tomography (CT) images [19, 20], and mammography images [20–23]. These researches have indicated the feasibility of using similar cases as a diagnostic assist. However, to the best of our knowledge, there are no studies on the feasibility of using similar planning cases for the determination of beam arrangements in the field of radiation therapy.

Computer-Aided Beam Arrangement Based on Similar Cases in Radiation Treatment Planning Databases

The authors developed a computer-aided decision making method for determination of beam arrangements based on similar cases in a radiotherapy treatment planning (RTP) database of the results from experienced treatment planners. Similar-case-based beam arrangements were automatically determined based on the following two steps. First, the five plans showing the greatest similarity to an objective case were automatically selected in the RTP database by considering the weighted Euclidean distance of geometrical feature vectors, i.e., related to the location, size, and shape of the planning target volume (PTV), lung, and spinal cord, between the objective case and each plan in the RTP database. Second, the five beam arrangements of an objective case were automatically determined by registering five cases similar to the objective case with respect to lung regions by means of an affine transformation.

Selection of Similar Treatment Plans Based on Geometrical Features

In the first step, the five plans most similar to an objective case were automatically selected in the RTP database by considering the weighted Euclidean distance of geometrical feature vectors between the objective case and each plan in the RTP database. The weighted Euclidean distance was considered a similarity measure. The weights of geometrical features were needed to give the geometrical features the appropriate degree of importance from the treatment planning point of view. Therefore, when applying the proposed method to their own databases, each institute should determine the appropriate weights of the geometrical features based on their own philosophy or policy of treatment planning. The weighted Euclidian distance d_{image} was calculated by the following equation:

$$d_{image} = \sqrt{\sum_{i=1}^{G} w_i(\alpha_i - \beta_i)^2}, \tag{4.1}$$

where G is the number of geometrical features, w_i is the weight of the i-th geometrical feature, α_i is the i-th geometrical feature for the objective case, and β_i is the i-th geometrical feature for each case in the RTP database. Note that each geometrical feature was divided by the standard deviation of all cases in the RTP database to normalize the range of each feature value. In this study, we defined ten geometrical features, i.e., the x, y, z coordinates of a PTV centroid, the effective diameter of the PTV, the sphericity of the PTV, the lung length in the left–right (LR), anterior–posterior (AP), and superior–inferior (SI) directions, the distance in the centroid between the PTV and spinal cord in the isocenter plane, and the angle from the spinal cord to the PTV in the isocenter plane. Weights for geometrical features were empirically determined by using the five training cases so that cases more similar to the objective case could be selected.

Determination of Beam Arrangements Based on Similar Treatment Plans Using the Linear Registration Technique

In the second step, five beam angles of an objective case were automatically determined by registration of five similar treatment plans with the objective case with respect to lung regions using a linear registration technique, i.e., affine transformation [24]. First, the affine transformation matrix to register the lung regions of each similar plan with that of the objective case was calculated by using a least squares method based on eight feature points, which were automatically selected for the registration in vertices of the circumscribed parallelepiped of lung regions. Second, a beam direction, i.e., beam position vector, based on a gantry angle θ and couch angle φ was transformed from a spherical polar coordinate system to a Cartesian coordinate system as a unit position vector. Third, each beam position vector of similar cases was modified in the Cartesian coordinate system by using the same affine transformation matrix as a registration in terms of lung regions. Finally, the resulting position vector was converted from the Cartesian coordinate system to the spherical polar coordinate system as gantry angle θ' and couch angle φ'.

Evaluation of Beam Arrangements Determined Based on Similar Treatment Plans Using Planning Evaluation Indices

The most usable plan was selected by sorting the five plans based on an RTP evaluation measure with 11 planning evaluation indices, which was the Euclidean distance in a feature space between each plan and an ideal plan. In this study, the ideal plan was assumed to produce a perfect uniform irradiation with a prescription dose in the PTV and no irradiation in the surrounding organs and tissues. The usefulness of each plan was estimated by the following Euclidean distance d_{plan} of the planning evaluation vector between the ideal plan and each plan determined by a similar plan, and the Euclidean distance was considered the RTP evaluation measure:

$$d_{plan} = \sqrt{\sum_{j=1}^{J} \left(X_j - Y_j\right)^2}, \tag{4.2}$$

where J is the number of planning evaluation indices, X_j is the j-th planning evaluation index for the ideal plan, and Y_j is the j-th planning evaluation index for the plan based on the five most similar plans. Each planning evaluation index

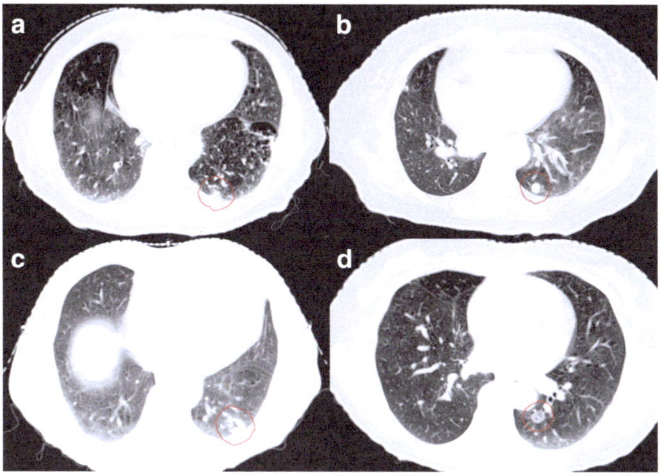

Fig. 4.2 An objective case with a tumor on the lung wall (**a**) and the first to third most similar cases (**b–d**) to the objective case

was normalized in the same manner as the geometrical features. The eight evaluation indices consisted of the D95, homogeneity index (HI), conformity index (CI) for the PTV, V5, V10, V20, mean dose for the lung, and maximum dose for the spinal cord, and their values for the ideal plan were set to 48 Gy (prescription dose), 1.0, 1.0, 0 %, 0 %, 0 %, 0 Gy, and 0 Gy, respectively.

Evaluation of Computer-Aided Beam Arrangement Based on Similar Cases

We applied the proposed method to ten test cases by using an RTP database of 81 cases with lung cancer and compared the eight planning evaluation indices between the original plan and the corresponding most usable similar-case-based plan. Figure 4.2 shows an objective case with a tumor on the lung wall (Fig. 4.2a) and the first to third most similar cases (Fig. 4.2b–d) to the objective case. The similar cases geometrically resemble the objective case (Fig. 4.2a), especially in terms of the geometrical relationship between the tumor and the spinal cord. Figure 4.3 shows a plan obtained by the original beam arrangement (Fig. 4.3a), and three plans determined by similar-case-based beam arrangements (Fig. 4.3b–d), which were sorted in descending order based on the RTP evaluation measure. The plans of Fig. 4.3b–d were derived from similar cases as shown in Fig. 4.2b–d, respectively. In this case, the beam arrangements consisted of seven to eight beams with three to four coplanar beams and three to four non-coplanar beams. The objective case (Fig. 4.3a) received an oblique lateral beam, which passed close to the spinal cord in order to increase the conformity of the PTV. On the other hand, the most usable similar-case-based beam arrangement (Fig. 4.3b) had no lateral beams for avoiding the spinal cord,

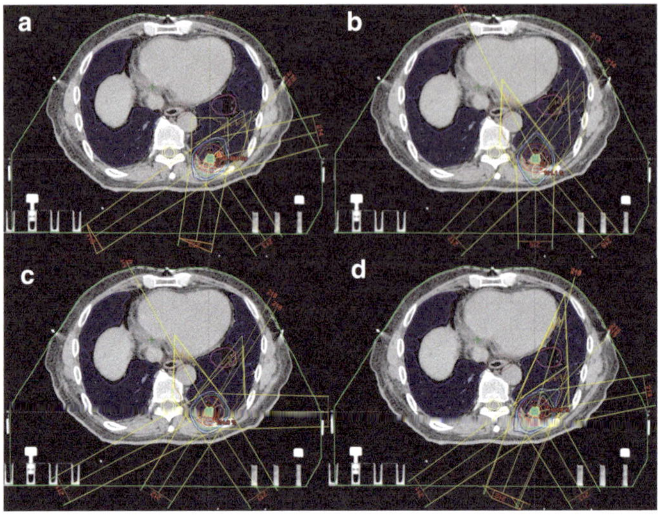

Fig. 4.3 A plan obtained by the original beam arrangement (**a**), and three plans determined by similar-case-based beam arrangements (**b**–**d**), which were sorted in descending order based on the RTP evaluation measure

but the second to third usable cases (Fig. 4.3c, d) had lateral beams due to prioritizing the PTV conformity rather than sparing the spinal cord. As a result, there were no statistically significant differences between the original beam arrangements and the most usable similar-case-based beam arrangements ($P > 0.05$) in terms of the eight planning evaluation indices including the D95, mean lung dose, and spinal cord maximum dose. In conclusion, the proposed method suggested usable beam arrangements with little difference from cases in the RTP database, and thus it could be employed as an educational tool for less experienced treatment planners.

Computer-Assisted Contouring of Tumor Regions in Radiation Treatment Planning

Background

To improve the outcomes of radiotherapy, stereotactic radiotherapy has been developed for the treatment of stable tumors such as brain tumors by delivering very higher doses in small irradiation fields. Moreover, SBRT has been applied to moving tumors such as lung tumors while immobilizing the body and monitoring tumor locations. In the SBRT technique, tumor dose is maximized while the normal tissue dose is minimized. However, it would be assumed that the tumor and OAR contours should be determined as accurately as possible. In fact, the accuracy of contouring or segmentation of tumors affects the precision of radiotherapy, because the prescribed dose distribution in RTP is determined based on the tumor regions, which are manually determined on planning CT images on a slice-by-slice basis by a treatment planner. However, the subjective manual contouring is tedious and its reproducibility would be relatively low, resulting in inter-observer variability and intra-observer variability of tumor regions [4, 25–28]. The tumor region is called the GTV, which is defined as the visible tumor volume in images. A number of automated contouring methods for the GTVs have been proposed for reducing the inter-observer variability and intra-observer variability, planning time, and increasing segmentation accuracy of the GTVs. The conventional methods are based on thresholding of the standardized uptake value (SUV) [29, 30], or on the region growing method [28], Gaussian mixture model [31], fuzzy c-means algorithm [32], fuzzy locally adaptive Bayesian approach [33, 34], gradient-based segmentation method [35], model-based method [36], and atlas-based method [37]. However, there have been a few studies on segmentation methods for tumor regions based on biological information as well as physical information, such as PET and CT images. 18F-FDG PET directly shows biological information of higher metabolic rates compared with normal tissues for the radiolabeled glucose, which is associated with malignant neoplasms. El Naqa et al. [38] developed a multimodality segmentation method using a multivalued level set method, which can provide a feasible and accurate framework for combining imaging data from different modalities (PET/CT), and is a potentially useful tool for the delineation of biophysical structure volumes in radiotherapy treatment planning. On the other hand, in this study, we tried to incorporate the tumor contours determined by radiation oncologists based on the PET biological information and CT morphological information into the proposed contouring method by using a machine learning method. Therefore, the aim of this study was to develop an automated method for contouring the GTVs of lung tumors with an SVM, which learned various contours determined on planning CT images by radiation oncologists while taking into account the PET/CT images.

Automated Method for Contouring the GTVs of Lung Tumors Using an SVM Classifier with Knowledge from Radiation Oncologists' Contours on Data Sets of Planning CT and FDG-PET/CT Images

The proposed method was composed of four steps. First, the planning CT, the PET/CT images, and GTV data were converted into isotropic images by using interpolation methods. Second, the PET images were registered with the planning CT images through the diagnostic CT images of PET/CT. Third, six voxel-based features including voxel values and magnitudes of image gradient vectors were derived from each voxel in the planning CT and PET /CT image data sets. Finally, lung tumors were extracted by using an SVM, which learned six voxel-based features inside and outside each true tumor region.

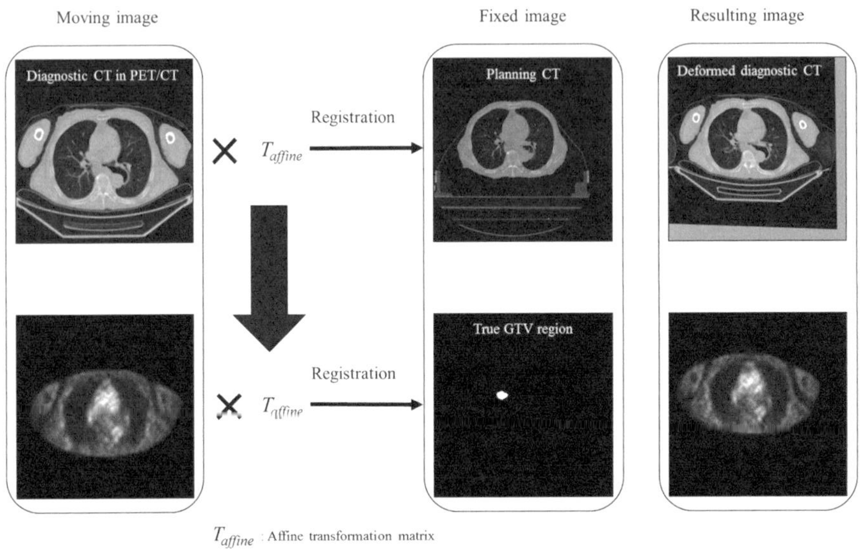

Fig. 4.4 An illustration for registration of a PET image to a planning CT image

Registration of the PET Image to the Planning CT Image

Prior to the registration, a diagnostic CT image of the PET/CT data set was registered with the PET image using an image position in a digital imaging and communications in medicine (DICOM) header information and a rigid registration based on normalized mutual information [39]. Figure 4.4 shows an illustration for registration of a PET image to a planning CT image. First, the diagnostic CT image of the PET/CT data set was registered with a planning CT image by using an affine transformation. Then, the PET image was registered with the planning CT image and a GTV region (radiation therapy structure data) in DICOM-RT (DICOM for radiation therapy) by using the same affine transformation matrix, because the PET image was scanned as the same coordinate system as the diagnostic CT image of the PET/CT data set.

Determination of Voxel-Based Image Features

Six voxel-based features were derived for the SVM from each voxel in the planning CT and PET/CT image data sets. All image data, including planning CT images, GTV regions, and PET/CT data sets were placed in the same coordinate system after the registration in the previous step. Therefore, each voxel value and its magnitude of image gradient vector were obtained as image features from each voxel in the planning CT image, diagnostic CT and PET images of a PET/CT data set. The image gradient was derived from the following one-order polynomial within a 5 × 5 × 5 voxel region, which was obtained by a least-square method:

$$f(x, y, z) = ax + by + cz + d, \tag{4.3}$$

where x, y, and z are coordinates in a three-dimensional image, $f(x, y, z)$ is the one-order polynomial, and a, b, c, and d are constants. The gradient magnitude was defined by the following equation:

$$G = \sqrt{\left(\frac{\partial f}{\partial x}\right)^2 + \left(\frac{\partial f}{\partial y}\right)^2 + \left(\frac{\partial f}{\partial z}\right)^2} = \sqrt{a^2 + b^2 + c^2}. \tag{4.4}$$

Segmentation of the GTV Region Using an SVM

The GTVs were extracted by using an SVM, which learned three or six voxel-based features inside and outside each true tumor region (gold standard). The teacher signal was plus one if the voxel was inside the GTV region, whereas the teacher signal was minus one if the voxel was outside the GTV. The outside region of the GTV was defined as the region dilated six times by a circle kernel with a radius of 1 mm. The training voxels were selected at various sampling intervals depending on the ratio between the numbers of inside and outside voxels so that the number of the inside voxels could be the same as that of outside voxels. We constructed an SVM classifier with a Gaussian kernel, i.e., $\exp(-\gamma||x-y||^2)$, by using the open source software package SVM light [40]. In this study, the value γ, the parameter C, and the threshold value were set as 0.0001, 12.5, and 0.50, respectively.

Performance of the Automated Method for Contouring GTVs of Lung Tumors Using SVM

Figure 4.5 shows a pair plot matrix between any two of the six image features, i.e., the voxel values of the planning CT image and diagnostic CT, and the SUV of PET images, and three gradients for the three kinds of images. In this pair plot matrix, each graph in the intersection shows the relationship between any two of the six image features. The gold standard of GTV voxels is indicated by red circles and the outside volume of GTV voxels is indicated by blue crosses. The aim of this feature analysis is to characterize a voxel (tumor or normal tissue) to be recognized by measurements based on a voxel whose feature value is very similar to those for objects in the same category, but as different or distinguishable as possible from those for objects in different categories. According to Fig. 4.5, the relationships related to the SUV obtained from the PET images seem to be relatively distinguishable between the tumor and normal tissue. The GTVs extracted by using the SVM,

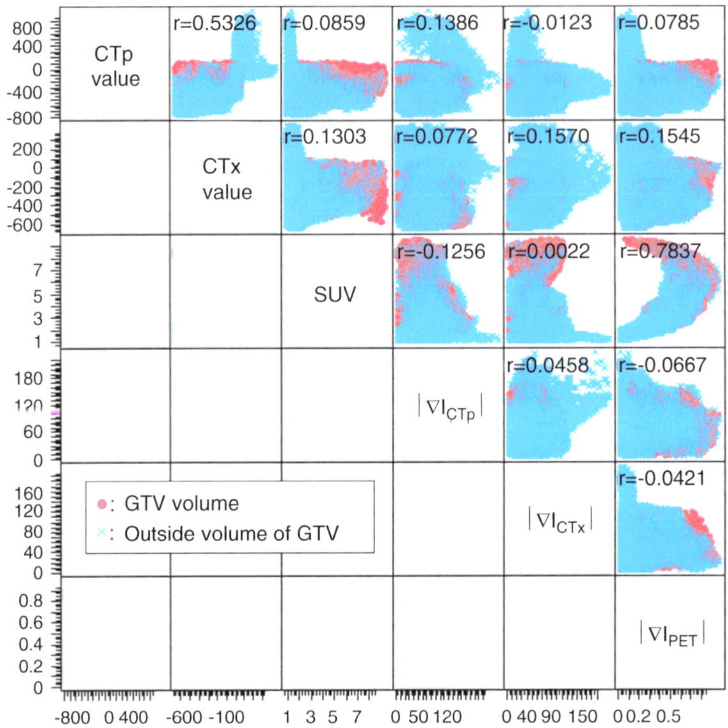

Fig. 4.5 Pair plot matrix between any two of the six image features. The gold standard of GTV voxels is indicated by *red circles* and the outside volume of GTV voxels is indicated by *blue crosses*. CTp value: CT value of the planning CT; CTx value: diagnosCc CT value of PET/CT; SUV: standardized uptake value obtained by PET of PET/CT; $|\nabla ICTp|$: magnitude of the gradient of the planning CT; $|\nabla ICTx|$: magnitude of the gradient of the diagnosCc CT of PET/CT; $|\nabla I_{PET}|$: magnitude of the gradient of PET of PET/CT

which learned three or six voxel-based features inside and outside each true tumor region, are shown in Fig. 4.6 with the Dice similarity coefficient (DSC) between the gold standard and regions segmented by the proposed method. The three features were the voxel values of the planning CT image and diagnostic CT, and the SUV of PET images. Estimated GTV regions are shown in green, and the borders of the GTV contoured by radiation oncologists are indicated with red lines. In addition, overlap lines between the GTV outline and the estimated GTV are shown in yellow. The results showed that the average DSCs for three and six features were 0.744 and 0.899, and thus the SVM may need six features to learn the distinguishable characteristics. In addition, it might be a little more difficult for the SVM to learn the mixed grad glass opacity (GGO) tumor compared with the solid tumors.

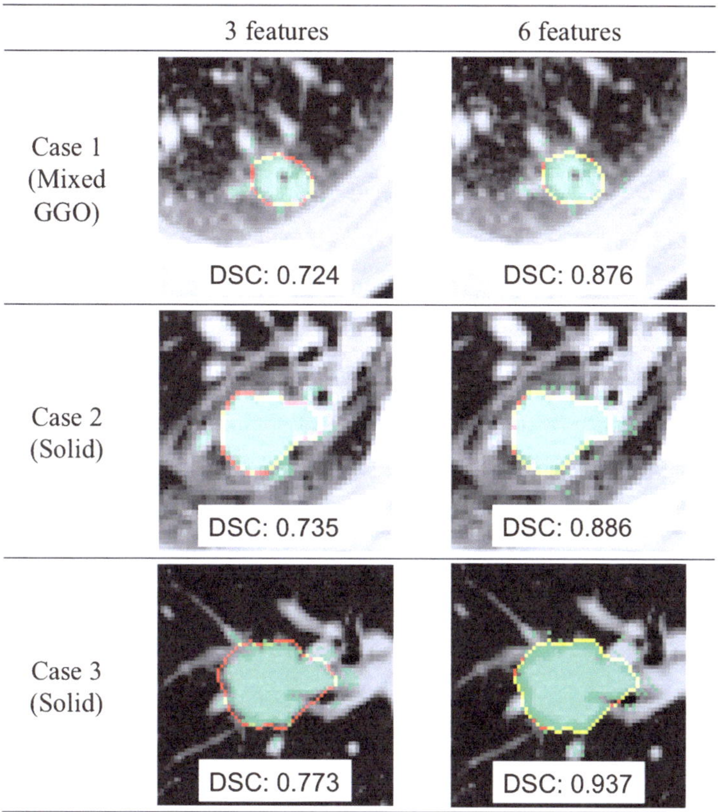

Fig. 4.6 GTVs extracted by using the support vector machine, which learned three or six voxel-based features inside and outside each true tumor region. Estimated GTV regions are shown in *green*, and the borders of GTV contoured by radiation oncologists are indicated by *red lines*. In addition, overlapping lines between the GTV outline and the estimated GTV are indicated in *yellow*

Computerized Method for Determination of Beam Directions in Hadron Particle Therapy

Background

Particle therapies such as proton therapy or heavy ion therapy (carbon ion) have the physical ability to better define and control the dose distribution produced with the particles, which have the Bragg peak, and to increase the high dose delivered to tumors while achieving a very low dose to normal tissue [41, 42]. Furthermore, the highly ionizing property of the heavy ion charged particles, i.e., higher linear energy transfer (LET), results in greater potential for killing tumor cells than conventional radiotherapy of X-rays or electrons from the biological point of view.

In the particle therapy, the shape of dose distribution is modulated by the following three steps in general, so that the three-dimensional (3D) dose distribution conforms to a target volume. First, mono-energetic particle beams were modulated to the target thickness range along each beam path (Spread-out of Bragg peak; SOBP) with a ridge filter. Second, the distal end of the SOBP can be conformed to each tumor by use of a range shifter and a patient-specific compensator in a depth dose shaping system, which is made based on lateral distributions in the beam's eye view (BEV) of a 3D electron density (ED) map of a computed tomography (CT) image for each patient. Third, the lateral radiation field edge was formed to the lateral outline of the target from the BEV by using a multi-leaf collimator. This method is called a passive beam shaping method. Another beam shaping method is called the active beam shaping method or the pencil beam scanning method, e.g., the spot scanning method and raster scanning method. In this method, the target volume is accurately painted by the pencil beam with modulating particle energy.

However, the accurate dose distributions produced by the hadron particles may be very sensitive to patient setup errors [43–49] occurring in a lateral direction orthogonal to the beam direction. In the conclusion of our previous study [50], we discussed the need to develop a method for finding robust beam directions for patient setup error in hadron particle therapy when there are abrupt lateral fluctuations of the electron density projection within the irradiation field.

Decision Making Method for Suggestion of Robust Beam Directions Against the Patient Setup Error Based on Power Spectra of Electron Density Images

If the patient setup errors are not taken into account during the treatment planning, the actual dose distribution that would occur in the patient during treatment could be strongly degraded compared with the planned dose distribution. In other words, due to patient setup errors, the distal end of the dose distribution in a beam direction could not be fitted with that of a tumor shape if the ED-based BEV in the beam direction changed more abruptly (high frequency fluctuation) with large amplitude fluctuation. This incident could lead to significant tumor underdose, but fatal overdose in OAR. Therefore, our goal in this study was to develop a computerized method for determination of robust beam directions against the patient setup error based on the ED-based BEV in the beam direction in the hadron therapy. The proposed method mainly consisted of the following two steps.

1. Production of a BEV image by projecting a 3D electron density image from a particle source to a planning target volume (PTV) distal end.
2. Determination of robust beam directions against patient setup errors by using the slope of the power spectrum.

Production of a BEV Image by Projecting a 3D Electron Density Image

A BEV image was produced by projecting a 3D electron density image in a beam direction from a particle source to the distal end of a planning target volume (PTV).

First, isotropic CT images were derived from original CT images by using a cubic interpolation.

Second, a 3D electron density image was obtained from a patient's CT image by using a conversion table from the CT value (Hounsfield unit) to the electron density relative to water using an experimental method [51]. The relationship between the CT values and the electron density relative to water was experimentally measured using a tissue characterization phantom.

Third, each patient body region was extracted in the isotropic CT image by the following method. The original CT image was binarized by using an automated thresholding technique [52] to obtain a patient body, but including other regions such as the couch or immobilizing devices. The patient body region was obtained from the binarized image by applying an opening filter followed by extraction of the largest region, and a closing filter, which was used for removing the other regions.

Fourth, the PTV region was defined by adding a 5 mm margin for the contour data of the CTV, which were delineated by a radiation oncologist and obtained from digital imaging and communications in medicine for radiation therapy (DICOM-RT) files. The isotropic PTV region was produced by use of a shape-based interpolation [53] for matching the voxel size of the PTV data with the isotropic electron density image.

The ED-based BEV was produced by projection of the 3D electron density image from a particle source to the distal end of a planning target volume (PTV). The vertical beam port of the heavy ion medical accelerator in Chiba (HIMAC) was virtually built as a particle source in this study. The SAD and SID were virtually set as 990 and 1,040 cm, respectively. The isocenter in the planning CT image obtained in a DICOM-RT file was placed at an SAD of 990 cm in the world coordinate system. For production of the ED-based BEV image, a divergent primary beam with a number of rays produced from a particle source was virtually delivered to a 3D ED image. Then, the ED values on each ray in the divergent beam in the 3D ED image were sampled at a certain interval, and accumulated for each pixel in a virtual imaging plane, which was the same pixel size of 0.59 mm as the planning CT, but a 512×512 matrix size. The ED values on the ray were interpolated by using a linear interpolation technique. The simulated irradiation field was considered as the irradiation field if the particle therapy was performed for the patient.

Determination of Robust Beam Directions Against Patient Setup Errors by Using the Slope of the Power Spectrum

The basic idea of our proposed method was to find the robust beam directions whose ED-based BEV images had spatial fluctuations with low special frequency and small amplitude. Power spectra of the ED-based BEV images in all directions, i.e., 0–355°, with an interval of 5° were calculated for evaluation of the spatial fluctuations in the ED-based BEV images in a beam direction. We assumed that as the average spatial frequency and amplitude of the fluctuation in the ED-based BEV images in a beam direction become lower and smaller, respectively, the absolute value of the slope of the power spectrum becomes larger. Therefore, the slope of one-order polynomial of the power spectrum was calculated for determination of the robust beam directions.

Prior to calculation of the power spectral images, the ED-based BEV images were preprocessed as follows. First, the pixel values outside the irradiation field were assigned the average pixel value of the ED-based BEV inside the simulated irradiation field for decreasing the difference in the pixel value between inside and outside of the irradiation field. Second, a Gaussian filter was applied to inner and outer narrow bands (ten pixels) apart from the edge of the ED-based BEV for reducing the higher frequency components in the power spectrum, which were not related to the ED-based BEV. Third, a mean value in the ED-based BEV image was subtracted from the image to remove the influence of the mean value of the power spectral image.

Fourth, a power spectral image was calculated by using two-dimensional Fourier transformation from the preprocessed image. The two-dimensional Fourier transformation and the power spectrum were calculated by the following equations:

$$F(u,v) = \int_{-\infty}^{\infty}\int_{-\infty}^{\infty} f(x,y)e^{-j2\pi(ux+vy)}dxdy, \tag{4.5}$$

$$P(u,v) = |F(u,v)|^2, \tag{4.6}$$

where $f(x, y)$ is the preprocessed ED-based BEV image, $F(u, v)$ is the Fourier transformed image, $P(u, v)$ is the power spectral image, x and y are the coordinates in the real space, and u and v are the coordinates in the spatial frequency space.

The power spectral image in the Cartesian coordinate system was converted to the polar coordinate system, which has the horizontal axis of the angle and the vertical axis of the spatial frequency. The power spectral image was integrated over a range of angles from 0° to 360° to calculate the slope of an average power spectrum by using the following equation:

$$G(f) = \int_{0}^{360} \ln P(f,\theta)\, d\theta, \tag{4.7}$$

where f is the spatial frequency (mm^{-1}) and θ is the angle (degree) in the power spectral image. The slope of the average power spectrum was evaluated as the slope of a one-order polynomial of the power spectrum from 0.0195 mm^{-1} to a Nyquist frequency, which was calculated by a least-square method. The slopes were calculated in all directions (0–355°) with an interval of 5°. Finally, the robust beam directions

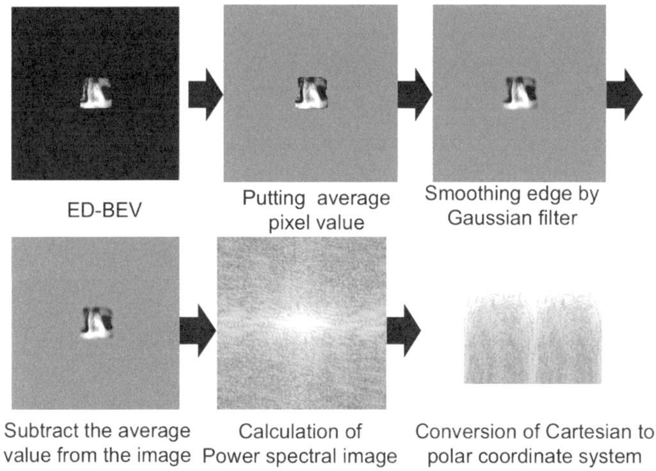

Fig. 4.7 Resulting images in the major steps of the proposed method

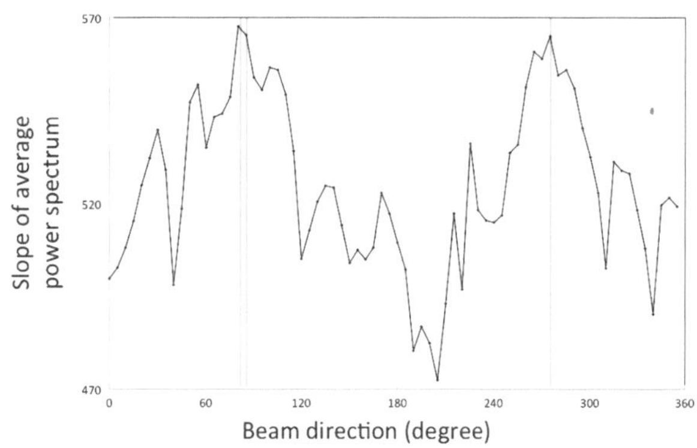

Fig. 4.8 Slope of average power spectral value as a function of the beam direction (0–355°). The *blue lines* show the three most robust beam directions, i.e., 80°, 85°, and 275°

against patient setup errors were determined by selecting the directions corresponding to the several largest gradients of average power spectra for all beam directions. Figure 4.7 shows the resulting images in the major steps of the proposed method.

Performance of the Decision Making Method for the Suggestion of Robust Beam Directions Against the Patient Setup Error

We applied the proposed method to four head and neck cancer cases and detected the beam directions. Figure 4.8 shows the slope of the average power spectra as a function of beam direction, and the detected beam directions of 0–355° are indicated by blue lines. The blue lines show the three most robust beam directions. Figure 4.9 shows the robust beam directions determined by the proposed method on three CT slices for a case. Each red region shows a PTV region, and each light blue

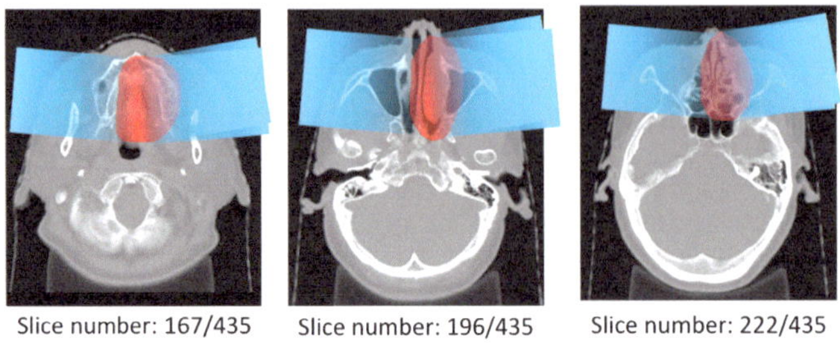

Fig. 4.9 Robust beam directions determined by the proposed method on three CT slices for a case by selecting the directions corresponding to the three largest slopes of average power spectra for all beam directions

region shows the beam path. In this case, 80°, 85°, and 275° were considered as the robust beam directions. In a discussion of the results with radiological oncologists, all the oncologists agreed with most of the beam directions determined by the proposed method, which seems to indicate that the method is robust against patient setup errors.

Acknowledgments The authors are grateful to all members of the Arimura Laboratory (http://www.shs.kyushu-u.ac.jp/~arimura), whose comments made an enormous contribution to this chapter. This research was partially supported by the Ministry of Education, Culture, Sports Science, and Technology (MEXT), Grant-in-Aid for Scientific Research (C), 22611011, 2011to 2012, and Grant-in-Aid for Scientific Research on Innovative Areas, 24103707, 2012.

References

1. National Cancer Center (2010) Cancer statistics in Japan http://ganjoho.jp/public/statistics/backnumber/2010_en.html
2. Dawson LA, Sharpe MB (2006) Image-guided radiotherapy: rationale, benefits, and limitations. The Lancet Oncol 7(10):848–858
3. Evans PM (2008) Anatomical imaging for radiotherapy. Phys Med Biol 53(12):R151–R191
4. ICRU (1999) ICRU report 62, Prescribing, recording and reporting photon beam therapy. (supplement to ICRU report 50)
5. Onishi H et al (2011) Stereotactic body radiotherapy (SBRT) for operable stage I non-small-cell lung cancer: can SBRT be comparable to surgery? Int J Radiat Oncol Biol Phys 81:1352–1358
6. Ploquin N, Rangel A, Dunscombe P (2008) Phantom evaluation of a commercially available three modality image guided radiation therapy system. Med Phys 35(12):5303–5311
7. Wang Z, Nelson JW, Yoo S et al (2009) Refinement of treatment setup and target localization accuracy using three-dimensional cone-beam computed tomography for stereotactic body radiotherapy. Int J Radiat Oncol Biol Phys 73(2):571–577
8. Shirato H, Shimizu S, Kitamura K et al (2000) Four-dimensional treatment planning and fluoroscopic real-time tumor tracking radiotherapy for moving tumor. Int J Radiat Oncol Biol Phys 48:435–442
9. Su M, Miften M, Whiddon C, Sun X, Light K, Marks L (2005) An artificial neural network for predicting the incidence of radiation pneumonitis. Med Phys 32(2):318–325

10. Kakar M, Seierstad T, Røe K, Olsen DR (2009) Artificial neural networks for prediction of response to chemoradiation in HT29 xenografts. Int J Radiat Oncol Biol Phys 75(2):506–511
11. El Naqa I, Bradley JD, Lindsay PE, Hope AJ, Deasy JO (2009) Predicting radiotherapy outcomes using statistical learning techniques. Phys Med Biol 54(18):S9–S30
12. Jayasurya K, Fung G, Yu S, Dehing-Oberije C, De Ruysscher D, Hope A, De Neve W, Lievens Y, Lambin P, Dekker AL (2010) Comparison of Bayesian network and support vector machine models for two-year survival prediction in lung cancer patients treated with radiotherapy. Med Phys 37(4):1401–1407
13. Atsumi K, Shioyama Y, Arimura H, Terashima K, Matsuki T, Ohga S, Yoshitake T, Nonoshita T, Tsurumaru D, Ohnishi K, Asai K, Matsumoto K, Nakamura K, Honda H (2012) Esophageal stenosis associated with tumor regression in radiation therapy for esophageal cancer: frequency and prediction. Int J Radiat Oncol Biol Phys 82(5):1973–1980
14. Nagata Y, Wulf J, Lax I, Timmerman R, Zimmermann F, Stojkovski I, Jeremic B (2011) Stereotactic radiotherapy of primary lung cancer and other targets: results of consultant meeting of the international atomic energy agency. Int J Radiat Oncol Biol Phys 79:660–669
15. Takayama K, Nagata Y, Negoro Y, Mizowaki T, Sakamoto T, Sakamoto M, Aoki T, Yano S, Koga S, Hiraoka M (2005) Treatment planning of stereotactic radiotherapy for solitary lung tumor. Int J Radiat Oncol Biol Phys 61:1565–1571
16. Meyer J, Hummel SM, Cho PS, Austin-Seymour MM, Phillips MH (2005) Automatic selection of non-coplanar beam directions for three-dimensional conformal radiotherapy. Br J Radiol 78:316–327
17. dePooter JA, Méndez Romero A, Wunderink W et al (2008) Automated non-coplanar beam direction optimization improves IMRT in SBRT of liver metastasis. Radiother Oncol 88:376–381
18. Aisen AM, Broderick LS, Winer-Muram H, Brodley CE, Kak AC, Pavlopoulou C, Dy J, Shyu CR, Marchiori A (2003) Automated storage and retrieval of thin-section CT images to assist diagnosis. System description and preliminary assessment. Radiology 228:265–270
19. Li Q, Li F, Shiraishi J, Katsuragawa S, Sone S, Doi K (2003) Investigation of new psychophysical measures for evaluation of similar images on thoracic CT for distinction between benign and malignant nodules. Med Phys 30:2584–2593
20. Kumazawa S, Muramatsu C, Li Q, Li F, Shiraishi J, Caligiuri P, Schmidt RA, MacMahon H, Doi K (2008) An investigation of radiologists' perception of lesion similarity: observations with paired breast masses on mammograms and paired lung nodules on CT images. Acad Radiol 15:887–894
21. Muramatsu C, Li Q, Suzuki K, Schmidt RA, Shiraishi J, Newstead GM, Doi K (2005) Investigation of psychophysical measure for evaluation of similar images for mammographic masses: preliminary results. Med Phys 32:2295–2304
22. Muramatsu C, Li Q, Schmidt RA, Shiraishi J, Doi K (2009) Determination of similarity measures for pairs of mass lesions on mammograms by use of BI-RADS lesion descriptors and image features. Acad Radiol 16:443–449
23. Muramatsu C, Schmidt RA, Shiraishi J, Li Q, Doi K (2010) Presentation of similar images as a reference for distinction between benign and malignant masses on mammograms: analysis of initial observer study. J Digit Imaging 23:592–602
24. Burger W, Burge MJ (2007) Digital image processing: an algorithmic introduction using java, 1st edn. Springer, New York
25. Steene JV et al (2002) Definition of gross tumor volume in lung cancer: inter-observer variability. Radiother Oncol 62:37–49
26. Bradley JD, Perez CA, Dehdashti F et al (2004) Implementing biologic target volumes in radiation treatment planning for non-small cell lung cancer. J Nucl Med 45:96S–101S
27. Nakamura K, Shioyama Y, Tokumaru S et al (2008) Variation of clinical target volume definition among Japanese radiation oncologist in external beam radiotherapy for prostate cancer. Jpn J Clin Oncol 38(4):275–280
28. Day E, Betler J, Parda D et al (2009) A region growing method for tumor volume segmentation on PET images for rectal and anal cancer patients. Med Phys 36(10):4349–4358

29. Biehl JB, Kong FM, Dehdashti F et al (2006) ^{18}F-FDG PET definition of gross tumor volume for radiotherapy of non-small cell lung cancer: is a single standardized uptake value threshold approach appropriate? J Nucl Med 47(11):1808–1812
30. Zhang T, Tachiya Y, Sakaguchi Y et al (2010) Phantom study on three-dimensional target volume delineation by PET/CT-based auto-contouring. Fukuoka Acta Media 101(11):238–246
31. Aristophanous M, Penney BC, Martel MK et al (2007) Gaussian mixture model for definition of lung tumor volumes in positron emission tomography. Med Phys 34(11):4223–4235
32. Belhassen S, Zaidi H (2010) A novel fuzzy C-means algorithm for unsupervised heterogeneous tumor quantification in PET. Med Phys 37(3):1309–1324
33. Hatt M, Rest CC, Turzo A et al (2009) A fuzzy locally adaptive Bayesian segmentation approach for volume determination in PET. IEEE Trans Med Imaging 28(6):881–893
34. Hatt M, Rest CC, Nidal A et al (2011) PET functional volume delineation: a robustness and repeatability study. Eur J Nucl Med Mol Imaging 38:3663–3672
35. Geets X, Lee JA, Bol A et al (2007) A gradient-based method for segmenting FDG-PET images: methodology and validation. Eur J Nucl Med Mol Imaging 34:1427–1438
36. Rousson M, Khamene A, Diallo M et al (2005) Constrained surface evolutions for prostate and bladder segmentation in CT images. In: Liu Y, Jiang T, Zhang C (eds) Lecture notes in computer science (LNCS), vol 3765. Springer, New York, pp 251–260
37. Strassmann G, Abdellaoui S, Richter D et al (2010) Atlas-based semiautomatic target volume definition (CTV) for head-and-neck tumors. Int J Radiat Oncol Biol Phys 78(4):1270–1276
38. El Naqa I, Yang D, Apte A et al (2007) Concurrent multimodality image segmentation by active contours for radiotherapy treatment planning. Med Phys 34(2):4738–4749
39. Pluim JP, Maintz JB, Viergever MA (2003) Mutual-information-based registration of medical images: a survey. IEEE Trans Med Imaging 22(8):986–1004
40. Joachims T (2008) SVMlight. Cornell University. http://svmlight.joachims.org/
41. Okada T, Kamada T, Tsuji H, Mizoe JE, Baba M, Kato S, Yamada S, Sugahara S, Yasuda S, Yamamoto N, Imai R, Hasegawa A, Imada H, Kiyohara H, Jingu K, Shinoto M, Tsujii H (2010) Carbon ion radiotherapy: clinical experiences at National Institute of Radiological Science (NIRS). J Radiat Res 51:355–364
42. Minohara S, Fukuda S, Kanematsu N, Takei Y, Furukawa T, Inaniwa T, Matsufuji N, Mori S, Noda K (2010) Recent innovations in carbon–ion radiotherapy. J Radiat Res 51:385–392
43. Hui Z, Zhang X, Starkschall G, Li Y, Mohan R, Komaki R, Cox JD, Chang JY (2008) Effects of interfractional motion and anatomic changes on proton therapy dose distribution in lung cancer. Int J Radiat Oncol Biol Phys 72:1385–1395
44. Inaniwa T, Kanematsu N, Furukawa T, Hasegawa A (2011) A robust algorithm of intensity modulated proton therapy for critical tissue sparing and target coverage. Phys Med Biol 56:4749–4770
45. Lomax AJ (2008) Intensity modulated proton therapy and its sensitivity to treatment uncertainties 2: the potential effects of inter-fraction and inter-field motions. Phys Med Biol 53:1043–1056
46. Pflugfelder D, Wilkens JJ, Oelfke U (2008) Worst case optimization: a method to account for uncertainties in optimization of intensity modulated proton therapy. Phys Med Biol 53:1689–1700
47. Sejpal SV, Amos RA, Bluett JB, Levy LB, Kudchadker RJ, Johnson J, Choi S, Lee AK (2009) Dosimetric changes resulting from patient rotational setup errors in proton therapy prostate plans. Int J Radiat Oncol Biol Phys 75:40–48
48. Unkelbach J, Bortfeld T, Martin BC, Soukup M (2009) Reducing the sensitivity of IMPT treatment plans to setup errors and range uncertainties via probabilistic treatment planning. Med Phys 36:149–163
49. Zhang X, Dong L, Lee AK, Cox JD, Kuban DA, Zhu RX, Wang X, Li Y, Newhauser WD, Gillin M, Mohan R (2007) Effect of anatomic motion on proton therapy dose distribution in prostate cancer treatment. Int J Radiat Oncol Biol Phys 67:620–629

50. Kakiuchi G, Arimura H, Shioyama Y, Nagano A, Minohara S, Mizoguchi A, Honda H, Toyofuku F, Ohki M, Hirata H (2011) Optimization of robust beam angles to patient setup errors for head and neck cancer in hadron particle therapy. ASTRO 2011, Abstract 3413
51. Saw CB, Loper A, Komanduri K, Combine T, Huq S, Scicutella C (2005) Determination of CT-to-density conversion relationship for image-based treatment planning system. Med Dosim 30:145–148
52. Otsu N (1979) A threshold selection method from gray level histograms. IEEE Trans Syst Man Cybern SMC-9:62–66
53. Herman GT, Zheng J, Bucholtz CA (1992) Shape-based interpolation. IEEE Comput Graph Appl 12:69–79

Part II
Computational Anatomy

Chapter 5
Computational Anatomy in the Abdomen: Automated Multi-Organ and Tumor Analysis from Computed Tomography

Marius George Linguraru and Ronald M. Summers

Abstract The interpretation of medical images benefits from anatomical and physiological priors to optimize computer-aided diagnosis (CAD) applications. Diagnosis also relies on the comprehensive analysis of multiple organs and quantitative measures of tissue. This chapter highlights our recent contributions to abdominal multi-organ analysis employing constraints typical to medical images and adapted to patient data. A new formulation for graph-based methods to segment abdominal organs from multi-phase CT data is first presented. The method extends basic graph cuts by using: multi-phases enhancement modeling, shape priors and location constraints. The multi-organ localization is also addressed using maximum a posteriori (MAP) probability estimations of organs' location, orientation, and scale. The probabilistic framework models the inter-organ spatial relations using a minimum volume overlap constraint. The liver, spleen, left kidney, right kidney and pancreas are concomitantly analyzed in the multi-organ analysis framework. Finally, the automated detection and segmentation of abdominal tumors (i.e., hepatic tumors) from abdominal CT images is presented using once again shape and enhancement constraints. Features are computed for the tumor candidates and machine learning is used to select the optimal features to separate true and false detections. The methods illustrate multi-scale analyses of the abdomen, from multi-organ to organ and tumors and promise to support the processing of large medical data in the clinically oriented integrated analysis of the abdomen.

M.G. Linguraru (✉)
Sheikh Zayed Institute for Pediatric Surgical Innovation, Children's National Medical Center, 111 Michigan Avenue NW, Washington, DC 20010, USA
e-mail: mlingura@cnmc.org

R.M. Summers
Imaging Biomarkers and Computer Aided Diagnosis Laboratory, Radiology and Imaging Sciences, Clinical Center, National Institutes of Health, 10 Center Drive, Bethesda, MD 20892, USA
e-mail: rms@nih.gov

K. Suzuki (ed.), *Computational Intelligence in Biomedical Imaging*,
DOI 10.1007/978-1-4614-7245-2_5,

Introduction

In CT-based clinical abdominal diagnosis, radiologists rely on analyzing multi-phase computed tomography (CT) data, as soft tissue enhancement can be an indicator of abnormality. Contrast-enhanced CT has proven exceptionally useful to improving diagnosis due to the ability to differentiate tumors from healthy tissue. For instance, the level of enhancement in the tumor is an important indication of malignancy and can be used to better classify abdominal abnormalities [1, 2]. This routine clinical acquisition protocol makes multi-phase data (with/without contrast) readily available.

Organ size and shape are additional image-based markers of disease that are commonly used in the radiological interpretation of the abdomen. Unusually sized organs flag infections, necrosis, or fatty infiltrations [3]. Although shape is locally variable in abdominal organs, global shape constraints remain valid. Similarly, tumor size and shape indicate cancer evolution, response to treatment, and the necessity of surgery. The enhancement of lesions is the primary biomarker used to classify them [1, 4, 5].

In traditional clinical practice, three-dimensional (3D) organ analysis is performed via time-consuming manual measurements or, as an alternative, the evaluation is incompletely based on two-dimensional (2D) projection images. Tumors are evaluated in a similar fashion. While size is approximated by a 2D measurement of the longest axis in a CT projection (typically the axial view), the intensity is estimated from 2D circular regions in the center of a tumor. These manual measurements show high intra- and inter-operator variability. In this context, computer-assisted radiology can improve the diagnosis of tumors by 3D quantifications of size, enhancement, and morphology from image analysis.

There are several advantages that automated methods have over manual or interactive techniques. An important aspect is the reproducibility of results, which in automated algorithms are not subjected to user interaction. Moreover, automated techniques may be faster, readily available, and can run in the background without interrupting the clinical workflow (do not require human presence).

Diagnosis also relies on the comprehensive analysis of groups of organs and quantitative measures of soft tissue. When presented with 3D patient data, such as CT, radiologists typically analyze them organ-by-organ and slice-by-slice until the entire image data are covered. This allows detecting multiple diseases from multiple organs.

Computer-aided diagnosis (CAD) and medical image analysis traditionally focus on organ- or disease-based applications. However there has been recent work toward the automated simultaneous segmentation and analysis of multiple organs for comprehensive diagnosis or pre-operative planning and guidance. Additionally, the interpretation of medical images should integrate anatomical and physiological priors, such as shape and appearance; synergistic combinations of priors were seldom incorporated in the optimization of CAD. The implementation of robust and automated 3D analysis techniques for multi-organs and tumors would allow radiologists and surgeons to have easy and convenient access to organ measurements and 3D visualization.

CT-Based Abdominal Organ Segmentation

A variety of methods have been proposed for the segmentation of individual abdominal organs from CT images, in particular CT with contrast enhancement. The liver enjoyed special attention in recent literature [6–12], kidneys were analyzed sporadically [13–15], while the spleen [8, 16, 17] and pancreas [18] were segmented less frequently. Model-driven approaches have been both popular and successful [10, 11], including active and statistical shape models [9, 12, 15] and atlas-based segmentation [8, 9, 18]. Level sets and geodesic active contours were frequently involved in these techniques [7, 8, 12]. Occasionally, graph cuts were employed [13, 14].

Recently, the simultaneous segmentation of multiple abdominal organs has been addressed in publications [18–23]. Most of these methods rely on some form of prior knowledge of the organs, for example probabilistic atlases [21, 23–25] and statistical models [20]. For instance, the relation between organs and manual landmarks was used in [21]. Also, an efficient optimization of level set techniques for general multi-class segmentation was proposed in [26], paving the way for the discrete optimization of graph cuts with nonsubmodular functions in [27].

Notably, a hierarchical multi-organ statistical atlas was developed by Okada et al. [20]. Also recently, Seifert et al. [22] proposed a semantic navigation for fast multi-organ segmentation from CT data. Decision forests were additionally proposed in [28] to classify multiple organs from CT volumes. Another interesting concept was presented in [29] for the scheduling problem of multi-organ segmentation to maximize the performance of CAD systems designed to analyze the whole human body. In addition, multi-phase contrast-enhanced CT data were employed in abdominal multi-organ analysis [19, 30, 31]. In [30], the segmentation was based on independent component analysis in a variational Bayesian mixture, while in [32], expectation-maximization and principal component analysis were combined. A 4D convolution was proposed in [19] constrained by a training model of abdominal soft tissue enhancement.

CT-Based Abdominal Organ Localization

Abdominal multi-organ segmentation remains a challenging task because the sizes, shapes, and locations of the organs vary significantly in different subjects. Moreover, these organs have similar appearance in CT images, especially non-contrast data, and are in close proximity to each other. Thus the successful segmentation requires a good initial identification and localization of individual organs, generally performed interactively [20, 21, 23]. Correct organ localization can also benefit other image processing tasks, including registration and computer-aided detection.

Among the most notable automated localization techniques for abdominal organs, Okada et al. [9] initialized the liver segmentation by estimating the abdominal cavity. In [33] a statistical location model was used, but the method was limited to estimating only the organ locations without considering the orientations and sizes. Yao et al. [34] simultaneously detected multi-organ locations by finding bounding boxes using principal component analysis and a probabilistic atlas. In [22] the organ location, orientation, and size were estimated using automatically detected anatomical landmarks, semantics, and machine learning techniques. Alternatively, regression techniques were used in [35] to detect multiple organs through the human body from MR data. Most recently, mouse abdominal organs were localized in CT using statistical atlases in [36].

Segmentation Competitions in the Abdomen

As already mentioned, the analysis of the liver has benefited from particular popularity in CAD research and has been at the forefront of validation techniques for medical image analysis. But importantly, according to the American Cancer Society, approximately 26,190 new cases of liver cancer are expected to occur in the USA in 2011 [37]. The incidence of liver cancer has been increasing by more than 3 % yearly. The liver is also a prime candidate for metastases from cancers in the breast, colon, prostate, lung, pancreas, stomach, esophagus, adrenal glands, or skin (melanoma) [38].

For a straightforward comparison of liver analysis techniques, a liver segmentation competition from mainly pathological CT data was held in conjunction with the International Conference on Medical Image Computing and Computer Assisted Intervention (MICCAI), in 2007 [7]. A variety of techniques were presented and their performance evaluated through a combination of metrics, including volume overlap and error, root-mean square error, and average surface distance. Among the ten automatic and six interactive methods for liver segmentation that were presented, the interactive methods achieved the best segmentation results [39, 40]. Statistical shape models were the best fully automated liver segmentation methods and performed competitively with the semiautomatic techniques [41]. Other notable participations in the competition employed region growing [42] and a semantic formulation of knowledge and context [43].

In 2008, another segmentation competition followed in conjunction with MICCAI, this time addressing the segmentation of liver tumors from CT data [44]. CT images covered a range of pathologies and were acquired with contrast enhancement to allow the differentiation of tumors from healthy liver parenchyma. As in the case of the liver segmentation, the highest scoring technique was interactive, using classic graph cuts and the watershed algorithm to accurately segment tumors [45]. The most successful semiautomatic approaches scored similarly and employed adaptive thresholding and morphological processing [46], voxel classification and propagational learning [47], and a level set with fuzzy pixel classification [48]. Automatically, tumors were best segmented via machine learning and classification techniques [49, 50].

In addition to the fully automated 3D segmentation of both the organs and tumors, CAD and surgical planning would benefit from the analysis of other types of abnormalities (i.e., fatty tissue), as well as the organ's vasculature [51–53]. Methods for the concurrent segmentations of liver structures remain mainly interactive [54].

Graph Cuts for Biomedical Data

Graph cuts [55] have become popular for image segmentation due to their ability to handle highly textured data via a numerically robust global optimization. As the segmentation techniques employed in this chapter rely on graph cuts, several other medical image analysis applications proposed in literature are using graph cuts are presented below.

To segment abdominal organs, in [13, 56–58] model-based information was included for the segmentation of the heart, spleen, and kidneys. The models were aligned using markers in [13, 58], manual placements in axial slices in [57], and intra-model constraints given in the first frame of the cardiac cycle in [56]. Shape priors were employed in [59, 60] to reconstruct the liver vasculature and lung airways; the cuts in the graph were constrained by a tubular filter. Probabilistic shape-based energies for graph cuts were combined with image intensity in a non-parametric iterative model in [61] for the segmentation of the kidneys. Also, in [62], shape priors and neighboring constraints were incorporated using signed distances from boundaries to segment the liver.

Graph-cut techniques were also used in brain segmentation and registration [15, 63–66], breast tumor analysis [67], and orthopedics [68]. Using an acquisition protocol for plaque reconstruction, carotid plaques were segmented semiautomatically from ultrasound images in [69]. In other types of biomedical applications, a multi-level automated graph-cut algorithm was used in [70] to segment cell nuclei. A graph-cut optimization was presented in [71] for the parcellation of the brain from functional MRI. In [72], a data-driven graph approach was implemented to estimate the variability of neural responses on magnetoencephalography or electroencephalography data. Finally, a study of the effect of weights and topology on the construction of graphs can be found in [73].

Contributions

Abdominal multi-organ segmentation remains a challenging task because the sizes, shapes, and locations of organs vary significantly between subjects. Moreover, organs have similar appearance in CT images, even in contrast-enhanced data, and are in close proximity to each other. The remainder of this chapter synthesizes our recent contributions to the automated multi-organ analysis from CT data developed at the National Institutes of Health Clinical Center. Besides the simultaneous detection, segmentation, and quantification of multiple abdominal organs, we also present contributions to the integrated analysis of single organs, exemplified through the liver, which can be seen as a multi-scale or hierarchical analysis from the abdomen to organ and tumor.

Methodologically, an integrated statistical model for medical data is described in this chapter and incorporated into a graph-based approach. An advantage in the handling of medical data is the available prior information regarding organ location, shape, and appearance. Although highly variable between patients and in the presence of disease, abdominal organs satisfy basic rules of anatomy and physiology. Hence, the incorporation of statistical models into algorithms for medical data analysis greatly benefits the segmentation of abdominal images.

In order, we first propose a new formulation of a 4D directional graph to automatically segment abdominal organs, at this stage the liver, spleen, and left and right kidneys, using graph cuts [74, 75]. The statistical priors comprise location probabilities that are intrinsic to medical data, an enhancement constraint characteristic to the clinical protocols using abdominal CT and an unbiased shape measure. We further present a maximum a posteriori (MAP) framework for automated abdominal multi-organ localization [76, 77]. Our method finds the poses of multiple abdominal organs, which include not only the locations but also the orientations and scales. The method was applied to five organs: liver, spleen, pancreas, and left and right kidneys. Finally, graph cuts are employed once more to detect and segment hepatic tumors using shape and enhancement constraints [78, 79]. The chapter ends with a short discussion of some of the current research directions designed to integrate multi-organ interaction and anatomical abnormality towards an integrated analysis of the entire abdomen.

Abdominal Multi-Organ Segmentation

This section describes the technique for abdominal multi-organ segmentation using graph cuts with embedded statistical anatomical and physiological information [75].

Data

Twenty-eight random abdominal CT studies with or without contrast enhancement from healthy subjects were used to create statistical models. Data were collected at high resolution (1 mm slice thickness). For testing the algorithm, 20 random abdominal CT studies (normal and abnormal) were obtained with two temporal acquisitions (40 CT scans). The first image was obtained at non-contrast phase (NCP) and a second at portal venous phase (PVP) using fixed delays. An example of multi-phase CT data is shown in Fig. 5.1. Ten images were of low resolution (5 mm slice thickness) and were used for training and testing the algorithm using a leave-one-out strategy. Ten images were of high resolutions (1 mm slice thickness) and

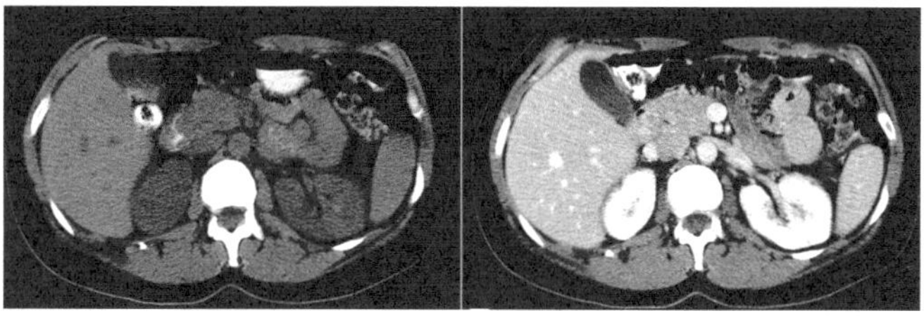

Fig. 5.1 An example of contrast-enhanced CT of the abdomen. The *left image* shows the non-contrast phase acquisition and the *right picture* shows the image of the same patient after contrast enhancement (portal venous phase)

used only for testing. The liver, spleen, and left and right kidneys were manually segmented (by two research fellows supervised by a board-certified radiologist) in all CT cases [75].

Model Initialization

The statistical models of location and appearance were built from the 28 CT cases described in the previous section. The 28 CT data were further used to build shape constraints via a Parzen window distribution, as explained later in the construction of the 4D graph.

For location models, a probabilistic atlas (PA) was constructed for each organ: liver, spleen, left kidney, and right kidney [8]. Organ locations were normalized to an anatomical landmark (xiphoid process) to preserve spatial relationships and model organs in the anatomical space. A random image set was used as reference and the other images registered to it. The registration was performed for each organ separately. Structural variability, including the size of organs, was conserved by a size-preserving affine registration adapted from [80]. The PA was constructed independently from the segmentation algorithm and it is shown in Fig. 5.2.

Appearance statistics were computed from the training data (the 28 cases used in the model). Histograms of the segmented organs (objects) and background at NCP and PVP were computed and modeled as sums of Gaussians, as in Fig. 5.3.

Preprocessing

Although multi-phase CT images were acquired during the same session and intrapatient, there was small, but noticeable abdominal inter-phase motion, especially associated with breathing. The preprocessing follows our work in [19].

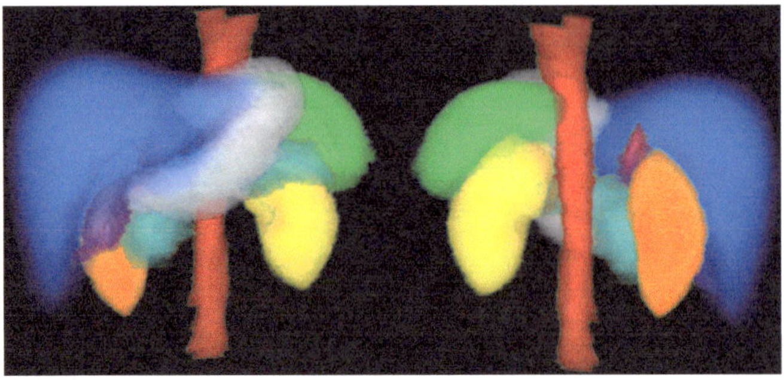

Fig. 5.2 The probabilistic atlas of the abdomen showing the liver (*blue*), spleen (*green*), left kidney (*yellow*), and right kidney (*orange*), the organs analyzed by our technique [24]. In addition, the pictures show the aorta (*red*), stomach (*green*), gallbladder (*purple*), pancreas (*light blue*), right adrenal gland (*magenta*), and left adrenal gland (*brown*)

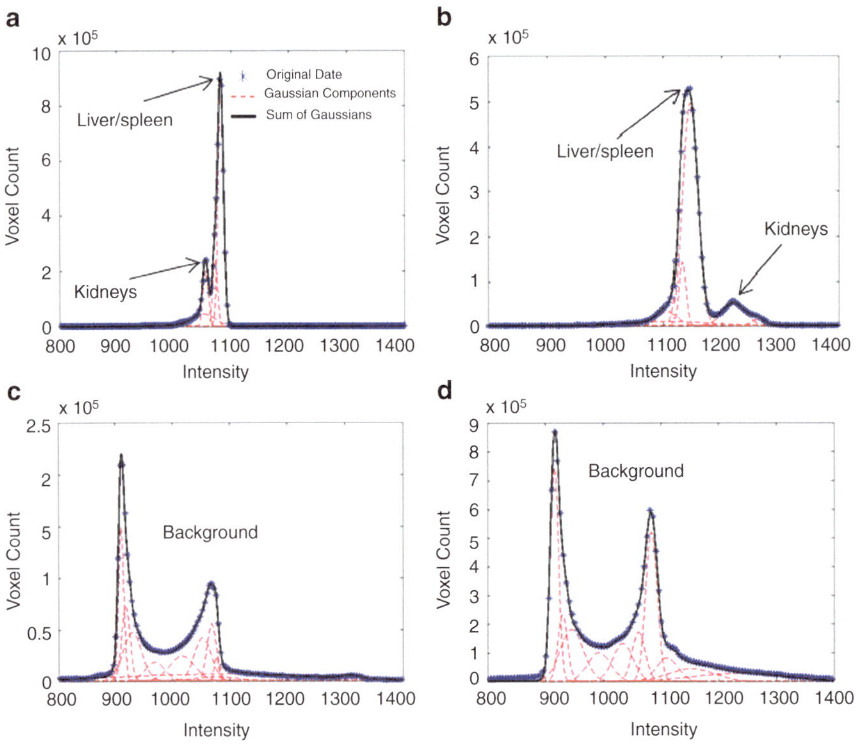

Fig. 5.3 Fitted sums of Gaussians to training data of organs/objects (**a** and **b**) and background (**c** and **d**) [75]. NCP intensity models are shown in (**a** and **c**) and PVP data in (**b** and **d**). Here, training data refers to the training cases in the leave-one-out strategy. The histogram peaks related to the liver/spleen and kidneys are marked

First, data were smoothed using anisotropic diffusion [81]. NCP data were registered to the PVP images. Then, the demons nonlinear registration algorithm was employed [82] to align NCP and PVP images, as the limited range of motion between acquisitions ensures partial overlaps between organs over multiple phases.

4D Convolution

From smoothed training data of multi-phase CT, the *min* and *max* intensities of organs were estimated: $min_{i,t} = \mu_{i,t} - 3\sigma_{i,t}$ and $max_{i,t} = \mu_{i,t} + 3\sigma_{i,t}$, where $i = 1\ldots3$ for liver, spleen, and kidneys, $\mu_{p,t}$ and $\sigma_{p,t}$ represent the mean and standard deviation, and $t = 1, 2$ for NCP and PVP. As in [19], a 4D array $K(x,y,z,t) = I_t(x,y,z)$ was created from multi-phase data. A convolution with a 4D filter f labeled only regions for which all voxels in the convolution kernel satisfied the intensity constraints

$$L(x,y,z) = (K \circ f)(x,y,z,t) = \begin{cases} l_j, if \bigcap_t \left(\min_{jt} \leq K(x,y,z,t) \leq \max_{jt}\right) \\ 0, \quad otherwise. \end{cases} \quad (5.1)$$

L represents the labeled image and l_j the labels ($j = 1\ldots4$ for liver, spleen, left kidney, and right kidney). Note that the labeled organs in L appear eroded as a result of the 4D convolution. In our method, L provided seeds for objects (I_o) in the 4D graph, as shown below, and was used to estimate the patient-specific histograms. The eroded inverted L provided the background (I_b) seeds and the related histograms. To report the segmentation results by 4D convolution, L was dilated to compensate for the undersegmentation of organs.

4D Graph

Graph cuts (GC) were chosen for the inherent capability to provide a globally optimal solution for segmentation [55]. Let $A = (A_1, A_2, \ldots, A_p, \ldots)$ be a vector that defines the segmentation. The component A_p associated with the voxel p in an image can be assigned a label of either object of interest/organ O_i (with $i = 1\ldots4$, for liver, spleen, left kidney, and right kidney) or background B, where $B \cap O = \emptyset$ and $O_i \cap O_j = \emptyset$ for $i \neq j$. In the classical graph-cut algorithm, A_p takes binary values for O and B. In our application, A_p can have a value from 0 to 4, where 0 denotes the background, 1 the liver, 2 the spleen, 3 the right kidney, and 4 the left kidney.

The inputs to our problem are two sets of registered abdominal CT scans per patient: the NCP and PVP sequences. Hence every voxel p in the graph has two intensity values: I^p_{ncp} and I^p_{pcp}. A simplified schematic representation of the 4D graph is shown in Fig. 5.4. Every voxel is connected to both O_i (sources) and B (sink) via

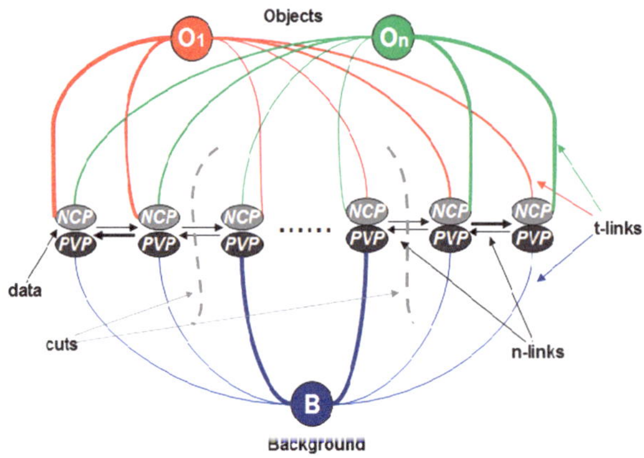

Fig. 5.4 A simplified schematic of the multi-object multi-phase graph [75]. Four-dimensional information is input from the NCP and PVP data. T-links are connected to the objects (O_1 to O_n) and background (B) terminals. Directional n-links connect neighboring nodes (the image shows only two neighbors for each voxel). The width of a line in the graph reflects the strength of the connection

t-links and to its neighbors via n-links (which can be directional). Source and sink are terminologies used in [55]. The costs of the connections determine the segmentation and weak links are good candidates for the cut.

We first extend the classical GC formulation to analyze 4D data and then incorporate penalties from the contrast enhancement of CT soft tissue, Parzen shape windows, and location from a priori probabilities. The energy E to minimize can be written generically as

$$E(A) = E_{data}(A) + E_{enhance}(A) + E_{location}(A) + \sum_{i=1}^{4} \left(E_{boundary}(A) + E_{shape}(A)\right), \tag{5.2}$$

with $i = 1\ldots4$ for liver, spleen, left kidney, and right kidney. The subparts of this cost function are described below.

T-Links

In our application, E_{data} is a regional term that computes penalties based on 4D histograms of O and B. The probabilities P of a voxel to belong to O or B are computed from patient-specific histograms of NCP and PVP data.

$$E_{data}(A) = \lambda \sum_{p \in O} R_p(O) + (1 - \lambda) \sum_{p \in B} R_p(B); \tag{5.3}$$

$$R_p(O_i) = -\ln\left(\frac{\sqrt{P_{ncp}\left(I^p_{ncp}|O_i\right)P_{pvp}\left(I^p_{pvp}|O_i\right)}}{\sum_i \sqrt{P_{ncp}\left(I^p_{ncp}|O_i\right)P_{pvp}\left(I^p_{pvp}|O_i\right)} + \sqrt{P_{ncp}\left(I^p_{ncp}|B\right)P_{pvp}\left(I^p_{pvp}|B\right)}}\right); \tag{5.4}$$

$$R_p(B) = -\ln\left(\frac{\sqrt{P_{ncp}\left(I^p_{ncp}|B\right)P_{pvp}\left(I^p_{pvp}|B\right)}}{\sum_i \sqrt{P_{ncp}\left(I^p_{ncp}|O_i\right)P_{pvp}\left(I^p_{pvp}|O_i\right)} + \sqrt{P_{ncp}\left(I^p_{ncp}|B\right)P_{pvp}\left(I^p_{pvp}|B\right)}}\right). \tag{5.5}$$

$E_{enhance}$ penalizes regions that do not enhance rapidly during the acquisition of NCP–PVP CT data (i.e., muscles, ligaments, and marrow). Liver, spleen, and kidneys are expected to enhance faster. $E_{enhance}$ can be seen as a gradient in the fourth dimension of the multi-phase data and σ_{ncp} and σ_{pvp} are the standard deviations of noise associated with the NCP and PVP images.

$$E_{enhance}(A) = \sum_{p \in P} 1/\left(1 + E_p^2\right) \quad \text{with} \quad E_p = \frac{\left(I^p_{pvp} - I^p_{ncp}\right)^2}{2\sigma_{ncp}\sigma_{pvp}}. \tag{5.6}$$

Due to the different enhancement patterns of abdominal organs, the peaks in the organs' histograms in Fig. 5.3 are distinguishable between liver/spleen (high peaks in Fig. 5.3a, b) and kidneys (low peaks in Fig. 5.3a, b). However, the probabilistic atlas used in $E_{location}$ allows separating the liver and spleen and the two kidneys. Location constraints from the normalized probabilistic atlas (PA) can be seen as

$$E_{location}(A) = -\sum_{p \in P} \ln\left(PA_p(p|O)\right). \tag{5.7}$$

PA_p represents the probability of p to belong to O. PA_p was obtained by registering PA to the test images by a sequence of coarse-to-fine affine registrations.

N-Links

$E_{boundary}$ assigns penalties for 4D heterogeneity between two voxels p and q with $q \in N_p$ a small neighborhood of p, and $dist(p, q)$ the Euclidean distance between p and q.

$$E_{boundary}(A) = \mu \sum_{\{p,q\}\in N_p} w_{\{p\to q\}} + (1-\mu) \sum_{\{p,q\}\in N_p} w_{\{q\to p\}}. \tag{5.8}$$

The directional penalties in $E_{boundary}$ are initialized symmetrically as

$$w_{\{p\to q\}} = w_{\{q\to p\}} = \begin{cases} 0, & \text{if } A_p = A_q \\ \exp\left(-\dfrac{\left|I^p_{ncp} - I^q_{ncp}\right| \cdot \left|I^p_{pvp} - I^q_{pvp}\right|}{2\sigma_{ncp}\sigma_{pvp}}\right) \dfrac{1}{dist(p,q)}, & \text{otherwise.} \end{cases} \tag{5.9}$$

Then the condition in (5.10) penalizes transitions from dark (less enhanced) to bright (more enhanced) regions to correct the edges of O, considering image noise. This is an intrinsic attribute of medical data (e.g., the visceral fluids and fat are darker than O).

$$\begin{aligned} &IF\left(\left(I^p_{pvp} - I^q_{pvp}\right) > \sigma_{pvp}\ OR\ \left(I^p_{ncp} - I^q_{ncp}\right) > \sigma_{ncp}\right) \\ &THEN\ w_{\{q\to p\}} = 1, \\ &ELSE\ w_{\{p\to q\}} = 1. \end{aligned} \tag{5.10}$$

Additionally, shape constraints were introduced in the n-links using Parzen shape (PS) windows [83] estimated from the reference organ shapes from the 28 CT data used for training/modeling. First, shape references were aligned to the result of the 4D convolution (L) using scaling, rotation, and the location of the centroids. An asymmetric normalized dissimilarity measure D (5.13) between two shapes (s_i and s_j) was used in the shape model to avoid the bias introduced by L, which is an approximation of the shape of the object/organ s. H is the Heaviside step function, s refers to the binary segmentation of an organ, and x to the integration over the image domain.

$$PS(s) = \sum\nolimits_{i=1}^{n} \exp\left(-D(s,s_i)/2\sigma^2\right)/n \tag{5.11}$$

with

$$\sigma^2 = \sum\nolimits_{i=1}^{n} \min_{j\neq i} D\left(s_j, s_i\right)/n \tag{5.12}$$

and

$$D\left(s_j, s_i\right) = \int \left(H\left(s_j\right) - H\left(s_i\right)\right)^2 H\left(s_j\right)dx \Big/ \int H\left(s_j\right)dx. \tag{5.13}$$

The penalties v used in E_{shape} are initialized symmetrically from PS.

$$v_{\{p\to q\}} = v_{\{q\to p\}} = \begin{cases} 0, & if\ A_p = A_q{}^q \\ \max(PS(s)^p, PS(s)^q)/dist(p,q), & otherwise \end{cases}. \tag{5.14}$$

and

$$\begin{array}{l} IF(PS(s)^{\mathrm{p}} > PS(s)^q) \\ THEN\ v_{\{q\to p\}}=1, \\ ELSE\ v_{\{p\to q\}}=1. \end{array} \tag{5.15}$$

The directionality of the n-link in (5.15) penalizes transitions from lower to higher shape probabilities to encourage cuts where there is a strong prior shape resemblance. The shape energy becomes

$$E_{shape}(A) = \delta \sum_{\{p,q\}\in N_p} v_{\{p\to q\}} + (1-\delta) \sum_{\{p,q\}\in N_p} v_{\{q\to p\}}. \tag{5.16}$$

Results

We compared results obtained after the 4D convolution to those achieved using intensity-based 4D GC (without shape and location constraints) and after including shape and location correction. We computed the Dice coefficient (symmetric volume overlap), volume error (absolute volume difference over the volume of the reference), root mean square error, and average surface distance from comparison with the manual segmentations. The influence of patient specific (from the patient CT) versus population (training data) statistics on the accuracy of organ segmentation was also analyzed. Non-parametric statistical tests (Mann–Whitney U test) were performed to assess the significance of segmentation improvement at different steps of the algorithm using the overlap measure at 95 % confidence interval.

Quantitative results from applying our method to the segmentation of liver, spleen, and kidneys are shown in Table 5.1 at different stages of the algorithm. The use of 4D intensity-based graph cuts improved the results significantly over those of the 4D convolution for all organs ($p < 0.05$ for all). Employing shape and location information brought a further significant improvement for the segmentation of the spleen and liver ($p < 0.05$ for both). Significantly better segmentations by using patient-specific data over training data were noted for both kidneys ($p < 0.03$ for both).

Figure 5.5 presents a typical example of liver, spleen, and kidneys segmentation from axial projections of the 3D CT. A 3D rendering is shown in Fig. 5.6 along with the errors between manual and automated segmentations.

Table 5.1 Statistics (mean ± std) for the liver, spleen, left kidney, and right kidney segmentation results from data of 5 mm slice thickness

	Organ	DC (%)	VER (%)	RMS (mm)	ASD (mm)
1. 4D C (Training data)	LKidney	88.7 ± 3.7	10.9 ± 8.9	2.3 ± 0.4	1.1 ± 0.3
	RKidney	89.6 ± 3.4	13.6 ± 6.8	2.1 ± 0.5	1.1 ± 0.3
	Spleen	79.9 ± 10.1	14.9 ± 16.9	4.5 ± 1.9	2.7 ± 1.7
	Liver	89.1 ± 3.7	7.3 ± 4.6	6.7 ± 1.5	3.4 ± 1.0
2. 4D GCI (Patient data)	*LKidney*	92.6 ± 2.4	5.4 ± 6.9	1.8 ± 1.2	0.8 ± 0.6
	RKidney	92.8 ± 1.9	5.6 ± 5.8	1.8 ± 0.8	0.8 ± 0.4
	Spleen	89.6 ± 2.7	11.4 ± 6.9	3.0 ± 1.4	1.5 ± 0.9
	Liver	94.0 ± 1.2	6.2 ± 2.8	4.4 ± 2.0	1.8 ± 0.7
3. 4D GCSL (Patient data)	LKidney	91.9 ± 3.0	6.7 ± 5.2	1.8 ± 0.8	0.8 ± 0.3
	RKidney	93.2 ± 1.5	5.5 ± 4.5	1.8 ± 0.8	0.8 ± 0.4
	Spleen	91.8 ± 1.5	6.6 ± 5.7	2.1 ± 0.9	1.0 ± 0.5
	Liver	95.6 ± 0.6	2.4 ± 1.1	3.0 ± 1.3	1.1 ± 0.4
4. 4D GCSL (Training data)	*LKidney*	90.8 ± 2.7	12.8 ± 7.1	2.6 ± 1.1	1.2 ± 0.6
	RKidney	92.6 ± 1.6	9.2 ± 4.3	2.0 ± 0.7	0.9 ± 0.3
	Spleen	91.9 ± 1.5	6.4 ± 5.0	1.9 ± 0.6	0.9 ± 0.4
	Liver	95.5 ± 0.7	2.1 ± 1.6	3.0 ± 1.3	1.2 ± 0.5

4D C represents the convolution, GCI is GC based solely on image intensity (including 4D appearance and enhancement) and 4D GCSL includes additional shape and location constraints

Italicized cells mark the organs where a significant improvement ($p < 0.05$) was obtained between consecutive steps of the segmentation algorithm, as indicated by numbers from 1 to 4 in the table. The metric used to test the significance of results was DC

Columns present the *DC* Dice coefficient, *VER* volume estimation error, *RMSE* root mean square error, *ASD* average surface distance

Abdominal Multi-Organ Localization

The automated segmentation of abdominal organs, as shown above, often benefits from a robust initialization, such as the localization of anatomical landmarks. In this section, we focus on the localization of five abdominal organs: liver, spleen, left and right kidneys, and pancreas, as means to initialize segmentation algorithms for abdominal multi-organs [77]. In particular, this method can help to initialize the segmentation of certain organs, such as the pancreas, which is less reliably handled by intensity-based methods.

Our multi-organ localization technique first computes statistical information from a set of N training images $\{\mathbf{I}_n\}_{n=1}^{N}$. The organs were manually segmented in each training image and statistically modeled by building an organ pose distribution model (OPDM), a probabilistic atlas (PA—see section "Model Initialization"), and a probabilistic intensity profile (IP). The statistical knowledge was then used to organ poses in a subject image using a MAP framework [76]. Additionally, we introduce a minimum volume overlap condition into the MAP formulation, which models the spatial inter-organ relationship and makes the method more robust to organ pose variations [77]. The technique is detailed as follows.

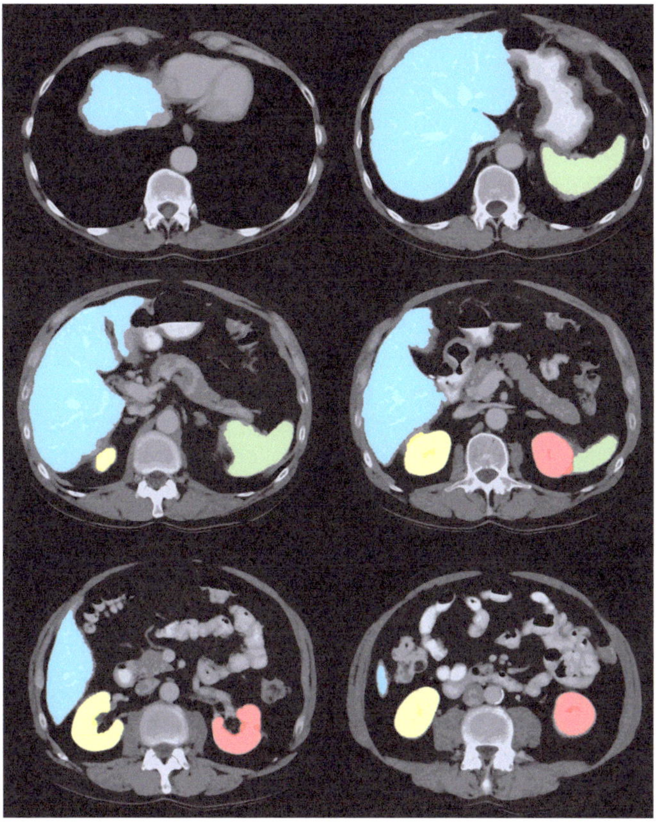

Fig. 5.5 A typical example of liver (*blue*), spleen (*green*), right kidney (*yellow*), and left kidney (*red*) automated segmentation on 2D axial views of the 3D CT data [75]. Images are shown in cranial to caudal order from top left to bottom right

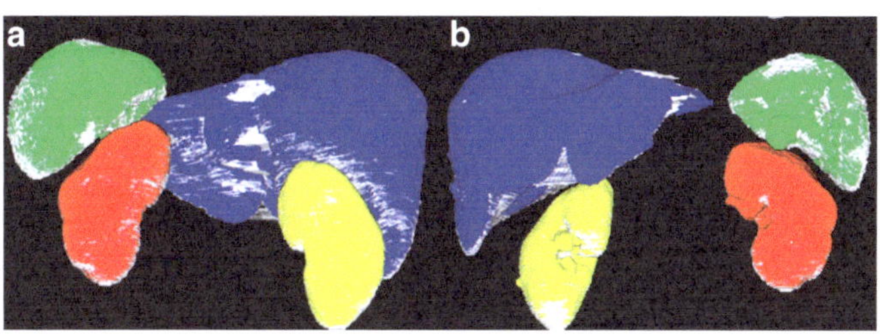

Fig. 5.6 3D images of the automatically segmented abdominal organs [75]; (**a**) is a posterior view and (**b**) an anterior view. The ground truth for the liver is *blue*, spleen is *green*, right kidney is *yellow*, left kidney is *red*. Segmentation errors are overlaid in white on each organ

The A Posteriori Probability

For a given organ $O^{(j)}$, its pose $\Theta^{(j)}$ is defined using nine parameters, which include the location c $= [c_x, c_y, c_z]$, orientation v $= [v_x, v_y, v_z]$ (Euler angles), and scale s $= [s_x, s_y, s_z]$. For a given abdominal subject CT image I in which the organs are to be localized, the a posteriori probability of the pose of $O^{(j)}$ is

$$p\left(\Theta^{(j)}|I,O^{(j)}\right) \propto p\left(I|\Theta^{(j)},O^{(j)}\right)p\left(\Theta^{(j)}|O^{(j)}\right), \tag{5.17}$$

where the prior $p(\Theta^{(j)}|O^{(j)})$ and the conditional probability $p(I|\Theta^{(j)}, O^{(j)})$ are computed using the statistical knowledge from training data sets after abdomen normalization based on anatomical landmarks extracted from bone segmentation [76]. For this, the vertebrae and the ribs are automatically segmented and identified from the CT scans using the method in [33]. A bounding box is then defined around the abdominal cavity. One standard image J_0 was chosen from the training images, and all the other images are then normalized to J_0 by aligning the abdominal bounding boxes [76].

The prior $p(\Theta^{(j)}|O^{(j)})$or OPDM models the organ pose distribution in the normalized abdomen. In our application, the OPDM of each organ was built independently. The pose of organ $O^{(j)}$ in the standard image J_0 was defined as the reference pose $\Theta_0^{(j)} = [\mathbf{c}_0^{(j)}, \mathbf{v}_0^{(j)}, \mathbf{s}_0^{(j)}]$ with $c_0^{(j)}$ being the center of gravity, $\mathbf{v}_0^{(j)} = [0,0,0]$ representing the orientations in the three dimensions, and $\mathbf{s}_0^{(j)} = [1,1,1]$being the three scales. The poses of $O^{(j)}$ in every other training image are computed by registering the manual segmentation of $O^{(j)}$ of the image to that of J_0 using a nine-parameter linear transformation. The pose of $O^{(j)}$ in the nth image is denoted as $\Theta_n^{(j)} = [\mathbf{c}_n^{(j)}, \mathbf{v}_n^{(j)}, \mathbf{s}_n^{(j)}]$. The nine pose parameters are assumed independently distributed and the OPDM can be estimated using Parzen windows [83]

$$p\left(\Theta^{(j)}|O^{(j)}\right) = \prod_{k=1}^{9} p\left(\theta_k^{(j)}|O^{(j)}\right) = \prod_{k=1}^{9} \frac{1}{N}\sum_{n=0}^{N-1} \frac{1}{\sqrt{2\pi h_k^{(j)}}} e^{-\frac{\left(\theta_k^{(j)}-\theta_{k,n}^{(j)}\right)^2}{2h_k^{(j)2}}} \tag{5.18}$$

where $\theta_k^{(j)}$ for $k = 1, \ldots, 9$ are the nine pose parameters, $\theta_{k,n}^{(j)}$ is the pose parameter value of organ $O^{(j)}$ computed from the nth training image, $h_k^{(j)}$ is the bandwidth and is estimated using the standard deviation of the sample data $\theta_{k,n}^{(j)}$ for $n = 0, \ldots, N-1$.

The conditional probability $p(I|\Theta^{(j)}, O^{(j)})$ for the given subject image I uses PA and IP, which are computed for each organ from the training data as shown in the previous section. The transformed PA, denoted as $p(\mathbf{x}|\Theta^{(j)}, O^{(j)})$, models the organ location and represents the probability that a point x belongs to the organ $O^{(j)}$ for a given pose parameter $\Theta^{(j)}$. The IP, denoted as $p(u|O^{(j)})$, describes the probability that any voxel in $O^{(j)}$ takes an intensity value of u. It can be shown that

$$p\left(I|\Theta^{(j)}, O_j\right) = \exp\left(\sum_{m=1}^{M} h\left(u_m|\Theta^{(j)}, O^{(j)}\right)\log p\left(u_m|O^{(j)}\right)\right). \tag{5.19}$$

with $h(u_m|\Theta^{(j)}, O^{(j)})$ being the conditional histogram

$$\begin{aligned} h\left(u_m|\Theta^{(j)}, O^{(j)}\right) &= \sum_{\mathbf{x}_i \in \mathbf{V}} f(u_m, \mathbf{x}_i) p\left(\mathbf{x}_i|\Theta^{(j)}, O^{(j)}\right), \\ \text{with } f(u_m, \mathbf{x}_i) &= \begin{cases} 1, & \text{if } u(\mathbf{x}_i) = u_m \\ 0, & \text{otherwise} \end{cases}. \end{aligned} \tag{5.20}$$

The exponent in (5.19) is the negative *cross entropy* between the two probability functions $h(u|\Theta^{(j)}, O^{(j)})$ and $p(u|O^{(j)})$, and is denoted as H. Thus, the logarithm of the a posteriori probability can be written as:

$$\begin{aligned} C_{AP}\left(O^{(j)}\right) = &-H\left(h\left(u|\Theta^{(j)}, O^{(j)}\right), p\left(u|\Theta^{(j)}, O^{(j)}\right)\right) \\ &+ \sum_{k=1}^{9} \log p\left(\theta_k^{(j)}|O^{(j)}\right) \end{aligned} \tag{5.21}$$

The Minimum Volume Overlap Condition

Experiments on non-contrast CT images [76] showed that the maximization C_{AP} failed to localize the kidneys in some cases. The reason is that the kidneys are located close to neighboring organs (liver and spleen), and they have similar intensity profiles in the non-contrast images. Therefore the second term in (5.21), which comes from OPDM, was not sufficient to guarantee that the MAP converges to the correct pose in some cases. As a result, the localized kidneys overlapped with the liver and spleen.

To prevent the localized organs from overlapping with each other, we explore the inter-organ spatial relationships. For the given pose parameters $\Theta^{(j)}$ of all organs, the normalized volume overlap of organ $O^{(j)}$ with all other organs is defined as

$$C_{VO}^{(j)} = \frac{\sum_{i \neq j} \sum_{\mathbf{x} \in \mathbf{V}} \left[p\left(\mathbf{x}|\Theta^{(i)}, O^{(i)}\right) p\left(\mathbf{x}|\Theta^{(j)}, O^{(j)}\right)\right]}{\sum_{\mathbf{x} \in \mathbf{V}} p\left(\mathbf{x}|O^{(j)}\right)}, \tag{5.22}$$

The denominator in (5.22) is the total volume of $O^{(j)}$ and is computed by adding up the PA at points x across the image volume V. By incorporating inter-organ relations in our method, the localization of abdominal organs is performed dependently instead of independently. Thus, we define a new cost function by combining the minimum volume overlap term in (5.22) with the logarithm of the a posteriori probability function in (5.21),

$$C = \sum_j C_{AP}^{(j)} - \lambda \sum_j C_{VO}^{(j)}, \tag{5.23}$$

where λ is a nonnegative weighting parameter.

For each organ, the maximization of (5.23) is performed using the steepest descent method [84] in an iterative fashion. A multi-resolution strategy is adopted for efficient computation. At each iteration, the poses of the five organs are computed in sequential order: liver, spleen, left kidney, right kidney, and pancreas. This order is adopted because it was found from experiments that liver and spleen are more likely to be successfully localized because they have relatively larger sizes, so that their intermediate localization can be used to better constrain the localization of kidneys and pancreas through the minimum volume overlap term. After the estimation of organ poses, the probabilistic atlas of each organ is transformed based on the computed pose and placed in the image volume to localize the organ.

Data and Analysis

We applied the method to 17 patients' contrast-enhanced CT data. The images were collected on four types of CT scanners from three manufacturers with 1 mm slice thickness. The five organs of interest were manually segmented from all images by a medical student supervised by a radiologist to create the ground truth. The symmetric volume overlap between the estimated organs and manual segmentations was measured using the Dice coefficient. In all the experiments, the weighting parameter λ was set to 2.

To validate the method to localize five abdominal organs, the liver, spleen, left and right kidneys, and pancreas, 17 experiments were performed using a leave-one-out strategy. In each experiment, one dataset was picked as the subject image, and the remaining 16 datasets served as the training data. After localization, the estimated organ was then compared with the ground truth.

Results

An example of pose distribution is shown in Fig. 5.7 for the liver. Figure 5.8 shows the localization results on a typical data set using the minimum overlap (MO) method. For comparison, we repeated the experiments using the independent localization (IL) approach in [76] in which all the organs were independently localized without considering the inter-organ relations. The results of both approaches are presented in Table 5.2. The two methods produced similar results

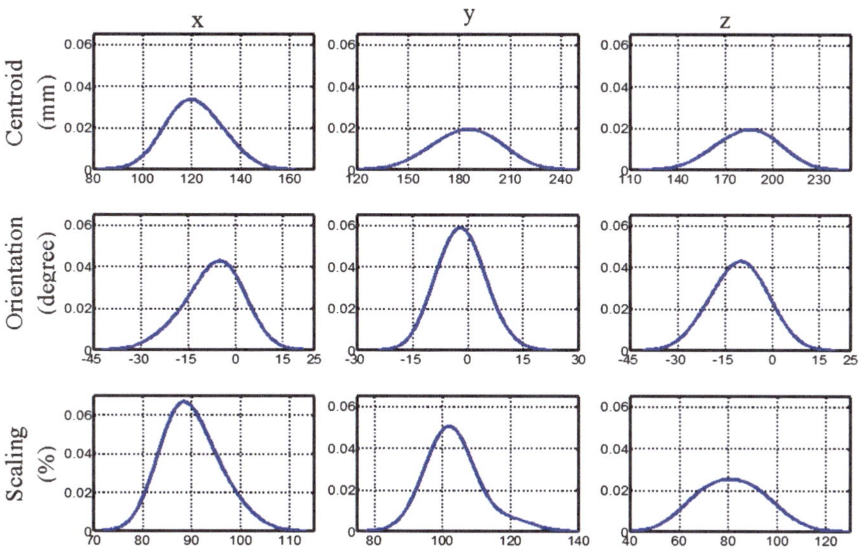

Fig. 5.7 The pose distribution functions of liver [76]. From *top* to *bottom* are the centroid, orientation, and scaling, respectively; the *x*, *y*, and *z* components are shown from *left* to *right*

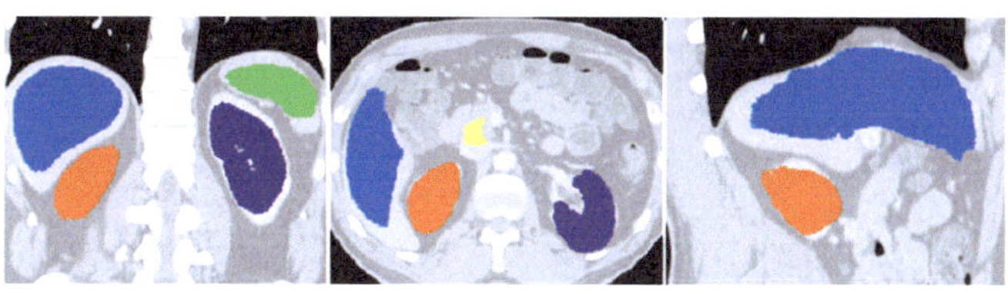

Fig. 5.8 The organ localization results, from *left* to *right*, on coronal, axial, and sagittal views of a contrast-enhanced data set [77]. The liver is shown in *blue*, the spleen in *green*, the left kidney in *purple*, the right kidney in *orange*, and the pancreas in *yellow*

Table 5.2 The average Dice coefficients between the organ localization results and manual segmentation

Method		Liver	Spleen	Left kidney	Right kidney	Pancreas
MO	Mean	0.80	0.65	0.75	0.79	0.42
	Std	0.03	0.06	0.05	0.03	0.15
IL	Mean	0.80	0.55	0.74	0.75	0.38
	Std	0.03	0.05	0.06	0.13	0.17
p-value		0.06	0.63	0.03	0.02	0.33

The p-values of the Wilcoxon sign rank test comparing the results of the minimum overlap (MO) and independent localization (IL) methods are presented

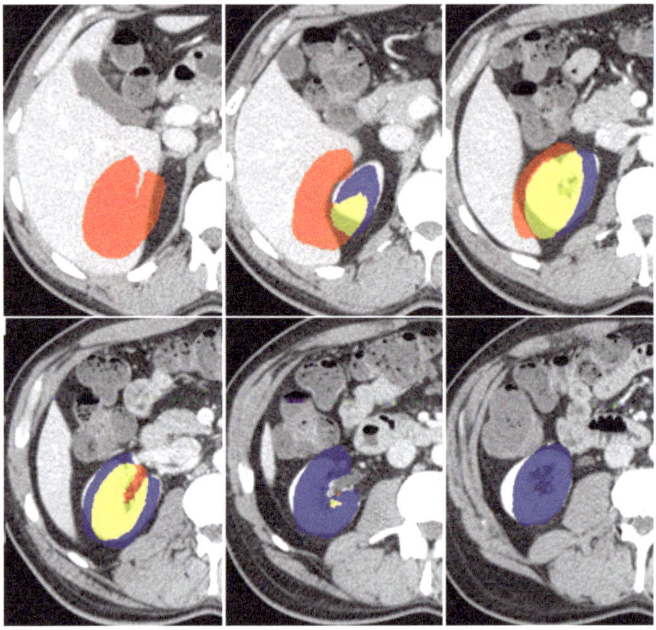

Fig. 5.9 Illustration of the localization results of the right kidney on one dataset in which the minimum overlap (MO) method succeeded and the independent localization (IL) method failed [77]. The results are shown on several slices from the 3D image volume. The results of the MO method are shown in *purple*, those of the IL method in *orange*, while the overlapping results from the two methods are presented in *yellow*

on the liver, and the MO method performed quantitatively better on all the other four organs. The non-parametric Wilcoxon sign rank test showed significant improvements for the localization of kidneys ($p < 0.05$). Qualitatively, all the five organs in all 17 experiments were successfully localized using the MO method. Using the IL approach, the right kidney was incorrectly localized on one data set where a large part of the right kidney was localized inside the liver, which resulted in a Dice coefficient of 0.24, as shown in Fig. 5.9. Note that these results do not reflect the segmentation of organs, but the enhanced localization using statistical models of data and inter-organ relationships.

Table 5.3 shows the localization error for the five abdominal organs using the MO method. The technique performed best on the left and right kidneys, which had an average location error less than 3 mm. The location error of the liver, a much larger organ with variable shape, was less than 5 mm. The pancreas, a thin and long organ with very large shape variability across subjects, had the largest localization error, especially in the y-axis.

Table 5.3 The errors (mean and standard deviation) of organ location using the minimum overlap (MO) method

Centroid (mm)		Liver	Spleen	Left kidney	Right kidney	Pancreas
x	Mean	4.77	5.30	0.83	1.22	8.72
	Std	4.96	8.72	0.61	0.98	7.66
y	Mean	3.96	5.32	1.02	1.75	7.86
	Std	3.37	3.56	0.63	1.56	14.3
z	Mean	3.17	4.22	2.69	2.36	6.62
	Std	2.18	3.04	1.60	1.77	6.47

Liver Tumor Segmentation

The purpose of this section is to change the scale of the analysis from multi-organ to organ and at even finer scale, inside the organ for the detection and segmentation of tumors. From organ detection and localization to organ segmentation and analysis and tumor detection, the combination of the techniques presented in this chapter illustrates the path toward the integrated and comprehensive analysis of abdominal radiological data via CAD. Our exemplification is done through the analysis of the liver, arguably the abdominal organ that received the highest level of interest from the medical image analysis community.

Data

Fourteen abdominal CT scans were collected from patients with prostate cancer at single/multiple time points on five different scanners with 5 mm slice thickness. Images were acquired with contrast at varying enhancement times, from early-arterial to late portal venous. Additional to the inconsistent enhancement, cases with imaging and movement artifacts were present in the database, as in the typical clinical scenario. Seventy-nine tumors larger than 10.0 mm in diameter were manually segmented in the 14 cases with liver cancer. Tumor size varied from 10.0 to 206.4 mm in the largest diameter [79].

Liver masks were obtained automatically using a method such as the one described in section "Abdominal Multi-Organ Segmentation" and [75]. Because the cases in the data exhibited artifacts and large abnormalities, a liver segmentation refinement was subsequently performed [78, 85]. The refinement was based on the robust parameterization of 3D shapes combined with an invariant shape feature to allow identifying organs (or parts of organs) from a training database that are similar to a given patient's data. This approach corrected the otherwise incomplete liver segmentations.

Graph Cuts for Tumor Segmentation

Once the liver was segmented, a graph-cut approach was applied to find the hepatic tumors. In the basic form, graph cuts [86] suffer from the shrinking bias problem, particularly for segmenting small structures, such as certain types of tumors. Graph cuts were shown to improve the segmentation of abdominal organs using training shapes [79], but tumors vary in size and shape between cases. However, liver tumors are generally round; hence, instead of using training tumor shapes, we define a roundness constraint.

Seed points for tumors were generated automatically by finding adaptive thresholds in the data. Additionally, the object seed points were also constrained to have nonzero Hessian-based shape response, as described below. Given a binary vector A where each element is associated with a voxel in the input image and each element's value is a binary label representing the object to be segmented or the background, the cost function of the graph E in our application can be written as

$$E(A) = E_{data}(A) + E_{enhance}(A) + E_{shape}(A) + E_{boundary}(A), \qquad (5.24)$$

More details on E_{data}, $E_{boundary}$, and $E_{enhance}$ can be found in section "Abdominal Multi-Organ Segmentation" of this chapter. The new term in the formulation is E_{shape}. E_{shape} is a Hessian-based shape condition to emphasize rounder tumors at multiple scales σ [87]. The eigenvalues of the Hessian ($\lambda_1 > \lambda_2 > \lambda_3$) at point p can be used to define unique shape constraints to optimize the segmentation of tumors. The following energy term was incorporated in the graph-cut definition:

$$\begin{aligned} E_{shape} &= -\ln \max_{\sigma} (w); \\ \text{with } \lambda_3 > 0; \text{and} \quad w &= e^{-(\lambda_1/\lambda_3 - 1)} \end{aligned} \qquad (5.25)$$

To account for the slight undersegmentation of tumors, a classic geodesic active contour [88] was employed to refine the segmentation.

Feature Selection and Classification

For each tumor candidate, 157 features were automatically computed to characterize the detection. They include the linear and volumetric size, roundness and elongation measures, intensity, the eigenvalues of the Hessian matrix, energy, entropy, inertia, correlation, cluster shade, cluster prominence, Haralick's correlation, inverse difference moment and statistics of these measures (see Table 5.4). Due to the large number of features used for classification, feature selection was used to retain the optimal combination of features for the separation of TP from FP detections.

Table 5.4 One hundred and fifty-seven automated tumor features were computed for the tumor candidates

3D Features	Descriptor	Explanation
Tumor volume	Size	Volumetric size
Tumor diameter	Size	Linear size
Tumor size region ratio	Shape	Ratio of the size of the object bounding box and the real size of the object
Tumor binary elongation	Shape	Ratio of the largest principal moment by the smallest principal moment
Tumor roundness	Shape	Sphericity
Tumor Hessian eigenvalues	Shape	Local extrema and stationary points
Tumor blobness measures	Shape	Roundness from the Hessian eigenvalues
Tumor intensity[a]	Enhancement	Enhancement of tumor
Edge intensity[a]	Enhancement	Enhancement of healthy parenchyma
Tumor cluster prominence[a]	Texture	Skewness/asymmetry
Edge cluster prominence[a]	Texture	Skewness/asymmetry
Tumor cluster shade[a]	Texture	Skewness/asymmetry
Edge cluster shade[a]	Texture	Skewness/asymmetry
Tumor correlation[a]	Texture	Correlation/complexity
Edge correlation[a]	Texture	Correlation/complexity
Tumor energy[a]	Texture	Uniformity
Edge energy[a]	Texture	Uniformity
Tumor entropy[a]	Texture	Randomness
Edge entropy[a]	Texture	Randomness
Tumor Haralick correlation[a]	Texture	Linear dependence between the voxels relative to each other
Edge Haralick correlation[a]	Texture	Linear dependence between the voxels relative to each other
Tumor inertia[a]	Texture	Local heterogeneity
Edge inertia[a]	Texture	Local heterogeneity
Tumor inverse difference moment[a]	Texture	Local homogeneity
Edge inverse difference moment[a]	Texture	Local homogeneity

Edge refers to the two pixel-wide band of liver tissue surrounding the tumor
For definitions of the texture features computed from the co-occurrence matrix, please refer to [89]
[a]The min, max, mean, standard deviation, variance, median, kurtosis and skewness were computed for the feature

By employing dimensionality reduction algorithms, we can extract useful information and build compact representations from the original data. We adopted the minimal-redundancy-maximal-relevance feature selection method [90]. In minimal-redundancy-maximal-relevance feature selection, the optimization criteria are affected by two factors: one is relevance between features and target classes and one is redundancy between features. Peng et al. [90] proposed a heuristic framework to minimize redundancy and maximize relevance at the same time.

Table 5.5 True Positives (TP) fraction and false positives (FP)/case are reported for the detection of hepatic tumors

Data	TP (%)	FP/case	DC (%)	JI (%)	VER (%)	ASD (mm)
79 tumors (n = 14)	100.0	2.3	74.1 ± 16.9	70.9 ± 17.7	12.4 ± 12.0	1.6 ± 1.5

Automated and manual segmentations of tumors were compared and we present *DC* Dice Coefficient, *JI* Jaccard index, *VER* volume errors, *ASD* average surface distances

Receiver operating characteristic curves for the hepatic tumor detection were generated with and without feature selection to record the effects of classification and feature selection on the reduction of false detections. The performances of the two classifiers (with and without feature selection) were compared using ROCKIT [91] to assess the statistical significance of differences between receiver operating characteristic curves and the areas under the curve (AUC).

The classification of detection into true and false positives is completed by support vector machines (SVM). SVM are a set of kernel-based supervised learning methods used for classification and regression [92] that minimize the empirical classification error and maximize the geometric margin simultaneously on a training set, which leads to a high generalization ability on the test samples. For training and testing purposes, a leave-one-patient-out strategy was employed.

Results

All the hepatic tumors were correctly identified (100 % TP) with 2.3 FP/case. FP occurred generally near the porta hepatis and coronary ligaments, where there is lack of enhancement (opacity) and high curvatures (roundness). The overlap between the manually and automatically segmented tumors was 74.1 % with a volume estimation error of 12.4 % and average surface distance of 1.6 mm. The results of the detection and segmentation of hepatic tumors are presented in Table 5.5. Figure 5.10 shows examples of tumor detection and segmentation from two patients, each with two time points.

The SVM classifier was employed after extracting 157 features for each true and false tumor candidate. Without feature selection, the AUC of the classifier was 0.62. The maximum AUC of 0.85 was achieved for a combination of eight tumor candidate features. Figure 5.11 shows the free-response receiver operating characteristic curves for tumor detection with and without feature selection. The eight selected features were a combination of statistics and texture inside and outside the tumor candidates. Namely, the selected tumor features were: the median intensity, roundness, mean λ_1, mean λ_3, and minimum value of the Haralick correlation. Additionally, the following features computed around the edge of the tumor were retained for classification: the median of the energy, kurtosis, and variance of the inverse difference moment.

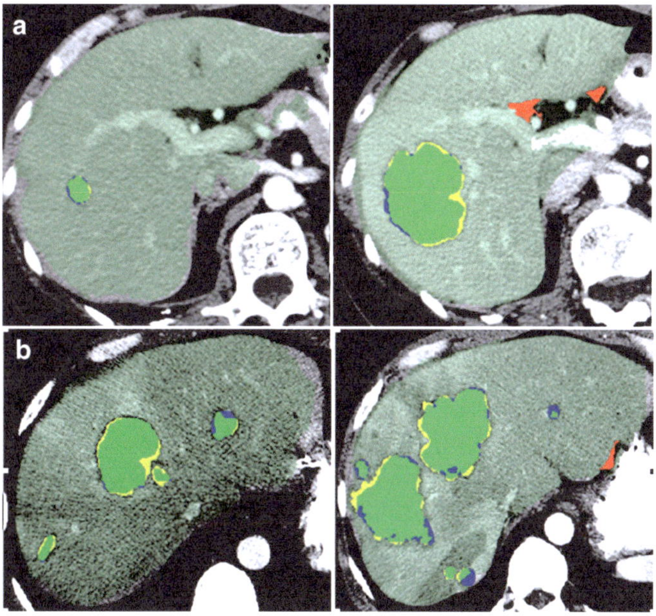

Fig. 5.10 Examples of hepatic tumor segmentation [75]: manual (*blue*), automated (*yellow*), and their overlaps in *green* overlaid on axial views of 3D CT of two patients (**a** and **b**), each at two time points (*left* and *right*). False positives from the automated segmentation are displayed in *red*. The two cases also illustrate the difference in the enhancement protocols: in (**a**) well-enhanced hepatic veins are visible at both time points; in (**b**) only the arteries are enhanced in the liver

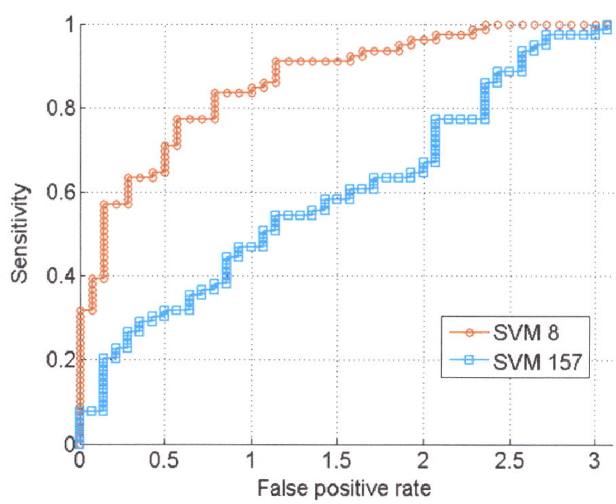

Fig. 5.11 Comparative free-response receiver operating characteristic curves using eight (SVM 8) and all 157 (SVM 157) features for classification [79]. The difference between the two classifiers was significant ($p < 0.001$)

The SVM classifier with eight features achieved a sensitivity of 100 % TP at 2.3 FP/case (or 94 % TP at 1.6 FP/case). There was a significant difference ($p < 0.001$) between the performances of the SVM classifiers with and without feature selection. Feature selection resulted in 32 % TP increase at 1.6 FP/case, as shown in Fig. 5.11.

Discussion

Medical image analysis benefits from models of anatomy and physiology. In CT-based clinical abdominal diagnosis, the concomitant analysis of multiple organs and information from contrast enhancement offer additional information to clinicians. In this chapter, we discussed our recent methods that incorporate anatomical and physiological priors into multi-organ CAD. From the localization, detection and segmentation of multiple organs in the abdomen, we also presented a technique for the detection and segmentation of tumors inside the organs (i.e., the liver) for a multi-scale comprehensive abdominal diagnosis.

Livers, spleens, and kidneys were segmented from multi-phase clinical data following the typical acquisition protocol of abdominal CT images. The cuts in the proposed 4D graph were based on globally minimizing an energy that included enhancement, location, and shape constraints. The method avoided the inclusion of heart segments in the segmentation of liver, but had the tendency to underestimate organ volumes, in particular that of the spleen. Parts of the inferior vena cava may be erroneously segmented in the mid-cephalocaudal liver region, especially when contrast enhancement is low, and represented one of the sources of error in the liver segmentation. Partial volume effects, small inter-phase registration errors and the estimation of object and background distributions may have also contributed to the undersegmentation.

For the robust initialization of segmentation and modeling techniques, we additionally presented a method for automated multi-organ localization from abdominal contrast-enhanced CT images. The algorithm found the locations, orientations, and scales of five abdominal organs (liver, spleen, pancreas, and left and right kidneys) by maximizing the a posteriori probabilities of organ poses. Additionally, the technique used a minimum volume overlap constraint to model inter-organ relations.

Once the organs were segmented (i.e., the liver) we applied a technique for tumor detection and segmentation based on graphs constrained by shape and enhancement models. This allowed to segment tumors of variable sizes with a reduced number of false positives. Additionally, we employed an extensive set of features computed for each tumor candidate (inside and outside the tumor) and demonstrated that through feature selection and classification using machine learning the number of false detections was significantly reduced. A clinical application of liver segmentation was proposed via the definition of normative values for detection hepatomegaly [93]. For examples of clinical studies of kidney tumors, please refer to [94, 95].

For a flavor of future developments, a number of notable recent advances in the field of computational anatomy in the abdomen and analysis of multi-organs should be mentioned. In [24, 96], a method for the automated analysis of organ shape variability in the abdomen was presented, based on a combination of statistical atlases, principal factor analysis, and a vector field clustering technique. The evaluation of deformation fields in [96] showed strong correlations with anatomical landmarks and known mechanical deformations in the abdomen. The automated hierarchical partitioning of organs identified relevant anatomical components that represent potentially important constraints for abdominal diagnosis and modeling and that may be used as a complement to multi-level statistical shape models. Also using hierarchical analysis, to explicitly incorporate the spatial inter-relations among abdominal organs, the method in [97] represented these inter-relations based on canonical correlation analysis in conjunction with the construction and utilization of a statistical atlas. Finally, in [98] a method for modeling abdominal organ shifts due to surgical procedures was introduced. This technique that accounts for pathology also detects the occurrence of missing organs. The resulting missing organ detection can be integrated within the multi-organ segmentation scheme to improve its accuracy for targeted diseased populations.

As the trend in multi-organ analysis shows, future work will include more organs for a holistic segmentation of radiological data. Additionally, the inclusion of data with a variety of pathologies in the abdomen and outside will allow developing segmentation techniques robust to physiological and clinical variability.

Conclusion

With the evolution of medical image analysis, more complex models of anatomy and physiology are explored to enhance the quality of CAD. Location, orientation, size, shape, and enhancement are only some of the clinical descriptors used in diagnosis and interventions. Their translation into computerized models of the human body has been beneficial for the accuracy of image analysis techniques and the intuitive clinical translation of machine-based methods. To enhance the clinical utility of CAD, multi-organ models of anatomy are particularly useful, as clinicians analyze concomitantly all the organs shown in a particular type of radiological image. Multi-organ analysis promises to support more investigative diagnosis tools for complex multi-focal multi-disease clinical scenarios.

Acknowledgments This work was supported in part by the Intramural Research Program of the National Institutes of Health, Clinical Center. The authors would like to acknowledge the contributions of (in alphabetical order) Ananda S. Chowdhury, Zhixi Li, Xiaofeng Liu, Vivek Pamulapati, John A. Pura,William J. Richbrough, Jesse K. Sandberg, Shijun Wang, Jeremy M. Watt, and Jianhua Yao.

References

1. Fritz GA, Schoellnast H, Deutschmann HA, Quehenberger F, Tillich M (2006) Multiphasic multidetector-row CT (MDCT) in detection and staging of transitional cell carcinomas of the upper urinary tract. Eur Radiol 16(6):1244–1252
2. Voci SL, Gottlieb RH, Fultz PJ, Mehta A, Parthasarathy R, Rubens DJ, Strang JG (2000) Delayed computed tomographic characterization of renal masses: preliminary experience. Abdom Imaging 25(3):317–321
3. Tsushima Y, Endo K (2000) Spleen enlargement in patients with nonalcoholic fatty liver: correlation between degree of fatty infiltration in liver and size of spleen. Dig Dis Sci 45(1):196–200
4. Ellert J, Kreel L (1980) The role of computed tomography in the initial staging and subsequent management of the lymphomas. J Comput Assist Tomogr 4(3):368–391
5. Soyer P et al (1992) Hepatic metastases from colorectal cancer: influence of hepatic volumetric analysis on surgical decision making. Radiology 184(3):695–697
6. Delingette H, Ayache N (2005) Hepatic surgery simulation. Commun ACM 48(2):31–36
7. Heimann T et al (2009) Comparison and evaluation of methods for liver segmentation from CT datasets. IEEE Trans Med Imaging 28(8):1251–1265
8. Linguraru MG, Sandberg JA, Li Z, Shah F, Summers RM (2010) Atlas-based automated segmentation of spleen and liver using adaptive enhancement estimation. Med Phys 37(2):771–783
9. Okada T, Shimada R, Hori M, Nakamoto M, Chen YW, Nakamura H, Sato Y (2008) Automatic segmentation of the liver from 3D CT images using probabilistic atlas and multilevel statistical shape model. Acad Radiol 15:1390–1403
10. Soler L, Delingette H, Malandain G, Montagnat J, Ayache N, Koehl C, Dourthe O, Malassagne B, Smith M, Mutter D, Marescaux J (2001) Fully automatic anatomical, pathological, and functional segmentation from CT scans for hepatic surgery. Comput Aided Surg 6(3):131–142
11. Song Y, Bulpitt A, Brodlie K (2009) Liver segmentation using automatically defined patient specific B-spline surface models. In: Medical Image Computing and Computer Assisted Intervention 2009 Part II, LNCS, vol 5762, pp 43–50
12. Wimmer A, Soza G, Hornegger J (2009) A generic probabilistic active shape model for organ segmentation. Med Image Comput Comput Assist Interv 12(Pt 2):26–33
13. Ali AM, Farag AA, El-Baz AS (2007) Graph cuts for kidney segmentation with prior shape constraints. In: Proceedings of Medical Image Computing and Computer Assisted Intervention 2007, Part I, LNCS, vol 4791, pp 384–392
14. Shim H, Chang S, Tao C, Wang JH, Kaya D, Bae KT (2009) Semiautomated segmentation of kidney from high-resolution multidetector computed tomography images using a graph-cuts technique. J Comput Assist Tomogr 33(6):893–901
15. So RWK, Chung AC (2009) Multi-level non-rigid image registration using graph-cuts. In: IEEE International conference on acoustics, speech and signal processing, pp 397–400
16. Danelson KA, Stitzel JD (2008) Volumetric splenic injury measurement in CT scans for comparison with injury score. Biomed Sci Instrum 44:159–164
17. Linguraru MG, Sandberg JK, Li Z, Pura JA, Summers RM (2009) Atlas-based automated segmentation of spleen and liver using adaptive enhancement estimation. In: Yang GZ et al (eds) Medical Image Computing and Computer-Assisted Intervention – MICCAI 2009. Lecture notes in computer science, vol 5762. Springer, New York, pp 1001–1008
18. Shimizu A, Kimoto T, Kobatake H, Nawano S, Shinozaki K (2010) Automated pancreas segmentation from three-dimensional contrast-enhanced computed tomography. Int J Comput Assist Radiol Surg 5:85–98
19. Linguraru MG, Summers RM (2008) Multi-organ segmentation in 4D contrast-enhanced abdominal CT. In: IEEE symposium on biomedical imaging, pp 45–48

20. Okada T, Yokota K, Hori M, Nakamoto M, Nakamura H, Sato Y (2008) Construction of hierarchical multi-organ statistical atlases and their application to multi-organ segmentation from CT images. In: Medical Image Computing and Computer Assisted Intervention 2008, Part I, LNCS, vol 5241, pp 502–509
21. Park H, Bland PH, Meyer CR (2003) Construction of an abdominal probabilistic atlas and its application in segmentation. IEEE Trans Med Imaging 22(4):483–492
22. Seifert S, Barbu A, Zhou K, Liu D, Feulner J, Huber M, Suehling M, Cavallaro A, Comaniciu D (2009) Hierarchical parsing and semantic navigation of full body CT data. In: Proceedings of the SPIE Medical Imaging, vol 7259, pp 725902–725908
23. Shimizu A, Ohno R, Ikegami T, Kobatake H, Nawano S, Smutek D (2007) Segmentation of multiple organs in non-contrast 3D abdominal CT images. Int J Comput Assist Radiol Surg 2:135–142
24. Reyes M, Gonzalez Ballester MA, Li Z, Kozic N, Chin S, Summers RM, Linguraru MG (2009) Anatomical variability of organs via principal factor analysis from the construction of an abdominal probabilistic atlas. In: IEEE international symposium on biomedical imaging (ISBI), pp 682–685
25. Zhou Y, Bai J (2007) Multiple abdominal organ segmentation: an atlas-based fuzzy connectedness approach. IEEE Trans Inf Technol Biomed 11(3):348–352
26. Bae E, Tai XC (2009) Efficient Global minimization for the multi-phase Chan-Vese model of image segmentation. In: Energy minimization methods in computer vision and pattern recognition. Lecture notes in computer science, vol 5681, pp 28–41
27. El-Zehiry N, Grady L (2011) Discrete optimization of the multi-phase piecewise constant Mumford-Shah functional. In: Energy minimization methods in computer vision and pattern recognition. Lecture notes in computer science, vol 6819, pp 233–246
28. Montillo A, Shotton J, Winn J, Iglesias JE, Metaxas D, Criminisi A (2011) Entangled decision forests and their application for semantic segmentation of CT images. In: Information processing in medical imaging. Lecture notes in computer science, vol 6801, pp 184–196
29. Zhan Y, Zhou XS, Peng Z, Krishnan A (2008) Active scheduling of organ detection and segmentation in whole-body medical images. Med Image Comput Comput Assist Interv 11 (Pt 1):313–321
30. Hu X, Shimizu A, Kobatake H, Nawano S (2004) Independent analysis of four-phase abdominal CT images. In: Medical Image Computing and Computer Assisted Intervention 2004, LNCS, vol 3217, pp 916–924
31. Sadananthan SA, Zheng W, Chee MW, Zagorodnov V (2010) Skull stripping using graph cuts. Neuroimage 49(1):225–239
32. Sakashita M, Kitasaka T, Mori K, Suenaga Y, Nawano S (2007) A method for extracting multi-organ from four-phase contrasted CT images based on CT value distribution estimation using EM-algorithm. In: Proceedings of SPIE Medical Imaging, vol 6509, pp 1C1–1C12
33. Yao J, Summers RM (2009) Statistical location model for abdominal organ localization. Medical Image Computing and Computer Assisted Intervention 2009, Part II, LNCS, vol 5762, pp 9–17
34. Yao C et al (2006) Simultaneous location detection of multi-organ by atlas-guided eigen-organ method in volumetric medical images. Int J Comput Assist Radiol Surg 1:42–45
35. Pauly O, Glocker B, Criminisi A, Mateus D, Möller AM, Nekolla S, Navab N (2011) Fast multiple organ detection and localization in whole-body MR dixon sequences. Med Image Comput Comput Assist Interv 14(Pt 3):239–247
36. Wang H, Stount DB, Chatziioannou AF (2012) Estimation of mouse organ locations through registration of a statistical mouse atlas with micro-CT images. IEEE Trans Med Imaging 31(1):88–102
37. American Cancer Society (2011) Cancer facts and figures 2011. American Cancer Society, Atlanta
38. Lewis RL (2007) Liver and biliary tract tumors. In: Goldman L, Ausiello D (eds) Cecil medicine, 23rd edn. Saunders Elsevier, Philadelphia (Chapter 206)

39. Beck A, Aurich V (2007) HepaTux – a semiautomatic liver segmentation system. In: Medical Image Computing and Computer Assisted Intervention workshop on 3D segmentation in the clinic: a grand challenge, pp 225–233
40. Dawant BM et al (2007) Semi-automatic segmentation of the liver and its evaluation on the MICCAI 2007 grand challenge data set. In: Medical Image Computing and Computer Assisted Intervention workshop on 3D segmentation in the clinic: a grand challenge, pp 215–221
41. Kainmuller D, Lange T, Lamecker H (2007) Shape constrained automatic segmentation of the liver based on a heuristic intensity model. In: Medical Image Computing and Computer Assisted Intervention workshop on 3D segmentation in the clinic: a grand challenge, pp 109–116
42. Rusko L et al (2007) Fully automatic liver segmentation for contrast-enhanced CT images. In: Medical Image Computing and Computer Assisted Intervention workshop on 3D segmentation in the clinic: a grand challenge, pp 143–150
43. Schmidt G et al (2007) Cognition network technology for a fully automated 3D segmentation of the liver. In: Medical Image Computing and Computer Assisted Intervention workshop on 3D segmentation in the clinic: a grand challenge, pp 125–133
44. Deng X, Du G (2008) Editorial: 3D segmentation in the clinic: a grand challenge II – liver tumor segmentation. In: Medical Image Computing and Computer Assisted Intervention workshop on 3D segmentation in the clinic: a grand challenge II
45. Stawiaski J, Decenciere E, Bidault F (2008) Interactive liver tumor segmentation using graph-cuts and watershed. In: Medical Image Computing and Computer Assisted Intervention workshop on 3D segmentation in the clinic: a grand challenge II
46. Moltz J, Bornemann L, Dicken V, Peitgen H (2008) Segmentation of liver metastases in CT scans by adaptive thresholding and morphological processing. In: Medical Image Computing and Computer Assisted Intervention workshop on 3D segmentation in the clinic: a grand challenge II
47. Zhou J et al (2008) Semi-automatic segmentation of 3D liver tumors from CT scans using voxel classification and propagational learning. In: Medical Image Computing and Computer Assisted Intervention workshop on 3D segmentation in the clinic: a grand challenge II
48. Smeets D, Stijnen B, Loeckx D, Dobbelaer B, Suetens P (2008) Segmentation of liver metastases using a level set method with spiral-scanning technique and supervised fuzzy pixel classification. In: Medical Image Computing and Computer Assisted Intervention workshop on 3D segmentation in the clinic: a grand challenge II
49. Schmidt G, Binnig G, Kietzmann M, Kim J (2008) Cognition network technology for a fully automated 3D segmentation of liver tumors. In: Medical Image Computing and Computer Assisted Intervention workshop on 3D segmentation in the clinic: a grand challenge II
50. Shimizu A et al (2008) Ensemble segmentation using AdaBoost with application to liver lesion extraction from a CT volume. In: Medical Image Computing and Computer Assisted Intervention workshop on 3D segmentation in the clinic: a grand challenge II
51. Gonsalves CF et al (2011) Radioembolization as salvage therapy for hepatic metastasis of uveal melanoma: a single-institution experience. Am J Roentgenol 196(2):468–473
52. Pamulapati V, Venkatesan A, Wood BJ, Linguraru MG (2012) Liver segmental anatomy and analysis from vessel and tumor segmentation via optimized graph cuts. In: Yoshida H, Sakas G, Linguraru MG (eds) MICCAI 2011 workshop on abdominal imaging – computational and clinical applications. Lecture notes in computer science, vol 7029. Springer, New York, pp 189–197
53. Shevchenko N et al (2010) MiMed liver: a planning system for liver surgery. In: Proceedings of the IEEE engineering in medicine and biology society, pp 1882–1885
54. Peterhans A et al (2011) A navigation system for open liver surgery: design, workflow and first clinical applications. Int J Med Robotics Comput Assist Surg 7(1):7–16
55. Boykov Y, Jolly MP (2001) Interactive graph cuts for optimal boundary and region segmentation of objects in N-D images. In: International conference on computer vision, vol I, pp 105–112

56. Ben Ayed I, Punithakumar K, Li S, Islam A, Chong J (2009) Left ventricle segmentation via graph cut distribution matching. Med Image Comput Comput Assist Interv 12(Pt 2):901–909
57. Chen JH, Shapiro LG (2008) Medical image segmentation via min S-T cuts with sides constraints. In: International conference on pattern recognition, pp 1–4
58. Lin X, Cowan B, Young A (2005) Model-based graph cut method for segmentation of the left ventricle. In: Proceedings of the IEEE engineering in medicine and biology society, vol 3, pp 3059–3062
59. Bauer C, Pock T, Sorantin E, Bischof H, Beichel R (2010) Segmentation of interwoven 3D tubular tree structures utilizing shape priors and graph cuts. Med Image Anal 14(2):172–184
60. Esneault S, Lafon C, Dillenseger JL (2010) Liver vessels segmentation using a hybrid geometrical moments/graph cuts method. IEEE Trans Biomed Eng 57(2):276–283
61. Freiman M, Kronman A, Esses SJ, Joskowicz L, Sosna J (2010) Non-parametric iterative model constraint graph min-cut for automatic kidney segmentation. In: Med Image Comput Comput Assist Interv, LNCS, vol 6363, pp 73–80
62. Shimizu A, Nakagomi K, Narihira T, Kobatake H, Nawano S, Shinozaki K, Ishizu K, Togashi K (2010) Automated segmentation of 3D CT images based on statistical atlas and graph cuts. In: Med Image Comput Comput Assist Interv workshop on Medical Computer Vision, pp 129–138
63. García-Lorenzo D, Lecoeur J, Arnold DL, Collins DL, Barillot C (2009) Multiple sclerosis lesion segmentation using an automatic multimodal graph cuts. Med Image Comput Comput Assist Interv 12(Pt 2):584–591
64. van der Lijn F, den Heijer T, Breteler MM, Niessen WJ (2008) Hippocampus segmentation in MR images using atlas registration, voxel classification, and graph cuts. Neuroimage 43(4):708–720
65. Lötjönen JM, Wolz R, Koikkalainen JR, Thurfjell L, Waldemar G, Soininen H, Rueckert D (2010) Fast and robust multi-atlas segmentation of brain magnetic resonance images. Neuroimage 49(3):2352–2365
66. Wels M, Carneiro G, Aplas A, Huber M, Hornegger J, Comaniciu D (2008) A discriminative model-constrained graph cuts approach to fully automated pediatric brain tumor segmentation in 3-D MRI. Med Image Comput Comput Assist Interv 11(Pt 1):67–75
67. Zheng Y, Baloch S, Englande S, Schnall MD, Shen S (2007) Segmentation and classification of breast tumor using dynamic contrast-enhanced MR images. In: Med Image Comput Comput Assist Interv 2007, Part II, LNCS, vol 4792, pp 393–401
68. Liu L, Raber D et al (2008) Interactive separation of segmented bones in CT volumes using graph cut. In: Proceedings of Med Image Comput Comput Assist Interv 2008, Part I, LNCS, vol 5241, pp 296–304
69. Seabra JC, Pedro LM, Fernandes JF, Sanches JM (2009) A 3-D ultrasound-based framework to characterize the echo morphology of carotid plaques. IEEE Trans Biomed Eng 56(5): 1442–1453
70. Al-Kofahi Y, Lassoued W, Lee W, Roysam B (2009) Improved automatic detection and segmentation of cell nuclei in histopathology images. IEEE Trans Biomed Eng 57(4): 841–852
71. Deleus F, Van Hulle MM (2009) A connectivity-based method for defining regions-of-interest in fMRI data. IEEE Trans Image Process 18(8):1760–1771
72. Gramfort A, Keriven R, Clerc M (2010) Graph-based variability estimation in single-trial event-related neural responses. IEEE Trans Biomed Eng 57(5):1051–1061
73. Grady L, Jolly MP (2008) Weights and topology: a study of the effects of graph construction on 3D image segmentation. In: Med Image Comput Comput Assist Interv 2008, Part I, LNCS, vol 5241, pp 153–161
74. Linguraru MG, Pura JA, Chowdhury A, Summers RM (2010) Multi-organ segmentation from multi-phase abdominal CT via 4D graphs using enhancement, shape and location optimization. In: Jiang T et al (eds) Medical Image Computing and Computer-Assisted Intervention – MICCAI 2010. Lecture notes in computer science, vol 6363. Springer, New York, pp 89–96

75. Linguraru MG, Pura JA, Pamulapati V, Summers RM (2012) Statistical 4D graphs for multi-organ segmentation from multi-phase abdominal CT. Med Image Anal 16(4):904–914
76. Liu X, Linguraru MG, Yao J, Summers RM (2010) Organ pose distribution model and an MAP framework for automated abdominal multi-organ localization. In: Liao H et al (eds) Medical imaging and augmented reality – MIAR 2010. Lecture notes in computer science, vol 6326. Springer, New York, pp 393–402
77. Liu X, Linguraru MG, Yao J, Summers RM (2011) Abdominal multi-organ localization on contrast-enhanced ct based on maximum a posteriori probability and minimum volume overlap. In: IEEE international symposium on biomedical imaging (ISBI), pp 2083–1086
78. Linguraru MG, Richbourg WJ, Watt JM, Pamulapati V, Summers RM (2012) Liver and tumor segmentation and analysis from CT of diseased patients via a generic affine invariant shape parameterization and graph cuts. In: Yoshida H, Sakas G, Linguraru MG (eds) MICCAI 2011 workshop on abdominal imaging – computational and clinical applications. Lecture notes in computer science, vol 7029. Springer, New York, pp 198–206
79. Linguraru MG, Richbourg WJ, Pamulapati V, Wang S, Summers RM (2012) Robust automated detection, segmentation and classification of hepatic tumors from CT Data. In: SPIE medical imaging, vol 8317, 83170J-1-8
80. Studholme C, Hill DLG, Hawkes DJ (1999) An overlap invariant entropy measure of 3D medical image alignment. Pattern Recognit 32(1):71–86
81. Perona P, Malik J (1990) Scale-space and edge detection using anisotropic diffusion. IEEE Trans Pattern Anal Mach Intell 12:629–639
82. Thirion JP (1998) Image matching as a diffusion process: an analogy with Maxwell's demons. Med Image Anal 2(3):243–260
83. Parzen E (1962) On estimation of a probability density function and mode. Ann Math Stat 33:1065–1076
84. Burden RL, Faires JD (1993) Numerical analysis, 5th edn. PWS-Kent Publishing Company, Boston
85. Watt J, Linguraru MG, Summers RM (2011) Affine invariant shape parameterization to assess local 3D shape in abdominal organs. In: SPIE medical imaging, vol 7965, 79650F
86. Boykov Y, Kolmogorov V (2003) Computing geodesics and minimal surfaces via graph cuts. In: International conference on computer vision, pp 26–33
87. Sato Y et al (1997) 3D multi-scale line filter for segmentation and visualization of curvilinear structures in medical images. Lecture notes in computer science, vol 1205, pp 213–222
88. Caselles V, Kimmel R, Sapiro G (1997) Geodesic active contours. Int J Comput Vis 22(1):61–97
89. Haralick RM, Shanmugam K, Dinstein I (1973) Textural features for image classification. IEEE Trans Syst Man Cybern 3(6):610–621
90. Peng HC, Long FH, Ding C (2005) Feature selection based on mutual information: criteria of max-dependency, max-relevance, and min-redundancy. IEEE Trans Pattern Anal Mach Intell 27:1226–1238
91. Metz CE, Herman BA, Roe CA (1998) Statistical comparison of two ROC curve estimates obtained from partially-paired datasets. Med Decis Making 18:110–121
92. Burges CJC (1998) A tutorial on support vector machines for pattern recognition. Data Min Knowl Discov 2:121–167
93. Linguraru MG, Sandberg JK, Jones E, Petrick N, Summers RM (2012) Assessing hepatomegaly: automated volumetric analysis of the liver. Acad Radiol 19(5):588–598
94. Linguraru MG, Yao J, Gautam R, Peterson J, Li Z, Linehan WM, Summers RM (2009) Renal tumor quantification and classification in contrast-enhanced abdominal CT. Pattern Recognit 42(6):1149–1161 (special issue on cancer detection, Elsevier)
95. Linguraru MG, Wang S, Shah F, Gautam R, Peterson J, Linehan WM, Summers RM (2011) Automated noninvasive classification of renal cancer on multi-phase CT. Med Phys 38(10):5738–5746

96. Reyes M, Gonzalez Ballester MA, Kozic N, Sandberg JK, Summers RM, Linguraru MG (2010) Hierarchical patch generation for multi-level statistical shape analysis by principal factor analysis decomposition. In: SPIE Medical Imaging, vol 7626, p 762617
97. Okada T, Linguraru MG, Yoshida Y, Hori M, Summers RM, Chen YW, Tomiyama N, Sato Y (2012) Prediction-based statistical atlas and its application to abdominal multi-organ segmentation in CT Images. In: Yoshida H, Sakas G, Linguraru MG (eds) MICCAI 2011 workshop on abdominal imaging – computational and clinical applications. Lecture notes in computer science, vol 7029. Springer, New York, pp 173–180
98. Suzuki M, Linguraru MG, Summers RM, Okada K (2012) Analyses of missing organs in abdominal multi-organ segmentation. In: Yoshida H, Sakasm G, Linguraru MG (eds) MICCAI 2011 workshop on abdominal imaging – computational and clinical applications. Lecture notes in computer science, vol 7029. Springer, New York, pp 256–263

Chapter 6
Liver Volumetry in MRI by Using Fast Marching Algorithm Coupled with 3D Geodesic Active Contour Segmentation

Hieu Trung Huynh, Ibrahim Karademir, Aytekin Oto, and Kenji Suzuki

Abstract In this chapter, we present an accurate automated 3D liver segmentation scheme for measuring liver volumes in MR images. Our scheme consisted of five steps. First, an anisotropic diffusion smoothing filter was applied to T1-weighted MR images of the liver in the portal-venous phase to reduce noise while preserving the liver boundaries. An edge enhancer and a nonlinear gray-scale converter were applied to enhance the liver boundary. This boundary-enhanced image was used as a speed function for a 3D fast marching algorithm to generate an initial surface that roughly approximated the liver shape. A 3D geodesic active contour segmentation algorithm refined the initial surface so as to more precisely determine the liver boundary. The liver volume was calculated based on the refined liver surface. The MR liver volumetry based on our automated scheme agreed excellently with "gold-standard" manual volumetry (intra-class correlation coefficient was 0.98) and required substantially less completion time (our processing time of 1 vs. 24 min/case in manual segmentation).

Introduction

Medical and surgical advancements have brought the global success of liver transplantation with the increasing survival rates after transplantation in the past decades [1–3]. One of the important assessments contributing to the success of a

H.T. Huynh (✉)
Department of Radiology, The University of Chicago, Chicago, IL, USA

The Industrial University of Ho Chi Minh City, 12 Nguyen Van Bao, Go Vap District, Ho Chi Minh City, Vietnam
e-mail: hthieu@ieee.org

I. Karademir • A. Oto • K. Suzuki
Department of Radiology, The University of Chicago, Chicago, IL, USA
e-mail: k-suzuki@aoi.bsd.uchicago.edu

K. Suzuki (ed.), *Computational Intelligence in Biomedical Imaging*,
DOI 10.1007/978-1-4614-7245-2_6,

transplantation procedure is the estimation for total and segmental liver volumes. It is a major factor to predict the safe outcome for both donor and recipient. A minimum of 40 % of the standard liver mass is required by recipient while 30–40 % of the original volume is remained for donor to survive [4]. Hence, an accurate estimation of liver volumes is necessary for planning liver transplantation [5, 6]. Noninvasive measurement methods have been revealed by the advanced imaging technologies such as CT and MRI. Manual tracing of the liver on CT images is a current gold-standard method. Although the manual tracing method can obtain accurate results, it is subjective, tedious, and time-consuming. It takes 20–48 min to obtain the liver volume for one patient [7, 8]. In addition, the relatively large intraobserver and interobserver variations still occur in the manual method. To address this issue, the automated liver segmentation has been developed with image analysis techniques, and it has become an important research topic.

Several approaches to computerized liver segmentation on CT images have been published, including image-processing techniques such as thresholding, histogram analysis, morphological operations, and their combinations [9, 10]. A comparison between the semiautomatic liver volumetry and manual method in the living liver donors was presented by Hermoye et al. [11]. An automated scheme based on the combination of thresholding, feature analysis, and region growing was proposed by Nakayama et al. [8]. In comparison with manual tracing, it achieved a correlation coefficient of 0.883. Okada et al. [12] developed an automated scheme based on a probabilistic atlas and a statistical shape model, its performance was evaluated with eight cases. Selver et al. [13] developed a three-stage automated liver segmentation scheme consisting of preprocessing for excluding neighboring structures, k-means clustering, multilayer perceptron for classification, and postprocessing for removing mis-segmented objects and smoothing liver contours. The scheme was evaluated on 20 cases. An iterative graph-cut active shape model was developed by Chen and Bagci [14]. Their scheme combined the statistical shape information embodied in the active shape model with the globally optimal delineation capacity of the graph-cut method. Suzuki et al. [7, 15] developed a computer-aided liver volumetry scheme by means of geodesic active contour segmentation coupled with level set algorithms. They compared their automated scheme with manual segmentation and commercially available interactive software. Their scheme achieved the performance comparable to manual segmentation, while reducing the time required for volumetry by a factor of approximately 70.

In comparison with CT-based schemes, there are fewer publications for an automated liver segmentation scheme on MR images in spite of no risk for ionizing radiation, probably because it is believed that MR liver volumetry has more variations and more difficult than CT. Karlo et al. [16] compared the CT- and MRI-based volumetry of the resected liver specimens with intraoperative volume and weight measurements to calculate conversion factors. A semiautomated dual-space clustering segmentation method was proposed by Farraher et al. [17]. Their semiautomated method required manual drawing of a small region-of-interest (ROI) on the liver first; and then it iteratively evaluated temporal liver segmentations with the repeated adjustment of parameters to obtain the final liver segmentation result. Rusko and Bekes [18] proposed a partitioned probabilistic model to represent the liver. In this model, the liver was partitioned into multiple regions, and the different intensity statistical models were applied to these regions. The scheme was tested on eight cases. Gloger et al. [19] developed a three-step segmentation method based on a region-growing approach, linear discriminant analysis, and probability maps. Their method was evaluated with 20 normal cases and 10 fat cases. It achieved a true-positive volume error (TPVE) of 8.3 % with an average execution time of 11.2 min for each normal case, and a TPVE of 11.8 % with an average execution time of 15.4 min for each fat case.

Although the above studies showed a promise, there is still room for developing the computerized liver segmentation in MRI to make it a routine clinical use. In this chapter, we present an automated liver segmentation scheme in MRI based on geodesic active contour model and fast marching algorithm. The performance of our scheme was evaluated on 23 cases, and the comparison between the computerized volumetry and gold-standard manual volumetry was performed.

Materials and Methods

Liver MRI Datasets

In this study, 23 patients were scanned in the supine position with a 1.5T MRI scanners (Signa HDx/HDxt, GE Medical Systems, Milwaukee, WI; and Achieva, Philips Medical Systems, Cleveland, OH) at the University of Chicago Medical Center. Intravenous gadolinium contrast agent (8–20 mL; mean: 15.3 ± 4.2) was administrated. The post-contrast MRIs were obtained by using the T1-weighted liver acquisition with volume acceleration (LAVA) or T1-weighted high-resolution isotropic volume examination (THRIVE) sequence. The flip angle of 10° was used in context with TR and TE ranged from 3.48 to 3.92 ms and from 1.64 to 1.84 ms, respectively. The scanning parameters included collimation of 5 mm (for the GE system) or 4 mm (for the Philips system) and reconstruction intervals of 2.5 mm (for the GE system) or 2 mm (for the Philips system). Each MR slice had the matrix size of 256×256 pixels with an in-plane pixel size ranged from 1.17 to 1.72 mm. The 23 cases in our database had liver diseases.

The manual contours were traced carefully by a broad-certificated abdominal radiologist on each slice containing the liver. The number of slices in each case ranged from 88 to 120 (average: 97.9). The liver volume was calculated by multiplying the areas of the manually traced regions in each slice by the reconstruction interval. Note that the collimation was different from the reconstruction interval and that consecutive slices overlapped. The total liver volume of each case was obtained from the summation of volumes in all slices. We also recorded the time required for the completion of the manual contour tracing. The performance of our computerized liver extraction scheme was evaluated by using manual liver volumes as the "gold standard."

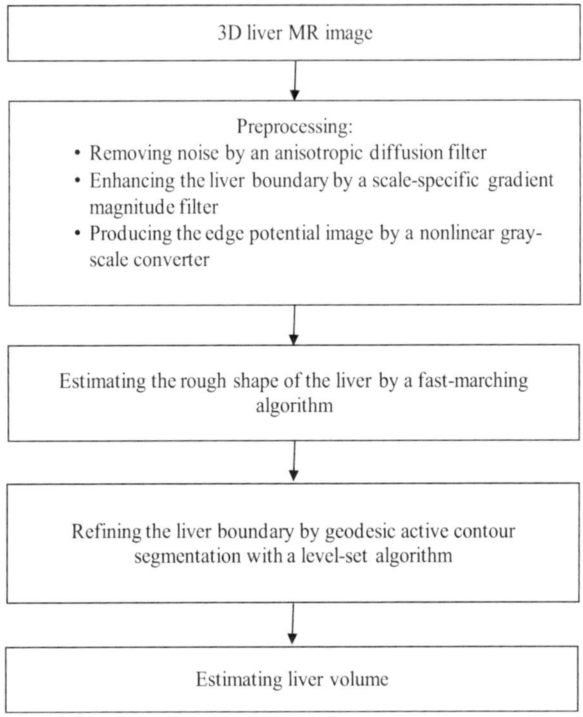

Fig. 6.1 Overview of our computerized MR liver volumetry scheme

Computer-Based Measurement Scheme for MR Liver Volumes

A computerized scheme employing level set algorithms coupled with geodesic active contour segmentation was proposed by our group for CT liver extraction. In this chapter, we present a scheme for the automated liver segmentation on MR images based on the knowledge and techniques acquired in the development of our CT liver extraction scheme. Our MR liver extraction scheme applied to the portal-venous-phase images in T1-weighted (T1w) sequences consists of five steps, as shown in Fig. 6.1. First, a 3D MR volume $I(x,y,z)$ consisting of portal-venous-phase images must be processed to reduce noise and enhance liver structures. This was accomplished by using an anisotropic diffusion algorithm (which is also called nonuniform or variable conductance diffusion proposed by Perona and Malik [20]). The algorithm based on the modified curvature diffusion equation is given by

$$I_N = \frac{\partial I}{\partial t} = |\nabla I| \nabla \cdot c(|\nabla I|) \frac{\nabla I}{|\nabla I|}, \tag{6.1}$$

where c(·) is a fuzzy cutoff function that reduces conductance at areas of large $|\nabla I|$. It can be any of a number of functions. The literature suggested

$$c(\nabla I) = e^{-\frac{|\nabla I|^2}{2\kappa^2}} \tag{6.2}$$

to be effective. Note that this term introduces a free parameter κ, the diffusion coefficient, which controls the sensitivity of edge contrast. The anisotropic diffusion algorithm smoothes noise in the image while preserving the major liver structures such as major vessels and the liver boundaries. The noise-reduced image was then passed through a Gaussian gradient magnitude filter to enhance the boundaries. This filter is given by

$$I_G = I_N * \frac{1}{(2\pi)^{1/2}\sigma} \exp\left(-\frac{x^2 + y^2 + z^2}{2\sigma^2}\right), \tag{6.3}$$

and

$$I_M = |I_G| \sqrt{\left(\frac{\partial I_G}{\partial x}\right)^2 + \left(\frac{\partial I_G}{\partial y}\right)^2 + \left(\frac{\partial I_G}{\partial z}\right)^2}, \tag{6.4}$$

where * denotes a convolution operator, σ is the standard deviation of the Gaussian filter controlling the scale of the edges to be enhanced. It was set to 0.5 in our scheme. The enhanced image was used to produce the edge potential image from the gradient magnitude image by using a sigmoid function defined by

$$f(x) = \frac{1}{1 + e^{-(x-\beta)/\alpha}}, \tag{6.5}$$

where α and β are parameters specifying the range and center, respectively, of intensity to be enhanced. They were set to -2.5 and 8.0 in our scheme. The normalized output image of the sigmoid gray-scale converter was used as a speed function for level set segmentation and fast marching algorithms.

In the following step, the shape of the liver was estimated roughly by a fast marching algorithm [21, 22]. This algorithm was initially proposed as a fast numerical solution of the Eikonal equation:

$$|\nabla T|F = 1, \tag{6.6}$$

where F is a speed function and T is an arrival time function. The algorithm requires five to eight initial seed points. From the initial location ($T = 0$), the algorithm propagates the information in one way from the smaller values of T to larger values based on the first order scheme. This algorithm consists of two main processes. First, all grid points generated from the entire region were categorized into three categories: seed points corresponding to the initial location were categorized into *Known*; the neighbors of *Known* points were categorized into *Trial* with the computed arrival time; and all other points were categorized into *Far* that the

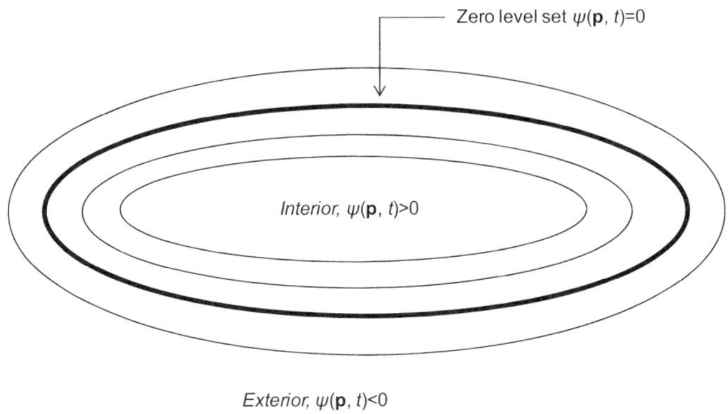

Fig. 6.2 Concept of level set method

arrival time was set to infinity. An iterative process served points in the *Trial* and *Far* list. The *Trial* point **p** with the smallest T value was chosen and moved to the *Known*. The arrival time of neighbors of **p** was recomputed based on the first order scheme, and the *Far* points that are neighbors of **p** were moved to the *Trial*. This iterative process was terminated when the maximum number of iterations was reached. The salient point of this algorithm is to use a heap data structure that can locate points with the smallest T value rapidly. The output of the fast marching algorithm is a time-crossing map indicating the time traveling to each point. It forms a rough shape of the liver in MR images.

A 3D geodesic active contour algorithm [23] was employed to refine the initial surface determined by the time-crossing map in order to determine the liver boundaries more precisely. This algorithm is based on the relation between active contours and the computation of geodesic or minimal distance curves, which allows boundary detection with large variations of gradients, including gaps. Let $\psi(\mathbf{p}, t)$ be a level set function with the initial surface corresponding to $\psi(\mathbf{p}, t) = 0$ (Fig. 6.2). This level set function is then evolved to fit the form of liver following the partial differential equation:

$$\frac{d\psi}{dt} = -\alpha \mathbf{A}(\mathbf{p}) \cdot \nabla\psi - \beta F(\mathbf{p})|\nabla\psi| + \gamma Z(\mathbf{p})\kappa|\nabla\psi|, \tag{6.7}$$

where $\mathbf{A}(\cdot)$ is an advection vector function, $F(\cdot)$ is a propagation (or expansion) function, and $Z(\cdot)$ is a spatial modifier function for the mean curvature κ. The scalar constants α, β, and γ allow trading off among three terms: advection, propagation, and curvature. The algorithm requires an initial zero level set containing an initial surface that roughly approximates the liver boundaries. The initial surface was propagated with speed and direction (outwards, inwards) controlled by the propagation function. The spatial modifier term controls the smoothness of the surface where regions of high curvature are smoothed out. The level set evolution was terminated when the convergence criterion or the maximum number of iterations

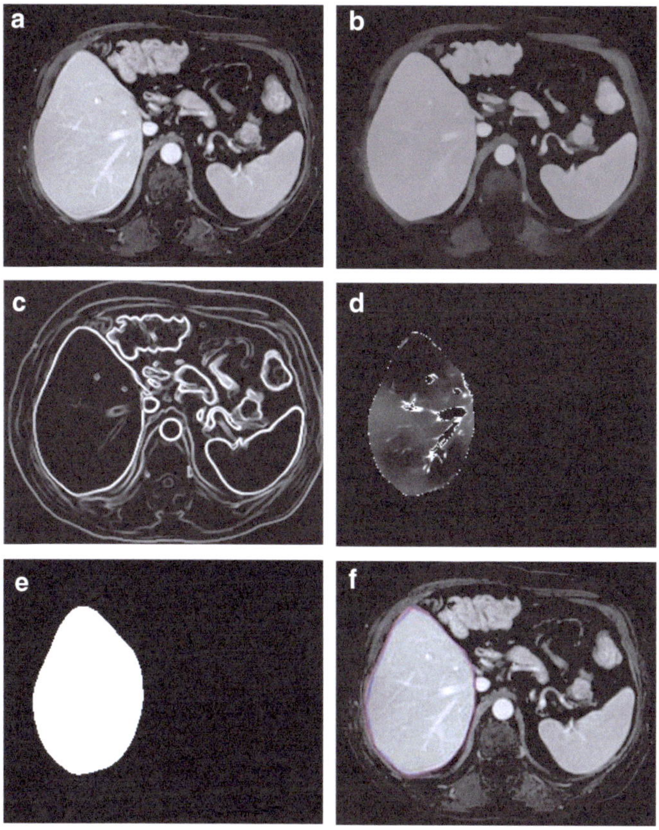

Fig. 6.3 Examples of the resulting images at each step in our automated volumetry scheme. (**a**) Original axial MR image of the liver. (**b**) 3D anisotropic diffusion noise reduction. (**c**) 3D gradient magnitude filter. (**d**) 3D fast marching algorithm. *Time-crossing map* indicates the traveling time to each voxel. The majority of vessels inside the liver are excluded at this stage. (**e**) 3D geodesic active contour segmentation. (**f**) Corresponding computer-based liver segmentation (*red contour*) and "gold-standard" manual liver segmentation (*blue contour*)

was reached. The convergence criterion was defined in terms of the root mean squared (RMS) change in the level set function. The evolution was considered to be converged if the RMS change is below a predefined threshold. The liver regions extracted by the geodesic active contour algorithm were used to calculate the liver volume. The intermediate results of our scheme for an example case are illustrated in Fig. 6.3. The original MR image in Fig. 6.3a was passed into the anisotropic diffusion filter to reduce noise while preserving the major liver structures such as the portal vein and liver boundary, as shown in Fig. 6.3b. The noise-reduced image was then passed through a Gaussian gradient magnitude filter to enhance the boundaries, as shown in Fig. 6.3c. The edge potential image generated from the enhanced image using the sigmoid gray-scale converter was applied to the fast

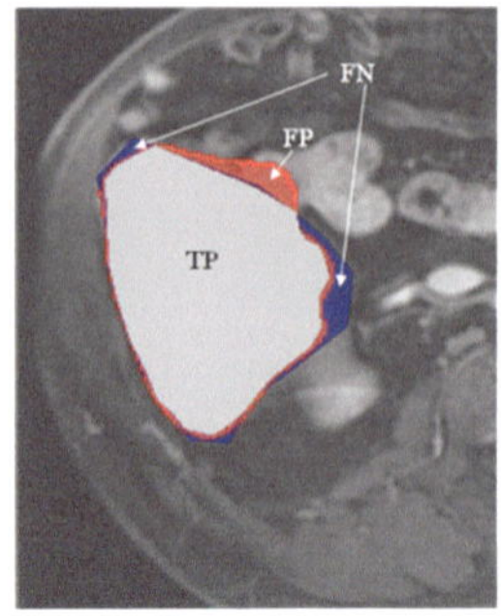

Fig. 6.4 Definitions of true-positive (TP) (*gray region*), false-positive (FP) (*red region*), and false-negative (FN) segmentation (*blue region*) in evaluation of computerized liver segmentation (*red contour*) compared to "gold-standard" manual segmentation (*blue contour*)

marching algorithm to generate the initial contour, as shown in Fig. 6.3d. The liver was extracted more precisely by using the geodesic active contour algorithm, as shown in Fig. 6.3e. Corresponding between computer-based liver segmentation (red contour) and "gold-standard" manual liver segmentation (blue contour) is shown in Fig. 6.3f. Liver volume was computed using the extracted regions.

Evaluation Criteria

The liver volumes obtained by using our computerized scheme were compared to the "gold-standard" manual volumes determined by the radiologist. The definitions used in evaluation of a computerized liver segmentation compared to the gold-standard manual liver segmentation are shown in Fig. 6.4. True-positive (TP) segmentation was defined as an overlapping region (gray color) between the computerized liver segmentation (indicated by a red contour), C, and a gold-standard manual segmentation (indicated by a blue contour), G; i.e., $TP = G \cap C$. False-positive (FP) segmentation (red region) was defined by $FP = C - TP$. False-negative (FN) segmentation (blue region) was defined by $FN = G - TP$. True-negative (TN) segmentation was defined by $TN = I - G \cup C$, where I is the entire image. We define accuracy, specificity, and sensitivity of the segmentation as

$$Accuracy = \frac{|TP| + |TN|}{|I|}, \tag{6.8}$$

$$Specificity = |TN|/(|TN| + |FP|), \tag{6.9}$$

$$Sensitivity = |TP|/(|TP| + |FN|). \tag{6.10}$$

The Dice measurement representing the fraction of the overlapping volume and the volume of two segmentation methods is given by

$$Dice = \frac{2|TP|}{2|TP| + |FP| + |FN|}. \tag{6.11}$$

We also determine the percentage volume error (E) for each computerized volume (V_c) and the gold-standard manual volume (V_m) as

$$E = |(V_c - V_m)/V_m|. \tag{6.12}$$

The association between the computerized volumetry and the manual volumetry was measured by the Pearson product–moment correlation coefficient (r). The significance of correlation coefficient was evaluated by using the Student t test. An agreement between two measurements was assessed by using the intraclass correlation coefficient (ICC) [24, 25]. The two-way random single measure model, $ICC(2,1)$, was used because we assumed that the cases were chosen randomly from population and each case was measured by two volumetric methods. The $ICC(2,1)$ was defined by the following equation:

$$ICC(2,1) = \frac{BMS - EMS}{BMS + (k-1) + k(RMS - EMS)/n}, \tag{6.13}$$

where n is the number of cases, k is the number of raters (i.e., volumetric methods), BMS is the between-cases mean square, EMS is the error mean square, and RMS is the between-raters mean square. The statistical significance was obtained by the analysis of variance. The post-hoc power analysis using the Walter–Eliasziw–Donner model [26] for ICC-based reliability studies was performed to determine the statistical power in this study. As done in [7], we assumed the type I error (α) of 0.05 and type II error (β) of 0.20 in this analysis. An additional agreement analysis for two measurements was performed by the Bland–Altman method [27] based on the mean difference (*bias*) and the standard deviation of difference (*SD*). The limits of agreement, which are given by *bias* $\pm$ 1.96 $\times$ *SD*, were used to consider the degree of agreement.

Results

The comparison on the liver volume between the two measurements is shown in Tables 6.1 and 6.2. The mean gold-standard manual volume was 1,710 cc with a standard deviation of 401 cc (range: 1,013–2,529 cc), while the mean volume of our computerized scheme was 1,697 cc with a standard deviation of 400 cc (range: 1,120–2,418 cc). The mean absolute difference and the percentage volume error (E) were 56 cc and 3.6 %, respectively.

The overall mean of the Dice coefficients was calculated as 93.6 $\pm$ 1.7 %, the accuracy was 99.4 $\pm$ 0.14 %, the sensitivity was 93.4 $\pm$ 3.3 %, and the specificity was 99.7 $\pm$ 0.12 %. The relationship between the computerized volumetry and the

Table 6.1 Comparison between computerized volumetry and "gold-standard" manual volumetry

	Average	Standard deviation
Computer volume (cc)	1,697	400
Manual volume (cc)	1,710	401

Table 6.2 Summary of quantitative evaluation of computerized liver extraction compared to "gold-standard" manual liver extraction

	Average	Standard deviation
Accuracy (%)	99.4	0.14
Sensitivity (%)	93.4	3.3
Specificity (%)	99.7	0.12
Percent volume error (%)	3.6	3.6
Dice coefficient (%)	93.6	1.7

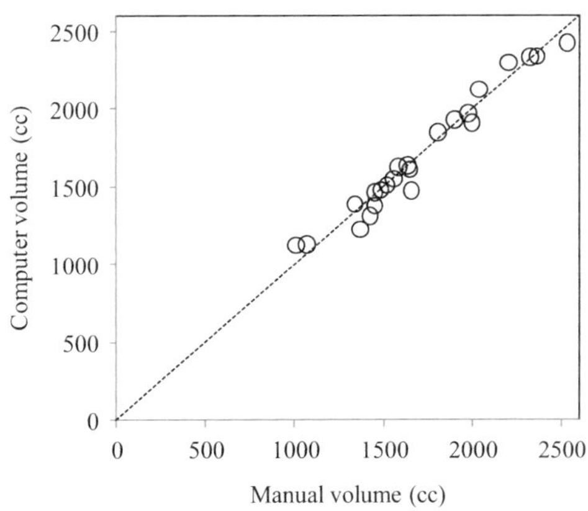

Fig. 6.5 Relationship between computer-based volumes and "gold-standard" manual volumes. Two volumetrics reached an excellent agreement (the intraclass correlation coefficient was 0.98)

Table 6.3 Analysis of variance table from intraclass correlation coefficient analysis

	Df	Sum of squares	Mean squares	F
Between raters	1	2,008	2,008	0.69
Between cases	22	6,999,296	318,150	108.5
Within cases	23	66,496	2,891	
Residual	22	64,488	2,931	
Total	45	7,065,792		

manual volumetry is shown in Fig. 6.5. The Pearson correlation coefficient was 0.98 at a level that was not statistically significant ($p = 23.65$). Table 6.3 presents the results from the ICC analysis. Two volumetric methods achieved an excellent agreement with an ICC of 0.98 and no statistically significant difference ($p = 0.42$). The statistical power in the study was evaluated by using the

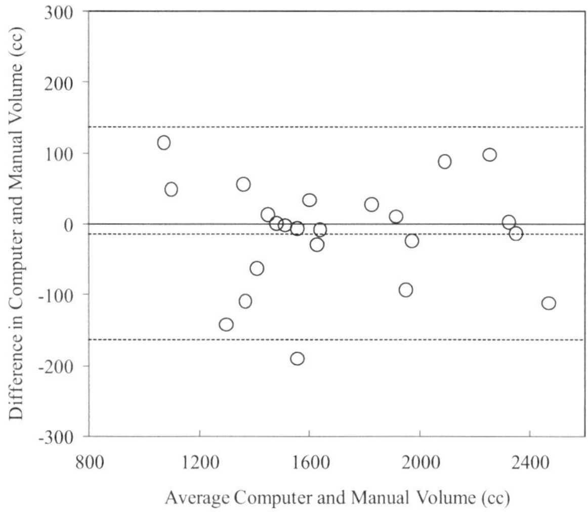

Fig. 6.6 Bland–Altman plot for agreement between computer and manual volumetry. The bias was 13.2 cc; 95 % limits of agreement were −163.7 and 136.9 cc

post-hoc power analysis based on the Walter–Eliasziw–Donner model [26]. The lowest ICC between the computer-based volumetry and the manual volumetry that we should have been able to detect with 23 cases was 0.95, and this study had the power to detect a bias of 0.03 in ICC. The Bland–Altman plot for assessing agreement is also presented in Fig. 6.6. Here the mean difference was −13.2. The limits of agreement with the 95 % confidence interval were −163 to 137 cc which were small enough to show a good agreement between two volumetric methods.

Figure 6.7 illustrates the computerized liver segmentation and manual liver segmentation for a case with a high accuracy (99.7 %). The computerized segmentation agreed almost perfectly with the gold-standard manual segmentation for slices through the superior portion of the liver, as shown in Fig. 6.7b, d. Two other cases with more typical results which have the accuracies close to the average accuracy are presented in Fig. 6.8. Overall, the computerized method was able to extract the livers very accurately. However, there were occasionally over- and under-extractions in the extracted livers. Major FP and FN extraction sources are illustrated in Fig. 6.9. The major FN sources included a lesion attaching to the liver boundary, a low-contrast liver boundary, and inhomogeneous density due to focal fatty and noise. The major FP sources included the heart, kidney, vena cava, and stomach, which abut the liver. They were also from artifact due to the partial volume effect. Other under- and over-extraction sources were convex and concave boundary parts with high curvatures.

The average processing time of our scheme for liver segmentation was 1.03 ± 0.13 min/case (range: 0.9–1.5 min/case) on a PC (CPU: Intel, Xeon, 2.66 GHz), whereas that for manual method was 24.0 ± 4.4 min/case (range: 18–30 min/case). The difference was statistically significant ($p < 0.001$).

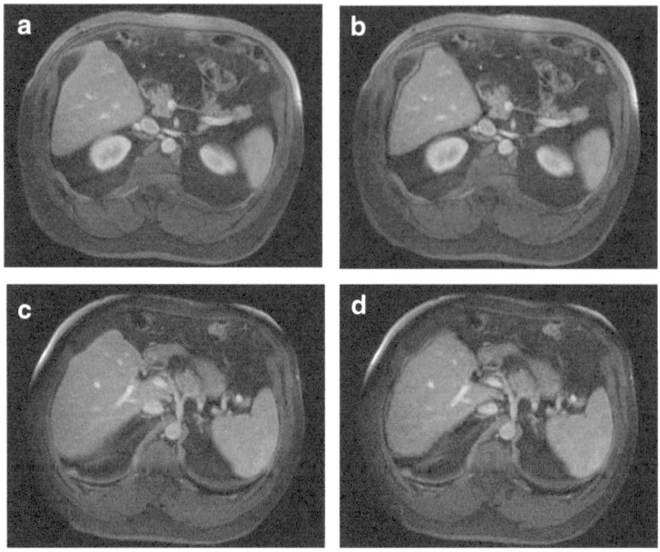

Fig. 6.7 Comparisons of computerized liver extraction with "gold-standard" manual liver extraction for the case with a high accuracy (99.7 %). (**a**) Original axial MR image from the case. (**b**) Computerized liver extraction (*red contour*) and "gold-standard" manual liver extraction (*blue contour*). (**c**) Original axial MR image (different slice) from the same case. (**d**) Computerized liver extraction (*red contour*) and "gold-standard" manual liver extraction (*blue contour*)

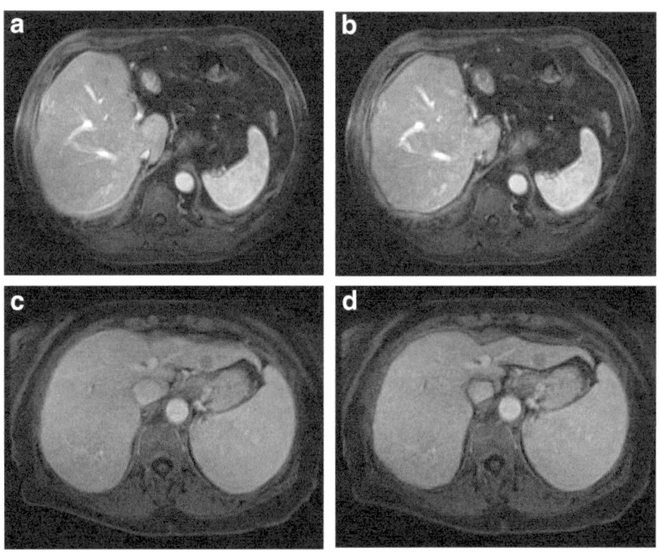

Fig. 6.8 Comparisons of the computerized liver extraction with "gold-standard" manual liver extraction for two cases with accuracies (99.5 % for the upper case; 99.2 % for lower case) close to the average accuracy (99.4 %). (**a**) Original axial MR image from one of the cases. (**b**) Corresponding computerized liver extraction (*red contour*) and "gold-standard" manual liver extraction (*blue contour*). (**c**) Original axial MR image from the other case. (**d**) Corresponding computerized liver extraction (*red contour*) and "gold-standard" manual liver extraction (*blue contour*)

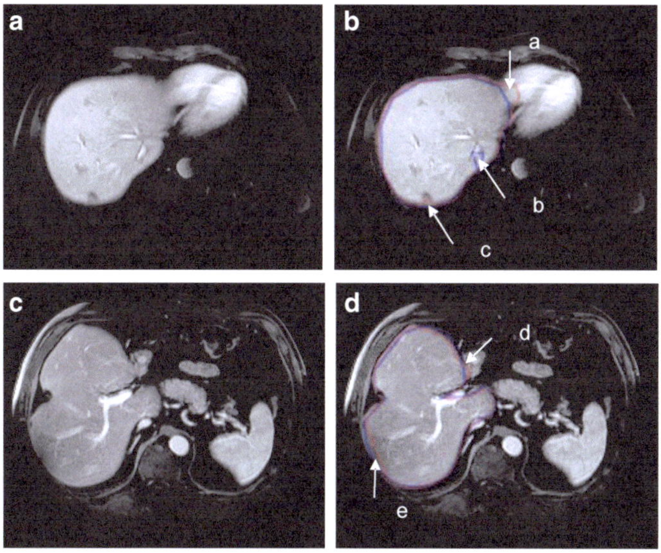

Fig. 6.9 Illustrations of major FP and FN sources. (**a**, **c**), Original axial MR images. (**b**, **d**) computerized liver extraction (*red contour*) and "gold-standard" manual liver extraction (*blue contour*). (**b**) There is an FP due to the heart (*a*), an FN due to vein (*b*), and an FN due to a lesion on the liver boundary (*c*). (**d**) There is an FP due to the duodenum (*d*), and an FN due to a low-intensity region (*e*)

Discussions

Liver volumetry is performed for hepatectomy to treat patients with liver tumors. Because the liver volume is reduced after hepatectomy, it must be ensured that the remaining liver volume is sufficient to maintain the liver function. In the case of complicated treatment such as chronic liver disease, a larger remaining liver volume is required [28]. Many researchers have tried to estimate the liver volume accurately based on CT images, such as the one using virtual hepatectomy [29]. However, fewer researchers have reported liver volumetry on MRI, probably because it is believed that MR liver volumetry has more variations, and manual MR liver volumetry is more difficult than CT. Furthermore, manual liver volumetry is very time-consuming and not cost-effective. Therefore, it is crucial to investigate the potential of a computerized volumetry for liver MR images. We believe that computerized MR liver volumetry is potentially very useful.

Although our computerized liver volumetry had an excellent agreement with the gold-standard manual liver volumetry (the ICC was 0.98), there were still occasional FNs and FPs which were mainly caused by the similar density of other organs abutting to the liver. The liver segmentation accuracy was also interfered by the partial volume effects and the liver intensity variation among different studies/ patients, as the intensity depends on acquisition timing and contrast material characteristics.

Although the volumes obtained by using our computerized method had a strong correlation with those by the gold-standard manual tracing method (Pearson's product–moment correlation coefficient was 0.98), it does not still reach the minimal variation in CT volumetry between expert radiologists that was reported as 0.997 [30] (Although we could not find a study reporting the variation in MR volumetry, we expect it would be larger than the one in CT). One can increase the overall accuracy by correcting FP and FN extractions manually. This can be accomplished rapidly with routine manipulations. The substantial amount of time saved by using the computerized method may justify the small error rate (average percentage volume error of 3.6 %) compared to the manual tracing method, which the average processing time was 24 min/case.

Direct comparisons of our method with existing methods in literature are not easy because different databases and quality measurements were used. Freiman et al. [31] achieved volume errors of 5.36 and 2.36 % in CT volumetry of their database and a publicly available database (i.e., SLIVER07), respectively. Florin et al. [32] obtained a volume error of 10.72 % in CT volumetry. For evaluation of liver MRI segmentation, Gloger et al. [19] obtained volume errors of 8.3 % for normal livers and 11.8 % for fat livers with runtime of 11.2 and 15.4 min, respectively. Besides volume errors, some researchers used the shape alignment measurement to evaluate the segmentation performance. A robust measurement based on the shape alignment is the modified Hausdorff distance (MHD) which overcomes the noise and outlier sensitivity of the original Hausdorff distance, defined by

$$MHD = \max\{d_H(X,Y), d_H(Y,X)\}, \tag{6.14}$$

$$d_H(X,Y) = \frac{1}{card(X)} \sum_{\mathbf{x}\in X} \min_{\mathbf{y}\in Y} \|\mathbf{x} - \mathbf{y}\|, \tag{6.15}$$

where X and Y are two sets of boundary positions of the liver extracted by a manual method and a computerized method, respectively. Our scheme achieved an average MHD of 12.8 ± 2.24 mm for livers with diseases, whereas an average original Hausdorff distance reported in [19] was 20.35 ± 8.66 mm for fat livers. Note that an MHD was not provided in [19].

The 95 % limits of agreement between our computerized volumes and the gold-standard manual volumes were −163.3 and 136.9 cc. These limits are smaller than the results reported by Nakayama et al. [8]: the limits between automated and manual volumes were −230.3 and 327.9 cc; and those between automated and measured liver volumes were −309.3 and 412 cc. In addition, these 95 % limits of agreement are smaller than those in our previous work on CT images [7] which were −211 and 278 cc for agreement between the automated and manual CT volumes. Note that the above comparisons were not direct comparisons due to different databases.

One of the limitations in this study is that the evaluation is performed with the gold-standard manual volumes determined by a single expert radiologist. Ideally, the gold-standard volumes are determined by multiple radiologists who are experts in liver diagnosis. However, this ideal evaluation would not be available at all institutions because not many institutions have a number of such radiologists who are sufficiently experienced in the liver diagnosis. Many publications reported the evaluation using the gold-standard manual volumes. However, none of them used the gold-standard volumes estimated from multiple radiologists. This may result from the above reason. Furthermore, it was shown that the correlation between two radiologists's manual volumes was 0.997 [30], which may infer that the interobserver variation is small and the difference among manual volumes determined by multiple radiologists and a single radiologist is not significant. We used the manual volumes determined from an experienced radiologist as the gold standard. We thought that the manual volumes from multiple inexperienced radiologists or mixture of inexperienced radiologists and experienced radiologists may be less reliable, compared to volumes determined by an experienced radiologist who traces liver boundaries very carefully.

Conclusions

In this chapter, we developed an automatic scheme for the liver volumetry in MR images by employing the fast marching algorithm combined with the geodesic active contour segmentation. MRI liver volumes obtained by using our scheme agreed excellently with those determined by the current "gold-standard" manual tracing method. With our computerized volumetry, the time required for volumetry was reduced significantly from 24 min per case to a min per case. Therefore, our computerized scheme would be useful for radiologists in liver volumetric analysis on MR images.

Acknowledgments The authors are grateful to members in the Suzuki Laboratory in the Department of Radiology at the University of Chicago for their valuable comments. This work was partly supported by the NIH S10 RR021039, P30 CA14599, and Vietnam Education Foundation. This work was partly 351 supported by the NIH S10 RR021039, P30 CA14599, Vietnam Education Foundation, and Vietnam National Foundation for Science and Technology Development (NAFOSTED).

References

1. Thuluvath PJ, Guidinger MK, Fung JJ, Johnson LB, Rayhill SC, Pelletier SJ (2010) Liver transplantation in the United States, 1999–2008. Am J Transplant 10:1003–1019
2. Biggins SW (2012) Futility and rationing in liver retransplantation: when and how can we say no? J Hepatol 56(6):1404
3. Monbaliu D, Pirenne J, Talbot D (2011) Liver transplantation using donation after cardiac death donors. J Hepatol 56:474–485

4. Lo CM, Fan ST, Liu CL et al (1997) Adult-to-adult living donor liver transplantation using extended right lobe grafts. Ann Surg 226:261–270
5. Radtke A, Sotiropoulos GC, Nadalin S et al (2007) Preoperative volume prediction in adult living donor liver transplantation: how much can we rely on it? Am J Transplant 7:672–679
6. Kamel IR, Kruskal JB, Warmbrand G, Goldberg SN, Pomfret EA, Raptopoulos V (2001) Accuracy of volumetric measurements after virtual right hepatectomy in potential donors undergoing living adult liver transplantation. AJR Am J Roentgenol 176:483–487
7. Suzuki K, Epstein ML, Kohlbrenner R et al (2011) Quantitative radiology: automated CT liver volumetry compared with interactive volumetry and manual volumetry. AJR Am J Roentgenol 197:W706–W712
8. Nakayama Y, Li Q, Katsuragawa S et al (2006) Automated hepatic volumetry for living related liver transplantation at multisection CT. Radiology 240:743–748
9. Gao L, Heath DG, Kuszyk BS, Fishman EK (1996) Automatic liver segmentation technique for three-dimensional visualization of CT data. Radiology 201:359–364
10. Bae KT, Giger ML, Chen CT, Kahn CE Jr (1993) Automatic segmentation of liver structure in CT images. Med Phys 20:71–78
11. Hermoye L, Laamari-Azjal I, Cao Z et al (2005) Liver segmentation in living liver transplant donors: comparison of semiautomatic and manual methods. Radiology 234:171–178
12. Okada T, Shimada R, Hori M et al (2008) Automated segmentation of the liver from 3D CT images using probabilistic atlas and multilevel statistical shape model. Acad Radiol 15:1390–1403
13. Selver MA, Kocaoglu A, Demir GK, Dogan H, Dicle O, Guzelis C (2008) Patient oriented and robust automatic liver segmentation for pre-evaluation of liver transplantation. Comput Biol Med 38:765–784
14. Chen X, Bagci U (2011) 3D automatic anatomy segmentation based on iterative graph-cut-ASM. Med Phys 38:4610–4622
15. Suzuki K, Kohlbrenner R, Epstein ML, Obajuluwa AM, Xu J, Hori M (2010) Computer-aided measurement of liver volumes in CT by means of geodesic active contour segmentation coupled with level-set algorithms. Med Phys 37:2159–2166
16. Karlo C, Reiner CS, Stolzmann P et al (2010) CT- and MRI-based volumetry of resected liver specimen: comparison to intraoperative volume and weight measurements and calculation of conversion factors. Eur J Radiol 75:e107–e111
17. Farraher SW, Jara H, Chang KJ, Hou A, Soto JA (2005) Liver and spleen volumetry with quantitative MR imaging and dual-space clustering segmentation. Radiology 237:322–328
18. Rusko L, Bekes G (2011) Liver segmentation for contrast-enhanced MR images using partitioned probabilistic model. Int J Comput Assist Radiol Surg 6:13–20
19. Gloger O, Kuhn J, Stanski A, Volzke H, Puls R (2010) A fully automatic three-step liver segmentation method on LDA-based probability maps for multiple contrast MR images. Magn Reson Imaging 28:882–897
20. Perona P, Malik J (1990) Scale-space and edge-detection using anisotropic diffusion. IEEE Trans Pattern Anal Mach Intell 12:629–639
21. Sethian JA (1999) Level set methods and fast marching methods, 2nd edn. Cambridge University Press, New York
22. Sethian JA (1996) A fast marching level set method for monotonically advancing fronts. Proc Natl Acad Sci U S A 93:1591–1595
23. Caselles V, Kimmel R, Sapiro G (1997) Geodesic active contours. Int J Comput Vis 22:61–79
24. Portney LG, Watkins MP (1993) Foundations of clinical research: applications to practice, 2nd edn. Appleton & Lange, Norwalk
25. Shrout PE, Fleiss JL (1979) Intraclass correlations: uses in assessing rater reliability. Psychol Bull 86:420–428
26. Walter SD, Eliasziw M, Donner A (1998) Sample size and optimal designs for reliability studies. Stat Med 17:101–110

27. Bland JM, Altman DG (1986) Statistical methods for assessing agreement between two methods of clinical measurement. Lancet 1:307–310
28. Okamoto E, Kyo A, Yamanaka N, Tanaka N, Kuwata K (1984) Prediction of the safe limits of hepatectomy by combined volumetric and functional measurements in patients with impaired hepatic function. Surgery 95:586–592
29. Yamanaka J, Saito S, Fujimoto J (2007) Impact of preoperative planning using virtual segmental volumetry on liver resection for hepatocellular carcinoma. World J Surg 31:1249–1255
30. Sandrasegaran K, Kwo PW, DiGirolamo D, Stockberger SM Jr, Cummings OW, Kopecky KK (1999) Measurement of liver volume using spiral CT and the curved line and cubic spline algorithms: reproducibility and interobserver variation. Abdom Imaging 24:61–65
31. Freiman M, Eliassaf O, Taieb Y, Joskowicz L, Azraq Y, Sosna J (2008) An iterative Bayesian approach for nearly automatic liver segmentation: algorithm and validation. Int J Comput Assist Radiol Surg 3:439–446
32. Florin C, Paragios N, Funka-Lea G, Williams J (2007) Liver segmentation using sparse 3D prior models with optimal data support. Inf Process Med Imaging 20:38–49

Chapter 7
Computer-Aided Image Analysis for Vertebral Anatomy on X-Ray CT Images

T. Hayashi, H. Chen, K. Miyamoto, X. Zhou, T. Hara, and H. Fujita

Abstract Osteoporosis has become an increasingly important public health problem because of the rapidly aging populations. To obtain the sophisticated knowledge on normal vertebral anatomy is essential to understand the vertebral fracture risk. Multi-detector row computed tomography (MDCT) method can be used for quantitative analysis of vertebral anatomy such as volumetric bone mineral density (vBMD), geometry, and alignment with high accuracy and precision from the same dataset. This chapter described our latest two findings on statistical analysis and image analysis for vertebral anatomy by use of the image processing technique on the MDCT scanning. One was the population-based statistical analysis on vBMD at vertebrae. It showed the trabecular vBMD distribution at healthy thoracic and lumbar vertebrae in Japanese subjects and specific differences in age and gender. The other presented a computerized scheme to quantify the vertebral geometry.

T. Hayashi
Department of Intelligent Image Information, Division of Regeneration and Advanced Medical Sciences, Graduate School of Medicine, Gifu University, 1-1 Yanagido, Gifu, Gifu 501-1194, Japan

Media Co., Ltd, NREG Hongo Sanchome Bldg 8F, 3-26-6 Hongo, Bunkyo-ku, Tokyo 113-0033, Japan

H. Chen
Department of Anatomy, Division of Disease Control, Graduate School of Medicine, Gifu University, Gifu, Japan

K. Miyamoto
Department of Reconstructive Surgery for Spine, Bone, and Joint, Graduate School of Medicine, Gifu University, Gifu, Japan

X. Zhou • T. Hara • H. Fujita (✉)
Department of Intelligent Image Information, Division of Regeneration and Advanced Medical Sciences, Graduate School of Medicine, Gifu University, 1-1 Yanagido, Gifu, Gifu 501-1194, Japan
e-mail: fujita@fjt.info.gifu-u.ac.jp

K. Suzuki (ed.), *Computational Intelligence in Biomedical Imaging*, DOI 10.1007/978-1-4614-7245-2_7,

The scheme provided appropriate values on the vertebral geometry with numerous CT cases. It is likely that such computer-based attempts will help us to achieve the sophisticated vertebral anatomy.

Introduction

Osteoporosis has become an increasingly important public health problem because of the rapidly aging populations. Early detection of bone loss is important for the prevention of vertebral fractures because therapeutic drug treatments are the most effective before the decrease of bone mineral density (BMD) affects bone fractures [1].

Dual X-ray absorptiometry (DXA) is the most widely used bone densitometry technique. Quantitative computed tomography (QCT) allows the selective assessment of skeletal status of trabecular bone of the vertebral bodies. Peripheral quantitative computed tomography (pQCT) measurements are typically obtained at the radius or the tibia. Also, there are quantitative ultrasound (QUS) approaches, which show substantial differences in performance [2]. In spite of having such technologies that estimate the magnitude of osteoporosis, its screening rates remain low [3, 4]. It is because osteoporosis is a silent disease with few symptoms in its early stage.

Panoramic radiography widely used in clinical dentistry may be useful to overcome its problem. Klemetti et al. [5] revealed that a decrease in the mandibular cortical thickness on the panoramic images was one of the radiographic signs of osteoporosis. This finding indicated that the panoramic images had a new potential to be used as a supplemental screening tool for early detection of osteoporosis. To verify its possibility, two clinical trials were conducted in Japan [6, 7]. These trials suggested that the screening by trained dentists was useful for identifying osteoporotic patients. Recently, triage screening for osteoporosis in dental clinics was advocated by Taguchi [8].

The question which we must consider here is whether general dental practitioners can play the new role. There are some specialized fields in dentistry such as dental radiologist, dental surgeon, endodontist, exodontist, and so on. Namely, not all dental practitioners are familiar with image interpretation. To facilitate the new role of identifying osteoporotic patients by the dental practitioners, the following computer-aided image analysis schemes (or systems) were presented: Taguchi et al. [9] have developed a diagnosis support device based on the evaluation of the morphology of the mandibular cortex; Asano et al. [10] have developed a diagnosis support device based on the measurement of the mandibular cortical thickness; Kavitha et al. [11] proposed a new approach on the basis of continuous measurements; Devlin et al. [12] presented an automated method for risk assessment of osteoporosis; Allen et al. [13] proposed a computerized scheme by use of statistical shape models; and Roberts et al. [14] proposed a computerized scheme by use of active appearance models.

We also presented a new screening pathway by cooperation of dental practitioners and computer-aided detection (CAD) system (see Fig. 7.1) [15–17]. Overview of the new screening pathway is as follows. In the routine work,

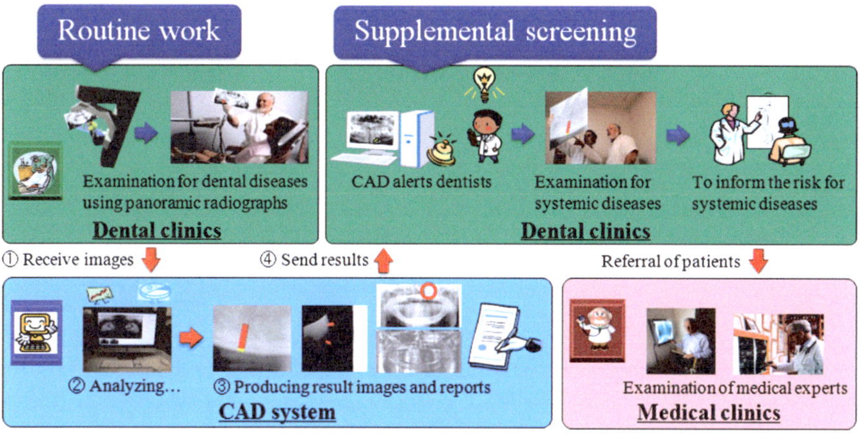

Fig. 7.1 New screening pathway via dental clinics with CAD system (adapted from [17])

panoramic radiographs are used to examine dental diseases in dental clinics. At this time, the dental practitioners send the images to CAD system as an extra task. Once upon receiving the images, our CAD system automatically runs the image analysis and the resulted images and reports are sent to the dental practitioners. If pathologic signs are detected, CAD alerts the dental practitioners. And then, refer to the CAD results, supplemental screening of osteoporosis is done by the dental practitioners. Finally, the dental practitioners inform patients of the risk for osteoporosis. If the patients desire, the dental practitioners will refer to the medical clinics. "The preliminary diagnosis by the dental practitioners" has a potential to afford some new perspectives on the osteoporosis treatment. Further technical innovations to drive such farsighted approach are encouraged.

Turning now to the topic of vertebral fracture, its risk is currently estimated on the basis of lumbar vertebral BMD in clinical practice. However, vertebral fractures can occur even when the BMD does not reach the osteoporotic threshold. There are some research findings on the vertebral fractures. For example, the compressive strength of vertebrae is determined not only by their bone density but also by their dimensions [18]. Reduced spinal sagittal curvature is an independent risk factor [19]. In spite of such discoveries, little is known about the role of vertebrae in fracture risk to date. It is likely that the sophisticated knowledge on normal vertebral anatomy is essential to understand the vertebral fracture risk.

Multi-detector row computed tomography (MDCT) scanning is widely used in clinical practice. It permits the acquisition of thin sections with isotropic voxel sizes. An example of body X-ray CT image is shown in Fig. 7.2. We see from Fig. 7.2 that human bone structures are radiologically visualized under high resolution. Namely, we can achieve the quantitative analysis of the vertebral anatomy such as volumetric BMD (vBMD), geometry, and alignment with high accuracy and precision from the same dataset by using the MDCT scanning. The problem is that such analysis takes a lot of time and effort. It is likely that computer-based image analysis is a key technology to overcome the above problem.

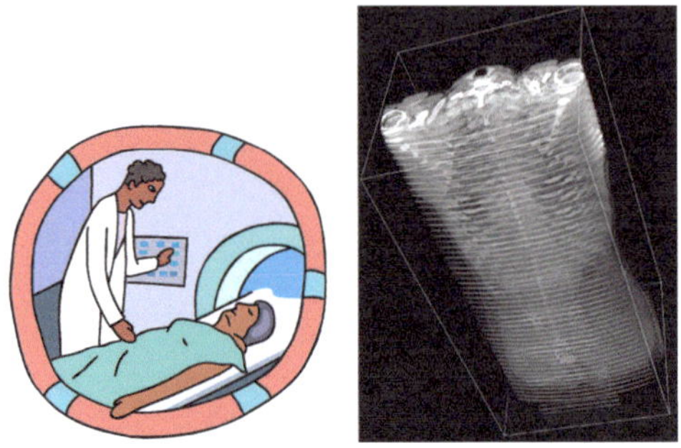

Fig. 7.2 An example of the body X-ray CT image

Here we present our latest studies of the computer-aided image analysis for vertebral anatomy by using the MDCT scanning. The second section describes a "Computer-Aided Analysis of vBMD at Trabecular Bones in Thoracic and Lumbar Vertebrae." Computer-based quantification of vertebral body geometry is described in the third section. The findings of our studies and follow-up prospects are summarized in the section "Summary."

Computer-Aided Analysis of vBMD at Trabecular Bones in Thoracic and Lumbar Vertebrae

The aims of this section were to investigate segmental variations in vBMD of thoracic and lumbar vertebral bodies and to show specific differences according to age and gender. First, a computer-assisted scheme to determine the volume of interest (VOI) at vertebrae was designed. And then, a large number of CT data set was employed to estimate the vBMD. On the basis of those results, we attempted to answer two key questions to improve our understanding of bone fragility: (1) Is there any vertebral level-dependent vBMD change? (2) Does the vBMD differ according to gender? This section summarized the publications in [20, 21] and it was beyond the scope of this section to discuss the clinical aspects.

Materials and Methods

Study Subjects

The study sample consisted of the first 1,750 enrolled Japanese men and women with CT images from 2002 to 2006, scanned for the purpose of examinations of various organs and tissues. The CT images included all thoracic and lumbar vertebrae [LightSpeed Ultra, GE Yokogawa Medical Systems Ltd, Tokyo, Japan] and were scanned for each subject using standard settings (120 kV, Auto mAs,

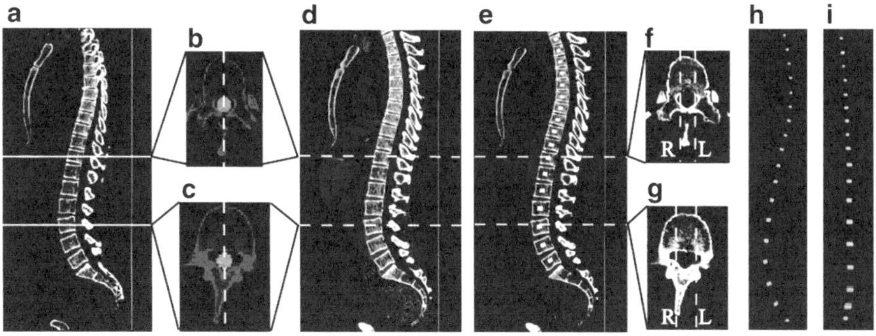

Fig. 7.3 Computer-assisted VOI decision. (**a**) One slice of sagittal section on CT images. (**b**, **c**) One slice of axial-sections of T11 and L3 on CT images, respectively (*White circle* denotes a segmented spinal canal). (**d**) Sagittal median plane image of the spine. (**e**) The VOI inputting on the sagittal median plane image of spine. (**f**, **g**) Input examples of the range of the right and left at T11 and L3 (*White dash lines* show the border of the VOI). (**h**, **i**) 3-D view of the inputted VOIs from the lateral and anterior sides, respectively (modified from [21])

1.25 mm-thick slice, pitch = 0.49–0.88 mm) routinely used clinically. Slice intervals were modified to the same value as the pitch using sinc interpolation to keep each voxel in an isotropic size in 3-D.

Of the 1,750 individuals with CT data available, 719 were excluded because of normal variants, bone pathology, vertebral fractures, or reasons other than mild degenerative changes at vertebrae, as confirmed by radiologists or anatomic experts. The study subjects consisted, therefore, of 1,031 individuals: 490 men and 541 women. The study subjects were then subdivided into five age categories (≦40, 41–50, 51–60, 61–70, ≧71) in order to observe age differences. Low vBMD was measured in the front and central regions at the lumbar vertebrae in [22]. For this reason, the vBMD of trabecular bones at the central region of the vertebral body was decided as the typical site.

Computer-Assisted VOI Decision

Each VOI from the first thoracic vertebra (T1) to the first sacral vertebra (S1) was determined as follows (Fig. 7.3).

1. The spinal canal regions were segmented based on the CT number and skeletal structures [23].
2. The central locations of the right and left sides of the spinal canal in each axial section were calculated, and a sagittal sectional image based on the center line of the spinal canal was generated. We defined the generated image as a sagittal median plane image of the spine. Figure 7.3b, c indicate the segmented spinal canal in one slice of axial sections of T11 and the third lumbar vertebra (L3), respectively (white circle denotes the segmented spinal canal). Figure 7.3d

shows an example of the sagittal median plane image of the spine. Although there is no guarantee that the vertebral bodies of T1–S1 can be seen in only one slice of the sagittal sections of the original CT image (see Fig. 7.3a), T1–S1 can always be seen in the sagittal median plane image of the spine (see Fig. 7.3d).

3. The VOIs of T1–S1 were manually inputted on the sagittal median plane image of the spine. Inputted VOIs are shown by the white regions in Fig. 7.3e.
4. Axial sectional images of the original CT image corresponding to the center of each vertebra were referenced, and then we determined the right and left range of the VOIs. Input examples of the range of the right and left at T11 and L3 are shown in Fig. 7.3f, g.
5. Each VOI inputted at the process 3 was extended to the range inputted at the process 4. Examples of the VOIs obtained by the above method are shown in Fig. 7.3h, i. They show a 3-D view of the inputted VOI from the lateral and anterior sides, respectively. The 3-D volumetric VOI can be checked from their figures.

Estimation of vBMD

It is impossible to measure BMD using the established method proposed by Cann and Genant [24] (e.g., QCT) because the purpose of our CT data was not the diagnosis of osteoporosis. Instead of using "traditional" QCT, we fixed the standard phantom (B-MAS 200, Kyoto Kagaku, Kyoto, Japan) under the human body phantom, and took exposed it to the same radiation dose as that used in diagnosis in order to calibrate the CT Hounsfield units to equivalent bone mineral concentrations. The standard phantom contained calibration cells of 0, 50, 100, 150, and 200 mg/cm^3 with equivalent concentrations of calcium hydroxyapatite. As a result, we estimated the vBMD as follows:

$$\mathrm{vBMD}\left[\mathrm{mg/cm^3}\right] = (\mathrm{CT\ number[HU]} - 3.55)/1.13. \tag{7.1}$$

Therefore, the mean CT number of the VOI determined in "Computer-Assisted VOI Decision" was computed. And then, the vBMD was estimated by using the calibration curve (i.e., Eq. 7.1).

Our New Findings on the Vertebral Trabecular vBMD

Vertebral Level-Dependent vBMD Change

The graph in Fig. 7.4 illustrates the vertebral level-dependent vBMD change in women between the ages of 51 and 60. We see from Fig. 7.4 that the vertebral level-dependent vBMD change is found and L3 has the lowest vBMD. Regardless of age and gender, similar level-dependent change was found in this study.

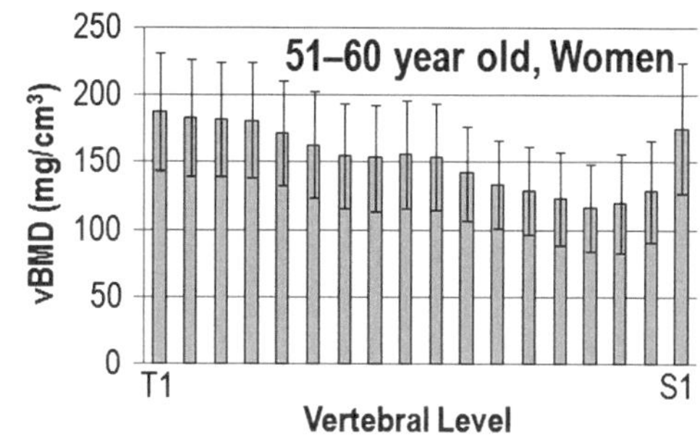

Fig. 7.4 Vertebral level-dependent vBMD change (modified from [21])

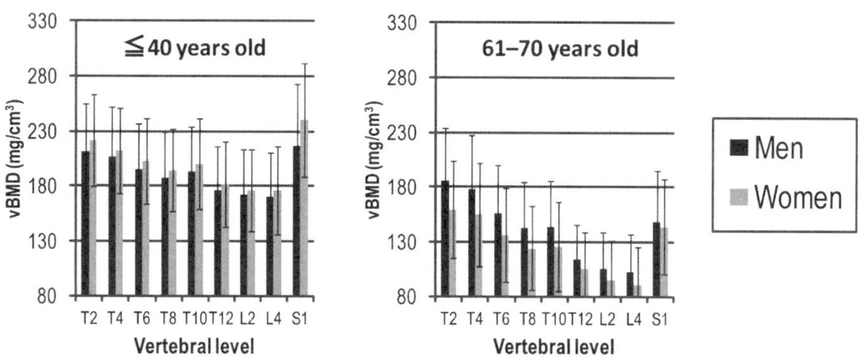

Fig. 7.5 Gender-dependent vBMD change (modified from [21])

Gender-Dependent vBMD Change

The graphs in Fig. 7.5 illustrate the gender-dependent vBMD change in the ages of 40 and 61–70. We see from Fig. 7.5 that gender-dependent vBMD change is found. Regardless of vertebral level, women in the ages of 40 had the highest vBMD. However, the women's vBMDs rapidly deteriorated with aging.

Deterioration of vBMD with Aging

Tukey multiple comparison test was used to understand the deterioration of vBMD with aging. Significant difference was defined as $p < 0.05$. Correlation value of the vBMDs between 41–50 years and other age categories is represented in Fig. 7.6. As for comparison with 51–60 years, a glance at Fig. 7.6a will reveal that the significant differences are found in all vertebral levels in women. In contrast, the significant differences are not found in all vertebral levels in men (see Fig. 7.6b). As for comparison with 61–70 years in men, the significant differences are found in the vertebral levels from T10 to L5 (see Fig. 7.6c). As for comparison with 71 years

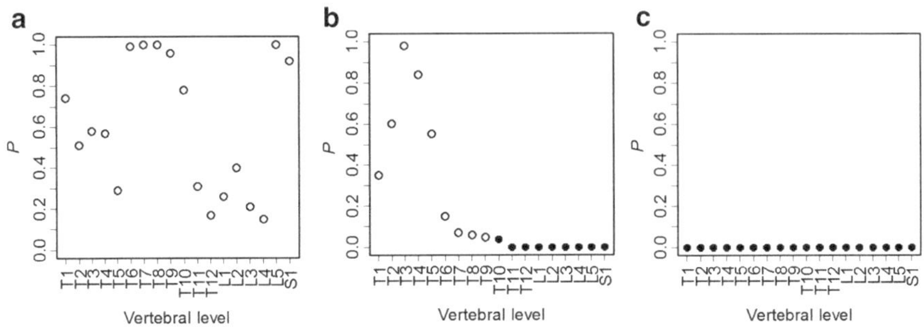

Fig. 7.6 Correlation value of the vBMDs between 41 and 50 years and other age categories by using Tukey multiple comparison test. Significant difference was defined as under 0.05 (as shown in *filled circle*) (**a**) Comparison with 51–60 years. (**b**) Comparison with 61–70 years. (**c**) Comparison with ≧71 years (modified from [21])

in men, the significant differences are found in all vertebral levels. Therefore, it is suggested that the deterioration of the vBMDs is similar in all vertebral levels in women, whereas it is faster at T11–L5 levels than at T1–T10 levels in men. It should be noted that its cause is not clear and further studies are required.

Computer-Based Quantification of Vertebral Body Geometry

We described in this section the computer-based quantification of the vertebral body geometry. For gaining a better understanding of bone quality, a great deal of attention has been paid to vertebral geometry in anatomy [18]. In order to accelerate such basic investigation, it may be helpful to develop a computer-assisted scheme for analyzing the vertebral geometry on body CT images.

It is thought that to design a sophisticated scheme for the localization of individual vertebral bodies would be helpful first to design a computer-assisted scheme to analyze the vertebral geometry. Although extraction of intervertebral discs (or end plates) is one of the effective approaches, missing an intervertebral disc leads to failure in the localization of vertebral bodies. Pattern matching or a registration-based approach can localize the vertebral bodies without extracting intervertebral discs. However, variations in the individual's posture during CT scans or individual differences in spinal curvature may contribute to the performance deterioration of such an approach. In terms of implicit anatomic knowledge, ribs and thoracic vertebrae are contiguous bones. For this reason, we assume that the detection of individual ribs contributes to the scheme's improved performance for the localization of individual vertebral bodies.

Our new scheme was designed to have the following key steps: (1) re-forming CT images on the basis of the center line of the spinal canal to visually remove the

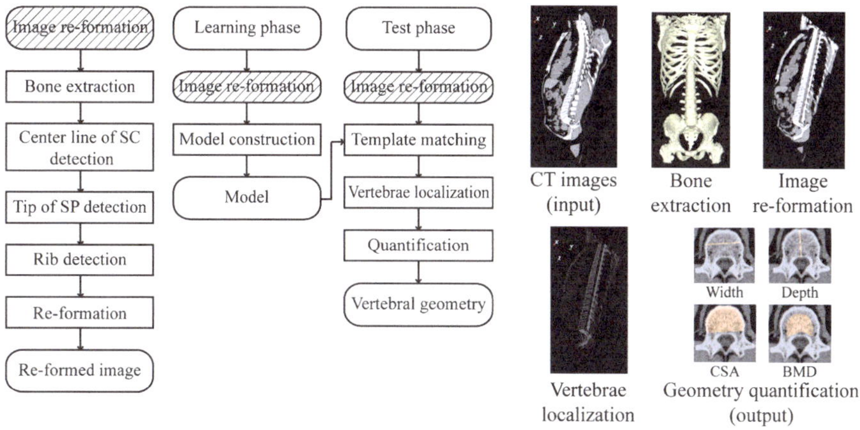

Fig. 7.7 Process flow of our scheme that quantifies the vertebral geometry (spinal canal: SC, spinous processes: SP) (modified from [25, 26])

spinal curvature, (2) using the information on the relative position between ribs and vertebral bodies, (3) the construction of a simple model (reference pattern) on the basis of the contour of the vertebral bodies on CT sections, (4) the localization of individual vertebral bodies by using a template matching technique, and (5) quantification of the vertebral body width, depth, cross-sectional area (CSA), and trabecular vBMD. This section summarized the publications in [25–27].

Computerized Scheme to Quantify the Vertebral Geometry

Overview of the Scheme

The proposed scheme is outlined in Fig. 7.7. It consists of the learning and test phases. The image re-formation technique, which is done on the basis of the detection/extraction of bone parts, is applied in both phases. The localization of vertebral bodies is carried out using a template matching technique. Afterward, the localization results are used to quantify the vertebral geometry. Each process is described below.

Image Re-Formation

At the beginning of the image re-formation technique, bone extraction and detection of the center line of the spinal canal, the tips of the spinous processes, and the ribs (boundary with vertebrae) are attempted. Examples of these extractions and detections are shown in Fig. 7.8.

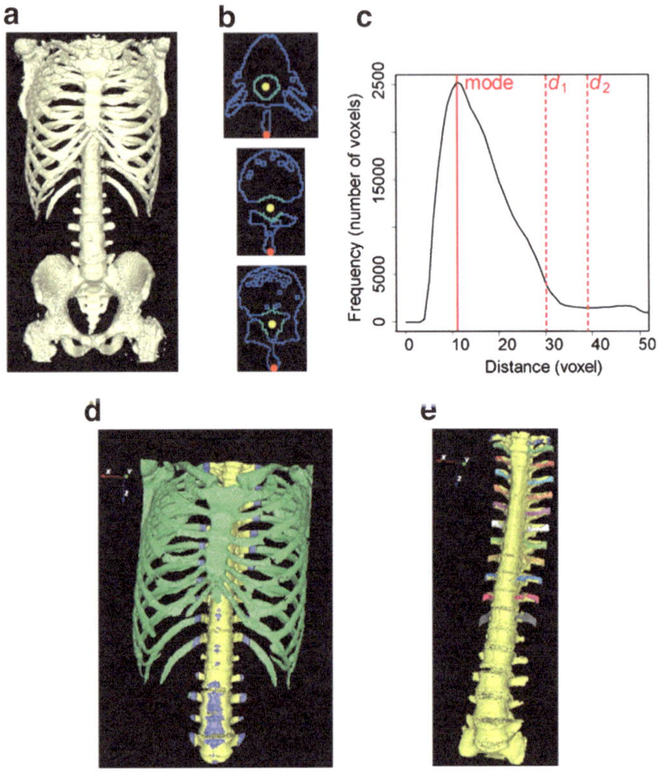

Fig. 7.8 Examples of bone parts detection/extraction in one case. (**a**) Surface view of bone voxels. (**b**) Three axial section views of bone voxels (*top* to *bottom*: T6, T11, and L3). *Yellow* and *red circles* denote centroids of the spinal canal and tips of spinous processes, respectively, and standard voxels and other bone voxels are indicated in *green* and *blue*, respectively. (**c**) The histogram of the distance map. d_1 and d_2 denote distance thresholds for dividing bone labels. (**d**) Surface view of bone voxels divided into three labels (*spine_label*, *boundary_label*, and *the_others_label* are indicated in *yellow*, *blue*, and *green*, respectively). (**e**) Surface view of bone voxels identified right and left ribs in each level (spine and ribs in each level are shown in *yellow* and the other *colors*, respectively) (adapted from [25])

CT numbers with bone voxels are higher than those of other internal organs. CT number thresholding or the region-growing method is used to extract bone voxels [28]. Figure 7.8a shows an example of extraction of bone voxels.

We can observe the spinal canal as a cave inside the spine. For that reason, the centroid of the cave on the Jacoby line (an upper boundary slice with a false pelvis) is determined. After that, it is tracked in the craniocaudal direction [29].

Spinous processes can be observed as tips of bone behind the spinal canal. Therefore, these tips of bone are detected on axial sections excluding the tail sections from the Jacoby line. Detection of the center line of the spinal canal and tips of spinous processes in three axial sections (from top to bottom: T6, T11, and L3) are shown in Fig. 7.8b. In these sections, yellow and red circles denote centroids of the spinal canal and tips of spinous processes, respectively.

Ribs are contiguous bones with the spine. In our scheme, ribs are detected on the basis of their distance from the spinal canal. The detailed process is as follows:

1. Bone voxels within r mm of the center line of the spinal canal are extracted as standard voxels. Extraction examples in three axial sections are illustrated in Fig. 7.8b. In these sections, standard voxels and other bone voxels are indicated with green and blue, respectively.
2. The distance map from standard voxels is generated. The distance is calculated by the shortest path through the bone voxels.
3. The histogram of the distance map is generated, and its mode and a standard deviation are computed. While frequency values increase with increasing distance within the spine, they decrease with increasing distance at the ribs because they are thinner than the spine. Therefore, the following equations are defined for dividing three bone labels (*spine_label*, *boundary_label*, and *the_others_label*) using the distance map:

$$0 < spine\_label \leq d_1, \tag{7.2}$$

$$d_1 < boundary\_label \leq d_2, \tag{7.3}$$

$$d_2 < the\_others\_label, \tag{7.4}$$

$$d_1 = move\_value + standard\_deviation \cdot b_1, \tag{7.5}$$

and

$$d_2 = move\_value + standard\_deviation \cdot b_2, \tag{7.6}$$

where d_1 and d_2 denote distance thresholds and b_1 and b_2 denote arbitrary variables. The histogram of the distance map and an example of the division into three bone labels are illustrated in Fig. 7.8c, d, respectively. In Fig. 7.8d, *spine_label*, *boundary_label*, and *the_others_label* are indicated in yellow, blue, and green, respectively. We can see the relation between distance map and bone labels in these figures.
4. Of the boundary labels, labels contiguous to both the *spine_label* and *the_others_label* are detected as *rib_candidate_labels*.
5. Of the *rib_candidate_labels*, 12 labels from the head are identified as the 1st–12th ribs. This identification is performed independently on the right and left sides. An example of 1st–12th ribs identification is demonstrated in Fig. 7.8e, in which the spine and the right and left ribs in each level are shown in yellow and the other colors, respectively.

To simplify the localization of vertebral bodies, CT images are re-formed on the basis of the spinal canal and spinous processes. The following three rules are applied to image re-formation.

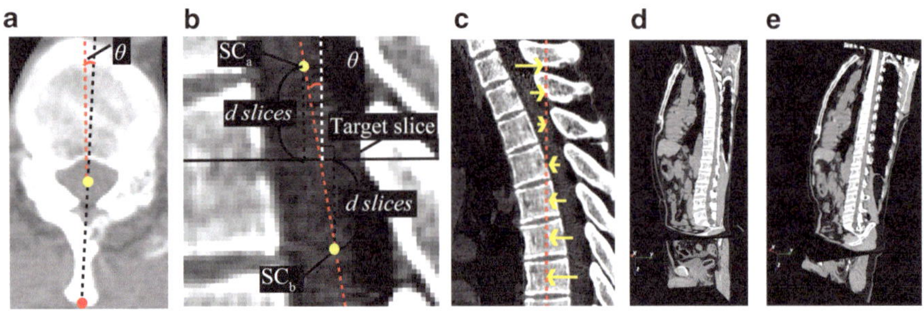

Fig. 7.9 CT images re-formation based on the spinal canal and spinous processes. (**a**) An axial section view of the spine. *Yellow* and *red circles* denote centroid of the spinal canal and the tip of spinous processes, respectively, and an axial rotation of this section is defined as the angle between the *black dashed line* via centroid of the spinal canal and the tip of spinous processes and *red dashed line* that indicates vertical line. (**b**) A sagittal section view of the spine. SC_a and SC_b denote centroid of the spinal canal on two axial sections. Sagittal rotation at a target slice is defined as the angle between the *red dashed line* via SC_a and SC_b and the *white dashed line* that indicates vertical line. (**c**) A sagittal section view of the spine. The translation is performed so that the center line of the spinal canal moves onto the straight line (*red dashed line*). (**d**) Section view of CT images. We can see the spinal curvature. (**e**) Section view of re-formed images. We can see the spine without its rotation and curvature (adapted from [25])

1. Axial rotation is adjusted in each slice so that the line via the center line of the spinal canal and tips of the spinous processes (that is, the black dashed line shown in Fig. 7.9a) becomes the center in the sagittal direction.
2. Sagittal rotation is adjusted in each slice. Sagittal curvature at a target slice (an axial section) is defined as the angle between the centroids of the spinal canal on two axial sections (that is, SC_a and SC_b shown in Fig. 7.9b). Two axial sections are determined as those that are far from the *d* slices of the target.
3. Translation is carried out in each slice so that the center line of the spinal canal moves onto a straight line (Fig. 7.9c).

Examples of CT images and re-formed CT images are demonstrated in Fig. 7.9d, e, respectively. We can see the spine in the reformed images without its rotation and curvature, as shown in Fig. 7.9e.

Learning Phase

CT images are re-formed to the beginning of a learning phase using the above-mentioned process. After that, the contour models of each vertebral body are built on the re-formed images as follows.

1. Contours of vertebral bodies (T1–L5) are tracked on the sagittal central section (Fig. 7.10a).
2. Contours of the vertebral bodies are tracked on axial and coronal sections through the center of the vertebral bodies that were tracked by the preceding

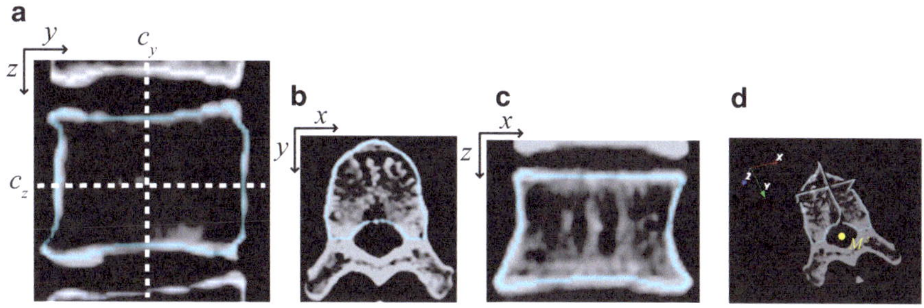

Fig. 7.10 Model building based on the contour tracking (tracked contours are indicated in *blue*). (**a**) An example of the tracked contour on the sagittal section. c_y and c_z denote the center position in the tracked contour on this section. (**b**) An example of the tracked contour on the axial section at c_z. (**c**) An example of the tracked contour on the coronal section at c_y. (**d**) Examples of tracked contours on three sections (adapted from [25])

process (that is, the axial section at c_z and the coronal section at c_y, as shown in Fig. 7.10a). Examples of tracked contours on the axial and coronal sections are illustrated in Fig. 7.10b, c, respectively.

3. Tracked contours are registered as relative coordinates from the center point (one from the center line, M^s) of the spinal canal. M^s, which is the centroid of the spinal canal on the axial section at c_z, is defined as the standard coordinate of the model. Examples of tracked contours on three sections are shown in Fig. 7.10d.

Test Phase (Localization)

CT images are re-formed to the beginning of a test phase using the above-mentioned process. After that, the vertebral bodies are localized as follows.

1. The morphological top-hat operation is applied to the target (re-formed) images, and voxels with >5 values are extracted as contour candidates of vertebral bodies. The target images, images after top-hat operation, and images after binarized operation are shown in Fig. 7.11a–c (left side), respectively.
2. Ribs are utilized for the localization of thoracic vertebrae. First, the shortest paths that connect the ribs on both sides via bone voxels for the k-th ribs ($k = 1, 2, \cdots, 12$) are computed. After that, axial sections of one point, S_z^k ($k = 1, 2, \cdots, 12$), nearest to the center line of the spinal canal for each path are detected. As for lumbar vertebrae, axial sections are predicted on the basis of the upper ribs:

$$S_z^k = S_z^{k-1} + \left(S_z^{k-1} - S_z^{k-2}\right)(k = 13, 14, \cdots, 18). \tag{7.7}$$

3. A template matching between the output of process 1 and models of vertebral bodies is performed to determine the precision between them. In the template matching, a rigid transformation is applied to the models, and the model whose

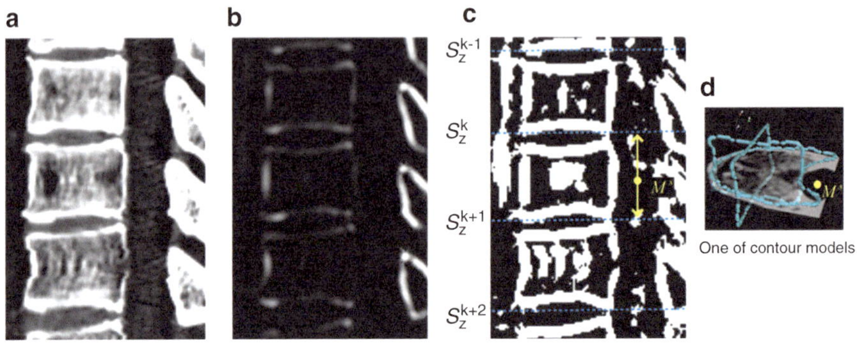

Fig. 7.11 Localizations of vertebral bodies by using a template matching technique. (**a**) Sagittal central section on the re-formed images. (**b**) Images after top-hat operation. (**c**) *Left*: Images after binarized operation. *Right*: One of the contour models indicates in *blue*. Blue voxels denote contours of the model (adapted from [25])

precision indicates the highest value is determined to be the target vertebral body. The rigid transformation is applied according to the following restrictions.

(a) Scaling, $s(0.9 \leq s \leq 1.1)$, is applied to the models.
(b) Rotation, $\gamma(-3.0^\circ \leq \gamma \leq 3.0^\circ)$, is applied to the models.
(c) Translation along the center line of the spinal canal is applied to the models. Ranges of translation are set for each vertebral body. For the k-th thoracic vertebral bodies, the standard coordinate of models should meet the following requirement:

$$S_z^k \leq M_z^s \leq S_z^{k+1} \ (k = 1, 2, \cdots, 12), \tag{7.8}$$

and for the k-th lumbar vertebral bodies, the standard coordinate of models should meet the following requirement:

$$S_z^{k+12} \leq M_z^s \leq S_z^{k+13} \ \ (k = 1, 2, \cdots, 5). \tag{7.9}$$

Translation of the model is illustrated in Fig. 7.11c. The percent of precision P of the template matching is calculated by the following equation:

$$P = \frac{P_A \cap P_B}{P_A}, \tag{7.10}$$

where P_A denotes voxels making up the model and P_B denotes voxels extracted by the process 1.

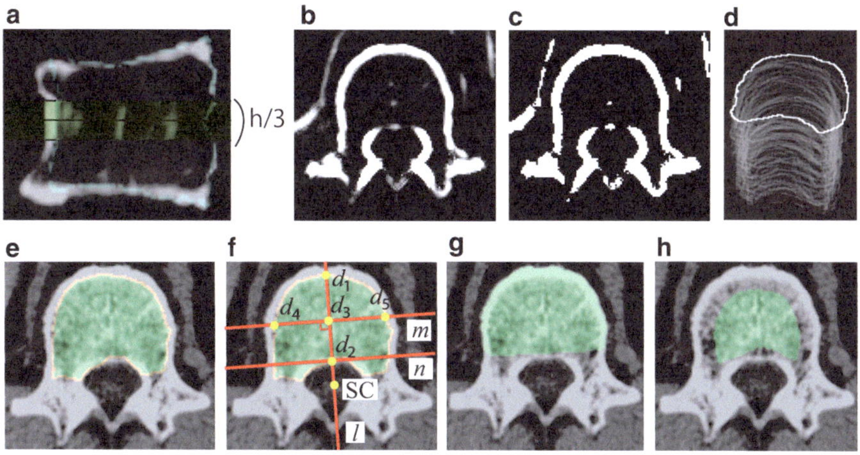

Fig. 7.12 The proposed scheme for vertebral body geometry. (**a**) Volume of interest (VOI) determination on the midsagittal section (the located vertebra is shown in *aqua*, and the VOI is shown in *green*). (**b**) A ray summation axial view of the VOI after applying the morphological top-hat operation. (**c**) Binarization. (**d**) Contour models of the target vertebra on a midaxial section with 100 cases. (**e**) Model fitting on a midaxial section (the fitted contour model is shown in *orange*, and inside of the vertebra is shown in *green*). (**f**) Geometric definition for vertebral body geometry on a midaxial section (SC denotes the spinal canal centroid). (**g**) One CSA example on a midaxial section (CSA is indicated in *green*). (**h**) One BMD measurement example on the ray summation axial view of the VOI without using morphological operation (the measurement region is indicated in *green*) (adapted from [26])

Test Phase (Quantification)

The computerized scheme for quantifying width, depth, CSA, and trabecular vBMD of vertebral bodies is described as follows.

1. Vertebral body height (h) is identified as the distance between the uppermost and lowermost slice, including the points produced using the localization scheme, and its central section is detected as the midaxial section of the target vertebral body. The h and the midaxial section of the target vertebra are detected, and then the axial sections of $h/3$ that belong to middle sections are selected as the VOI (Fig. 7.12a).
2. The morphological top-hat operation is applied to the VOI. After that, a ray summation image of the VOI is generated (Fig. 7.12b) and voxels with >20 values are extracted as contour candidates of vertebra (Fig. 7.12c).
3. The vertebral contour is determined by a template matching technique with contour models of the vertebral bodies built by manual tracking of the vertebral contour on the midaxial section (Fig. 7.12d). In the template matching technique, rigid transformation is applied according to the following restrictions:

   (a) Scaling, $s(0.9 \leq s \leq 1.1)$, is applied to the models.
   (b) Rotation, $r(-3.0^\circ \leq r \leq 3.0^\circ)$, is applied to the models.

Then, the precisions of the output of the process 2 and the transformed contour models are computed, and the transformed model with the highest indicated precision is selected as the target vertebral contour. The percent of precision P of the template matching is calculated by the following equation:

$$P = \frac{P_A \cap P_B}{P_A}, \tag{7.11}$$

where P_A denotes voxels that make up the model and P_B denotes voxels extracted by process 2. After that, voxels inside the vertebral contour are filled (Fig. 7.12e).

4. Line l, which divides equally the filled region that passes through the spinal canal centroid, is drawn. Next, two points, d_1 and d_2, are detected at the boundary of the line l with the filled region, and the distance between d_1 and d_2 is defined as "depth" (Fig. 7.12f).
5. Line m perpendicular to the line l that passes through point d_3, which is in the middle between d_1 and d_2, is drawn. Next, two points, d_4 and d_5, are detected at the boundary of the line m with the filled region, and the distance between d_4 and d_5 is defined as "width" (Fig. 7.12f).
6. Line n parallel to the line m that passes through point d_2 is drawn. Next, a cortical bone adjacent to the filled region is added as a part of the filled region. After that, the number of voxels that belongs to the filled region that is located anterior to the line n is defined as "CSA" (Fig. 7.12g).
7. To remove a cortical bone, voxels extracted by the process 2 are removed. After that, the morphological closing operation is applied to fill the voxels of the vertebral contour. To ensure that a cortical bone is not included, the morphological erosion operation is also applied to the extracted region.
8. A ray summation image of the VOI without using the morphological operation is generated, and the mean CT number of voxels overlapping with the extracted region from the process 7 is computed. Finally, "trabecular vBMD" is estimated on the basis of the mean CT number in a manner similar to the section "Estimation of vBMD" (Fig. 7.12h).

Performance Evaluation

Assessments

The Hausdorff distance [30], which is used to measure the boundary-based distance, was used to demonstrate the effect of the localization scheme. Given two finite point sets $A = \{a_1, a_2, \cdots, a_p\}$ and $B = \{b_1, b_2, \cdots, b_p\}$, the Hausdorff distance is defined as

$$H(A, B) = \max(h(A, B), h(B, A)), \tag{7.12}$$

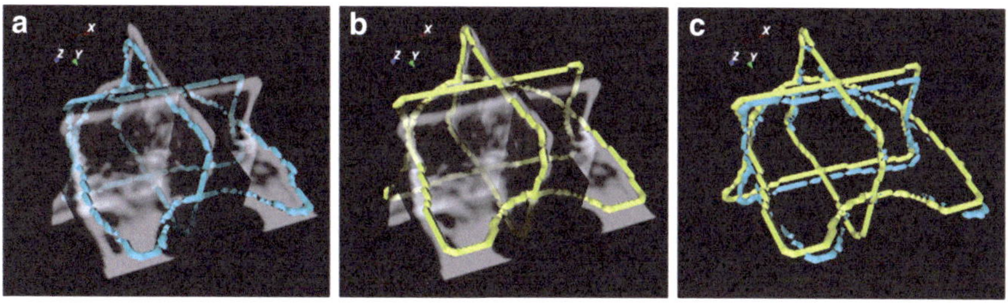

Fig. 7.13 Examples of the measurement by using the Hausdorff distance. (**a**) Points of contours of vertebral bodies by manual (*blue*). (**b**) Points produced using the localization scheme (*yellow*). (**c**) Overlaid image of two point sets. Hausdorff distance between two point sets is determined as the performance assessment (adapted from [25])

where

$$h(A, B) = \max_{a \in A} \min_{b \in B} \|a - b\|, \tag{7.13}$$

and $\|\cdot\|$ is some underlying norm on the points of A and B. In the experiment, the points of the contour of vertebral bodies tracked on re-formed images (ground truth) and points produced using the localization scheme were input as A and B, respectively, and the Euclidean norm was used as the underlying norm. One example of the measurement of the Hausdorff distance is illustrated in Fig. 7.13.

The performance of the quantification scheme was assessed by comparing it with the manual tracking done by an anatomic expert. For vertebral body width, depth, and CSA, manual tracking was carried out three times at the midaxial sections of L1 on "original" CT scans (not re-formed images), and mean values were determined to be the grand truth. Each tracking was set at a time interval of at least 1 week, and the position of the midaxial section of L1 was selected independently. For trabecular BMD, vBMD at the central site of the vertebral body measured in [20] was used as the grand truth. Pearson's product–moment correlation coefficient (r) and Bland–Altman analysis [31] were used to show relative and absolute reliability.

Vertebrae Localization

To assess the performance of the vertebrae localization scheme, it was applied to 104 body CT cases. Learning models were built with 103 samples except for the target case, and parameters were set as $r = 16$ mm, $d = 20$ slices, $b_1 = 3.0$, and $b_2 = 4.5$ for this experiment. These parameters were decided by trial and error. The localization performance from T2 to L5 was assessed in this study because T1 was outside of the CT scans with some cases. Experimental results from two cases are illustrated in Fig. 7.14.

The assessment result of the localization scheme is shown in Fig. 7.15, in which we can see the Hausdorff distance (mean and standard deviation) with 104 cases in

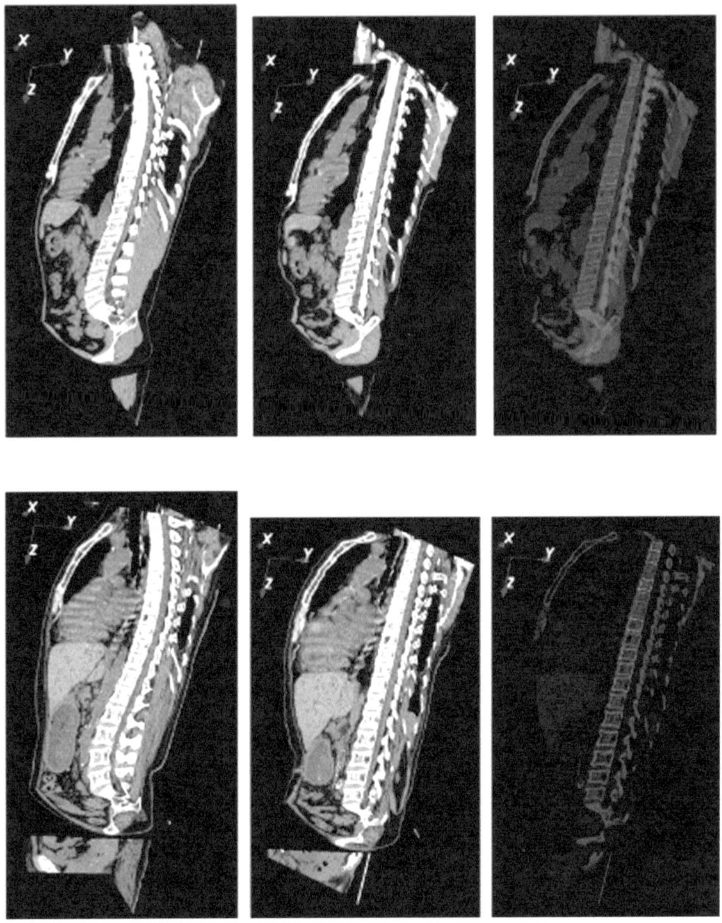

Fig. 7.14 Vertebrae localization results from two cases. *Left*: Section view of CT images. *Middle*: Section view of the re-formed images. *Right*: Section view of the overlaid images between the re-formed images and points produced using the localization scheme. Localization results of individual vertebral bodies are indicated in different *colors* (adapted from [25])

each vertebral level. The mean and standard deviations of the Hausdorff distance for the localization of vertebral bodies were 3.6–5.5 and 1.0–1.9 mm, respectively.

In addition, the following experiment was carried out to verify the effect of the learning models:

1. Samples were selected at random from 103 cases (except the target case).
2. Samples selected by the process 1 were used to build the learning models.
3. Localizations of vertebral bodies were carried out using models built by the process 2. After that, the Hausdorff distance between the localization result and the ground truth was measured.
4. The processes 1–3 were attempted 10 times, and the mean Hausdorff distance of their results was calculated.

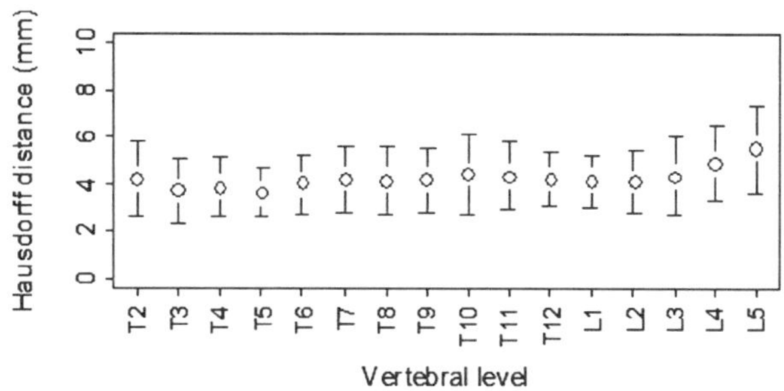

Fig. 7.15 Performance assessment by the Hausdorff distance. The mean and standard deviation of the Hausdorff distance for individual vertebral bodies by 104 cases are shown in *circle* and *error bar*, respectively (adapted from [25])

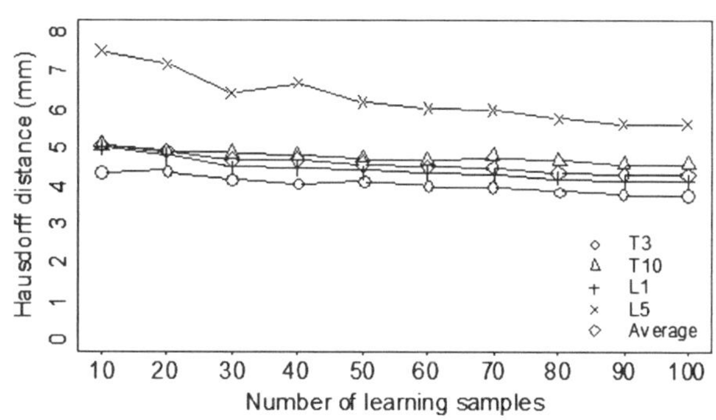

Fig. 7.16 The change in the mean Hausdorff distance according to the number of learning samples for the localization of vertebral bodies. The mean Hausdorff distances at T3, T10, L1, L5, and the average of T2–L5 are shown (adapted from [25])

The change in the mean Hausdorff distance according to the number of learning samples for the localization of vertebral bodies is shown in Fig. 7.16, which shows the mean Hausdorff distance at T3, T10, L1, L5, and the average of T2–L5. The average Hausdorff distance of T2–L5 from the learning models with 100 samples was 4.3 mm. On the other hand, the average Hausdorff distance with ten samples was 5.1 mm. In terms of vertebral level, the Hausdorff distance with L3–L5 was larger than that of other vertebrae.

Vertebral Geometry Quantification

To assess the performance of the quantification scheme, it was applied to ten body CT cases. Vertebral contour models were built with 100 samples except for the target case. Figure 7.17 illustrates the quantification scheme as well as measurement examples of vertebral body width, depth, and CSA taken by an anatomic expert. These measurements were done on the midaxial sections of L1. Figure 7.17 also enables us to understand intra-observer variability and to compare manual tracking with computerized tracking. Manual tracking done by an anatomic expert showed vertebral body width $= 37.1 \pm 1.07$ mm, depth $= 27.6 \pm 0.38$ mm, and CSA $= 920.4 \pm 60.7$ mm^2. In contrast, computerized measurements using the quantification scheme showed vertebral body width $= 33.5$ mm, depth $= 26.7$ mm, and CSA $= 818.2$ mm^2. A measurement example of the vertebral trabecular BMD

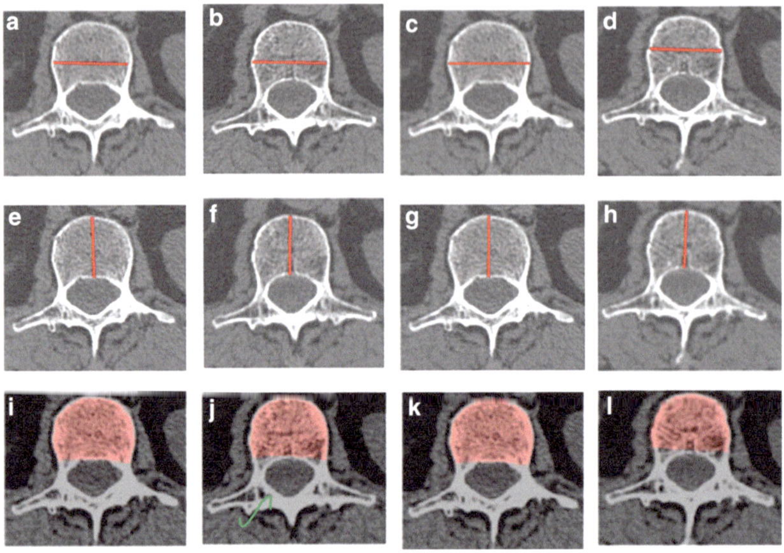

Fig. 7.17 Measurement examples of the vertebral body width (**a**–**d**), depth (**e**–**h**), and CSA (**i**–**l**) by an anatomy expert and the quantification scheme. These are the midaxial sections of L1 and measurement results of vertebral body width, depth, and CSA are shown in *red*. Manual tracking of first (**a**, **e**, **i**), second (**b**, **f**, **j**), third (**c**, **g**, **k**) and the points produced using the quantification scheme (**d**, **h**, **l**) are shown from *left* to *right* (adapted from [26])

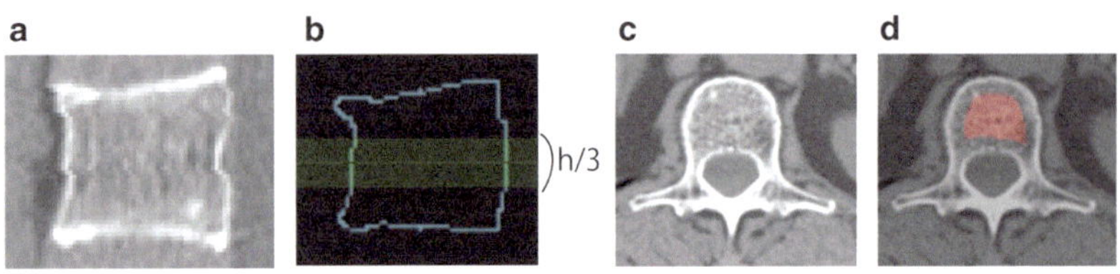

Fig. 7.18 Measurement example of the vertebral trabecular BMD at L1. (**a**) Midsagittal section on the re-formed CT images. (**b**) Volume of interest (VOI) determination on the midsagittal section (the located vertebra is shown in *aqua*, and the VOI is shown in *green*), (**c**) A ray summation axial view of VOI on the re-formed CT images, (**d**) BMD measurement on the ray summation axial view of the VOI (the measurement region is indicated in *red*) (adapted from [26])

at L1 is illustrated in Fig. 7.18, which also shows the process flow of the proposed scheme in measuring vertebral trabecular BMD. The vertebral trabecular BMD measured by [20] was 68.9 mg/cm^3, while that measured by the proposed scheme was 67.8 mg/cm^3.

The correlations of the vertebral geometries between the proposed scheme and manual tracking are shown in Fig. 7.19. As can be seen, moderate correlation was found in measuring depth [$r = 0.72$, $P = 0.02$, 95 % confidence interval (95 % CI) of the population correlation coefficient: 0.16–0.93], and high correlations were

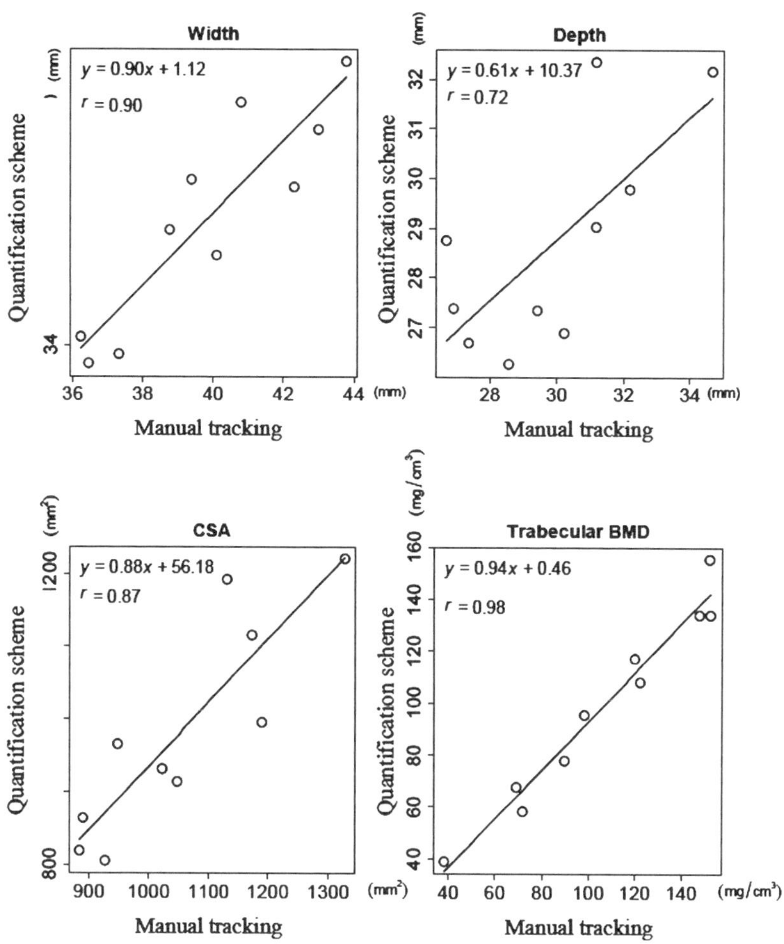

Fig. 7.19 The correlations of vertebral geometries between the quantification scheme and manual tracking by using Pearson's product–moment correlation coefficient (adapted from [26])

found in measuring width ($r = 0.90$, $P < 0.01$, 95 % CI: 0.63–0.98), CSA ($r = 0.87$, $P < 0.01$, 95 % CI: 0.54–0.97), and trabecular BMD ($r = 0.98$, $P < 0.01$, 95 % CI: 0.92–1.00), respectively.

Bland–Altman plots of vertebral geometries from the quantification scheme and the manual tracking are indicated in Fig. 7.20, which shows mean differences of width, depth, CSA, and trabecular BMD of 3.1 mm, 1.4 mm, 88.7 mm^2, and 7.3 mg/cm^3, respectively. No proportional biases were found for all four vertebral geometries between the proposed scheme and manual tracking when testing for no correlation. However, the 95 % CI of mean associated with width, depth, CSA, and BMD did not contain zero, as seen in Fig. 7.20. Namely, fixed biases in measuring these vertebral geometries between two methods were found. Therefore, it should be noted that careful checks by examiners will be required to use the measurement results of our scheme.

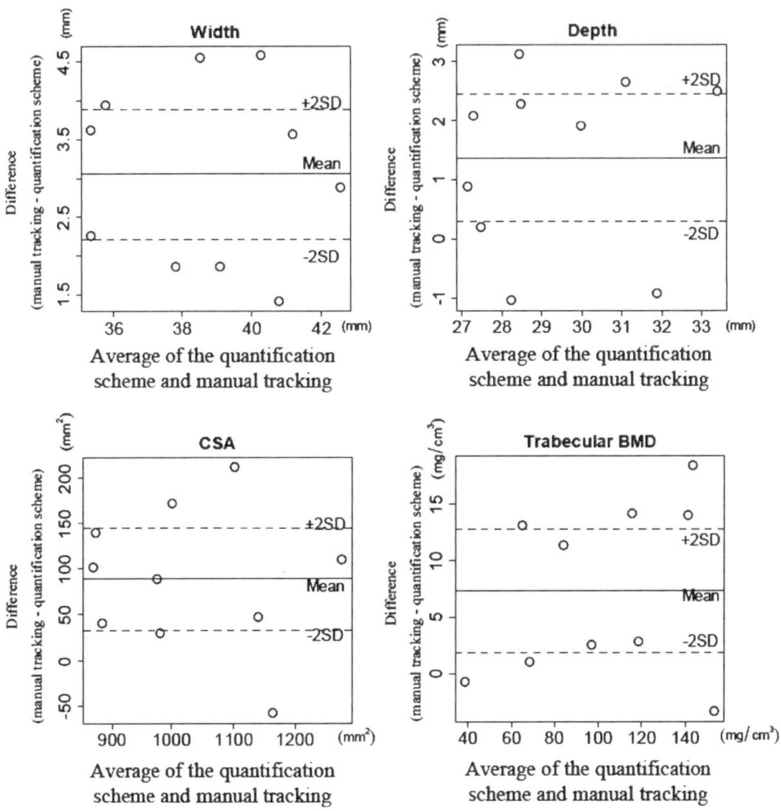

Fig. 7.20 Bland–Altman analysis of vertebral geometries between the quantification scheme and manual tracking. Three lines: mean, mean + 2 standard deviation (SD), and mean − 2 SD = limits of agreement (adapted from [26])

Summary

This chapter described our latest findings on image analysis and statistical analysis for vertebral anatomy by use of the image processing technique on MDCT scanning (Fig. 7.21). The population-based statistical analysis for vertebral trabecular vBMD was shown in the section "Computer-Aided Analysis of vBMD at Trabecular Bones in Thoracic and Lumbar Vertebrae." To the best of our knowledge, our retrospective analysis was the largest single-institutional study to investigate the vertebral trabecular vBMD. The section "Computer-Based Quantification of Vertebral Body Geometry" presented a computerized scheme to quantify the vertebral geometry. The scheme provided appropriate values on the vertebral geometry with numerous CT cases. Therefore, such successful CT cases were used to the preliminary study for statistical analysis on the vertebral geometry in [32].

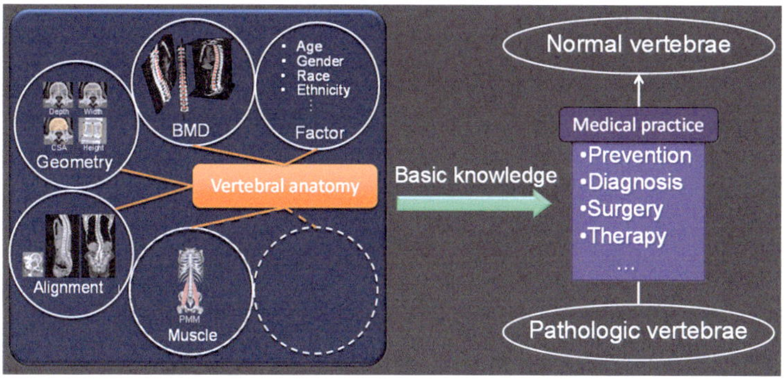

Fig. 7.21 Image analysis for obtaining sophisticated vertebral anatomy by use of the MDCT scanning (psoas major muscle: PMM, recuts abdominis muscle: RAM) (modified from [26, 27, 29, 32, 36, 37])

It is known that spinal sagittal curvature contributes to maintaining spinal balance and protecting impact. Alterations in the spinal sagittal curvature are deemed to be implicated in the development of various spinal disorders [33]. Furthermore, Sinaki et al. [34] state that stronger back muscles reduce the incidence of vertebral fractures. Namely, it is suggested that muscles are the important factor in determining the vertebral fracture as well as the vertebrae. Measurements of the vBMD, geometry, "zero load" alignment, and muscle mass from the same dataset are allowed by use of the MDCT scanning. It seems reasonable to suppose that a computer-based image analysis technology becomes increasingly important to obtain such a sophisticated vertebral anatomy.

In the field of medical imaging technology, numerous computer-based schemes have been proposed every year. For example, the computerized schemes to quantify the spinal curvature on the MDCT scanning were presented in [29, 35]. Muscle segmentation schemes by using MDCT scanning were also shown in [36, 37]. These technologies may be useful to improve our knowledge of vertebral anatomy. However, it is likely that the demand for the medical imaging technology will continue to grow. To achieve a further innovation of the medical imaging technology, the state-of-the-art project entitled "Computational anatomy for computer-aided diagnosis and therapy: Frontiers of medical image sciences" is currently in progress in Japan [38].

Acknowledgments The authors thank members of the Fujita Laboratory for their valuable discussion and are grateful to Gifu University Hospital staff for preparing the CT cases, especially to Dr. Kamiya N, Mr. Miyoshi T, Mr. Inoue Y, Dr. Yokoyama R, Dr. Kanematsu M, and Dr. Hoshi H. This research was supported in part by a research grant of Grant-in-Aid for Young Scientists B (21700462) from Japan Society for the Promotion of Science (JSPS), in part by a research grant from Japan Osteoporosis Foundation, and in part by a research grant of Grant-in-Aid for Scientific Research on Priority Areas (21103004) of the Ministry of Education, Culture, Sports, Science, and Technology, Japan.

References

1. McDonnell P, McHugh PE, O'Mahoney D (2007) Vertebral osteoporosis and trabecular bone quality. Ann Biomed Eng 35:170–189. doi:10.1007/s10439-006-9239-9
2. Geusens P, Sambrook P, Lindsay R (2004) Osteoporosis in clinical practice: a practical guide for diagnosis and treatment, 2nd edn. Springer, New York
3. Alan M (2010) Two-thirds of spinal fractures undiagnosed, untreated: report. HealthDay: News for Healthier Living (15 October 2010)
4. Gehlbach SH, Fournier M, Bigelow C (2002) Recognition of osteoporosis by primary care physicians. Am J Public Health 92:271–273. doi:10.2105/AJPH.92.2.271
5. Klemetti E, Kolmakov S, Kröger H (1994) Pantomography in assessment of the osteoporosis risk group. Scand J Dent Res 102:68–72. doi:10.1111/j.1600-0722.1994.tb01156.x
6. Taguchi A, Ohtsuka M, Nakamoto T, Naito K, Tsuda M, Kudo Y, Motoyama E, Suei Y, Tanimoto K (2007) Identification of post-menopausal women at risk of osteoporosis by trained general dental practitioners using panoramic radiographs. Dentomaxillofac Radiol 36:149–154. doi:10.1259/dmfr/31116116
7. Hashimoto M, Ito A, Yoneyama M, Takizawa H, Miyamura K (2007) Construction of osteoporosis identification system by panoramic radiographs. J Jpn Dent Assoc 60:626–633 (in Japanese)
8. Taguchi A (2010) Triage screening for osteoporosis in dental clinics using panoramic radiographs. Oral Dis 16:316–327. doi:10.1111/j.1601-0825.2009.01615.x
9. Taguchi A, Nakamoto T, Asano A (2011) Osteoporosis diagnosis support device using panorama X-ray image. US Patent 2006/0239532 A1, 24 Aug 2006
10. Asano A, Taguchi A, Nakamoto T, Tanimoto K, Arifin AZ (2011) Osteoporosis diagnosis support device. US Patent 7,916,921 B2, 29 Mar 2011
11. Kavitha MS, Samopa F, Asano A, Taguchi A, Sanada M (2012) Computer-aided measurement of mandibular cortical width on dental panoramic radiographs for identifying osteoporosis. J Investig Clin Dent 3:36–44. doi:10.1111/j.2041-1626.2011.00095.x
12. Devlin H, Allen PD, Graham J, Jacobs R, Karayianni K, Lindh C, van der Stelt PF, Harrison E, Adams JE, Pavitt S, Horner K (2007) Automated osteoporosis risk assessment by dentists: a new pathway to diagnosis. Bone 40:835–842. doi:10.1016/j.bone.2006.10.024
13. Allen PD, Graham J, Farnell DJ, Harrison EJ, Jacobs R, Nicopolou-Karayianni K, Lindh C, van der Stelt PF, Horner K, Devlin H (2007) Detecting reduced bone mineral density from dental radiographs using statistical shape models. IEEE Trans Inf Technol Biomed 11:601–610. doi:10.1109/TITB.2006.888704
14. Roberts MG, Graham J, Devlin H (2010) Improving the detection of osteoporosis from dental radiographs using active appearance models. In: IEEE international symposium on transactions on biomedical engineering: from nano to macro, pp 440–443. doi:10.1109/ISBI.2010.5490314
15. Matsumoto T, Hayashi T, Hara T, Katsumata A, Muramatsu C, Zhou X, Iida Y, Matsuoka M, Katagi K, Fujita H (2012) Automated scheme for measuring mandibular cortical thickness on dental panoramic radiographs for osteoporosis screening. In: van Ginneken B, Novak CL (eds) Proceedings of SPIE medical imaging 2012: computer-aided diagnosis, vol 8315, Bellingham, pp 83152L. doi:10.1117/12.912309
16. Hayashi T, Matsumoto T, Hara T, Katsumata A, Muramatsu C, Zhou X, Iida Y, Matsuoka M, Fujita H (2012) A computerized system for identifying osteoporotic patients on dental panoramic radiographs. ECR 2012, Vienna. doi:10.1594/ecr2012/C-1110
17. Hayashi T, Matsumoto T, Sawagashira T, Tagami M, Katsumata A, Hayashi Y, Muramatsu C, Zhou X, Iida Y, Matsuoka M, Katagi K, Fujita H (2012) A new screening pathway for identifying asymptomatic patients using dental panoramic radiographs. In: van Ginneken B, Novak CL (eds) Proceedings of SPIE medical imaging 2012: computer-aided diagnosis, vol 8315, Bellingham, p 83152K. doi:10.1117/12.911791

18. Ruyssen-Witrand A, Gossec L, Kolta S, Dougados M, Roux C (2007) Vertebral dimensions as risk factor of vertebral fracture in osteoporotic patients: a systematic literature review. Osteoporos Int 18:1271–1278. doi:10.1007/s00198-007-0356-6
19. Kobayashi T, Takeda N, Atsuta Y, Matsuno T (2008) Flattening of sagittal spinal curvature as a predictor of vertebral fracture. Osteoporos Int 19:65–69. doi:10.1007/s00198-007-0432-y
20. Hayashi T, Chen H, Miyamoto K, Zhou X, Hara T, Yokoyama R, Kanematsu M, Hoshi H, Fujita H (2011) Analysis of bone mineral density distribution at trabecular bones in thoracic and lumbar vertebrae using X-ray CT images. J Bone Miner Metab 29:174–185. doi:10.1007/s00774-010-0204-1
21. Hayashi T, Chen H, Miyamoto K, Zhou X, Hara T, Yokoyama R, Kanematsu M, Hoshi H, Fujita H (2011) Investigation of the new fracture risk prediction on the basis of the vertebral morphometry on X-ray CT images: interim report. Osteoporos Jpn 19:97–102 (in Japanese)
22. Hayashi T, Zhou Z, Chen H, Hara T, Fujita H, Yokoyama R, Kanematsu M, Hoshi H (2008) Investigation on the distribution of low bone-mineral-density locations at human vertebral trabecular bone from X-ray CT images. Trans Jpn Soc Med Biol Eng 46:451–457 (in Japanese)
23. Hayashi T, Zhou X, Hara T, Fujita H, Yokoyama R, Kiryu T, Hoshi H (2006) Automated segmentation of the skeleton in torso X-ray volumetric CT images. Int J Comput Assist Radiol Surg 1(Suppl 1):522–523. doi:10.1007/s11548-006-0030-z
24. Cann CE, Genant HK (1980) Precise measurement of vertebral mineral content using computed tomography. J Comput Assist Tomogr 4:493–500
25. Hayashi T, Chen H, Miyamoto K, Zhou X, Hara T, Yokoyama R, Kanematsu M, Hoshi H, Fujita H (2011) A computerized scheme for localization of vertebral bodies on body CT scans. In: Dawant BM, Haynor DR (eds) Proceedings of SPIE medical imaging 2011: image processing, vol 7962, p 796238. doi:10.1117/12.877511
26. Hayashi T, Chen H, Miyamoto K, Zhou X, Hara T, Yokoyama R, Kanematsu M, Hoshi H, Fujita H (2011) A decision support scheme for vertebral geometry on body CT scans. In: Dawant BM, Haynor DR (eds) Proceedings of SPIE medical imaging 2011: image processing, vol 7962, p 796245. doi:10.1117/12.877516
27. Fujita H, Hara T, Zhou X, Hayashi T, Kamiya N, Zhang X, Chen H, Hoshi H (2011) Model construction for computational anatomy. Med Imag Technol 29:116–121 (in Japanese)
28. Zhou X, Hayashi T, Han M, Chen H, Hara T, Fujita H, Yokoyama R, Kanematsu M, Hoshi H (2009) Automated segmentation and recognition of the bone structure in non-contrast torso CT images using implicit anatomical knowledge. In: Pluim JPW, Dawant BM (eds) Proceedings of SPIE medical imaging 2009: image processing, vol 7259, p 72593S. doi:10.1117/12.812945
29. Hayashi T, Zhou X, Chen H, Hara T, Miyamoto K, Kobayashi T, Yokoyama R, Kanematsu M, Hoshi H, Fujita H (2010) Automated extraction method for the center line of spinal canal and its application to the spinal curvature quantification in torso X-ray CT images. In: Dawant BM, Haynor DR (eds) Proceedings of SPIE medical imaging 2010: image processing, vol 7623, p 76233F. doi:10.1117/12.843956
30. Huttenlocher DP, Klanderman GA, Rucklidge WJ (1993) Comparing images using the Hausdorff distance. IEEE Trans Pattern Anal Mach Intell 15:850–863. doi:10.1109/34.232073
31. Bland JM, Altman DG (2003) Statistical methods for assessing agreement between two methods of clinical measurement. Lancet 1:307–310. doi:10.1016/S0140-6736(86)90837-8
32. Hayashi T, Fujita H, Chen H, Tajima Y, Miyamoto K, Zhou X, Hara T, Yokoyama R, Kanematsu M, Hoshi H (2011) Correlation between vertebral body geometry and trabecular volumetric bone mineral density (vBMD) using X-ray CT images. Osteoporos Int 22(Suppl 1): S181. doi:10.1007/s00198-011-1567-4
33. Keller TS, Colloca CJ, Harrison DE, Harrison DD, Janik TJ (2005) Influence of spine morphology on intervertebral disc loads and stresses in asymptomatic adults: implications for the ideal spine. Spine J 5:297–309. doi:10.1016/j.spinee.2004.10.050
34. Sinaki M, Itoi E, Wahner HW, Wollan P, Gelzcer R, Mullan BP, Collins DA, Hodgson SF (2002) Stronger back muscles reduce the incidence of vertebral fractures: a prospective 10 year follow-up of postmenopausal women. Bone 30:836–841. doi:10.1016/S8756-3282(02)00739-1

35. Vrtovec T, Likar B, Pernuš F (2008) Quantitative analysis of spinal curvature in 3D: application to CT images of normal spine. Phys Med Biol 53:1895–1908. doi:10.1088/0031-9155/53/7/006
36. Kamiya N, Zhou X, Chen H, Muramatsu C, Hara T, Yokoyama R, Kanematsu M, Hoshi H, Fujita H (2011) Automated segmentation of recuts abdominis muscle using shape model in X-ray CT images. In: Conference proceedings of the IEEE Engineering Medical Biological Society, pp 7993–7996. doi:10.1109/IEMBS.2011.6091971
37. Kamiya N, Zhou X, Chen H, Muramatsu C, Hara T, Yokoyama R, Kanematsu M, Hoshi H, Fujita H (2012) Automated segmentation of psoas major muscle in X-ray CT images by use of a shape model: preliminary study. Radiol Phys Technol 5:5–14. doi:10.1007/s12194-011-0127-0
38. Computational anatomy for computer-aided diagnosis and therapy: frontiers of medical image sciences. http://comp-anatomy.org. Accessed 6 Mar 2012. This is funded by Grant-in-Aid for Scientific Research on Innovative Areas, MEXT, Japan

Chapter 8
Robust Segmentation of Challenging Lungs in CT Using Multi-stage Learning and Level Set Optimization

Neil Birkbeck, Michal Sofka, Timo Kohlberger, Jingdan Zhang, Jens Wetzl, Jens Kaftan, and S. Kevin Zhou

Abstract Automatic segmentation of lung tissue in thoracic CT scans is useful for diagnosis and treatment planning of pulmonary diseases. Unlike healthy lung tissue that is easily identifiable in CT scans, diseased lung parenchyma is hard to segment automatically due to its higher attenuation, inhomogeneous appearance, and inconsistent texture. We overcome these challenges through a multi-layer machine learning approach that exploits geometric structures both within and outside the lung (e.g., ribs, spine). In the coarsest layer, a set of stable landmarks on the surface of the lung are detected through a hierarchical detection network (HDN) that is trained on hundreds of annotated CT volumes. These landmarks are used to robustly initialize a coarse statistical model of the lung shape. Subsequently, a region-dependent boundary refinement uses a discriminative appearance classifier to refine the surface, and finally a region-driven level set refinement is used to extract the fine-scale detail. Through this approach we demonstrate robustness to a variety of lung pathologies.

Introduction

Thoracic CT images are clinically used for screening, diagnosis, and treatment planning of lung diseases [13, 14, 16]. Computer aided diagnosis (CAD) tools built for CT imaging rely on a segmentation of the lung as the first step [24].

N. Birkbeck (✉) • M. Sofka • T. Kohlberger • J. Zhang • J. Wetzl • S.K. Zhou
Siemens Corp., Corporate Technology, 755 College Road East, Plainsboro, NJ, 08540, USA
e-mail: neil.birkbeck@siemens.com; michal.sofka@siemens.com; timo.kohlberger@siemens.com; jingdan.zhang@siemens.com; shaohua.zhou@siemens.com

J. Kaftan
Siemens Molecular Imaging, 23–38 Hythe Bridge Street, Oxford, OX1 2EP, UK
e-mail: jens.kaftan@siemens.com

K. Suzuki (ed.), *Computational Intelligence in Biomedical Imaging*,
DOI 10.1007/978-1-4614-7245-2_8,

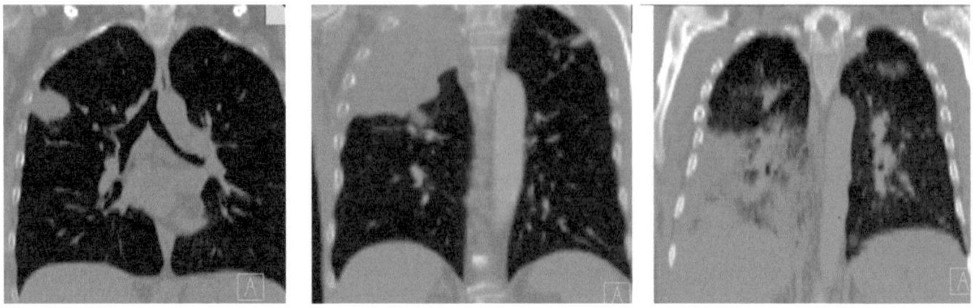

Fig. 8.1 Examples of how diseases, such as tumors or interstitial lung disease, affect the appearance of lung in CT

For example, algorithms for detection of malignant nodules [1, 15] and classification of lung tissue into various diseases [34, 37, 38, 40] restrict processing to within the lung regions only.

Further semantic decomposition of the lung tissue into lobes, e.g., [35, 41], and methods to visualize dynamic motion of lung function through respiratory cycles [8] also rely on a segmentation of the lung. As lung segmentation is an important prerequisite for these applications, it is important for it to be robust to abnormalities. Failures in the segmentation algorithm propagate to failures in further processing. In CAD applications, these failures mean a clinician may not be warned about a potential cancerous tumor [1].

Automatically segmenting healthy lung in CT is relatively easy due to low attenuation of lungs compared to surrounding tissue. Pathologies, such as interstitial lung disease (ILD), pleural effusion, and tumors, on the other hand, significantly change the shape, appearance, or texture of lung parenchyma (Fig. 8.1). In a clinical setting, pathologies are often no longer an exception but rather the norm, and methods robust to these variations are necessary.

In this article, we address the automatic segmentation of challenging cases described above and illustrated in Fig. 8.1. We first review the basic algorithms for segmenting healthy lung parenchyma and demonstrate the limitations of these algorithms in the presence of pathologies (Section "Segmenting Healthy Lungs"). We then discuss how texture cues, anatomical information, and statistical shape models, have been leveraged to improve robustness in the presence of disease. This is followed by the presentation of a method that utilizes machine learning with both texture cues and anatomical information from outside the lung to obtain a robust lung segmentation that is further improved with level set refinement (Section "Multi-Stage Learning for Lung Segmentation"). These algorithms are implemented in a modular software framework that promotes reuse and experimentation (Section "A Software Architecture for Detection and Segmentation").

Segmenting Healthy Lungs

As healthy lung parenchyma has lower attenuation than the surrounding tissue, simple image processing techniques often achieve good results. The attenuation of healthy lung tissue in CT varies across the lung, depends on the phase of respiratory cycle [25] and image acquisition settings [2], with mean values being around − 860 to − 700 HU [25]. However, as illustrated in Fig. 8.2, the intensity distribution within the lung region is often completely disjoint from that of the higher density body tissue. Thus simple image processing operations, such as region growing, edge tracking [10], or simple thresholding [4, 11, 23], can be used to separate lung from body tissue.

For example, thresholding methods first separate body tissue from surrounding background tissue by removing large connected components touching the edges of the images. Lung tissue can then be separated from the body tissue with a threshold. Hu et al. propose to use a dynamic threshold, τ, that is iteratively updated to be the mean of the average intensities between the lung and body, $\tau_t = (\mu^{t-1}_{\text{lung}} + \mu^{t-1}_{\text{body}})/2$, where μ^{t}_{lung} and μ^{t}_{body} are the mean HU values of the lying below and above τ_t, respectively [11]. The initial threshold, τ_0, is estimated with $\mu^{0}_{\text{lung}} = -1{,}000$ and μ^{0}_{body} is the average intensity of all HU values greater than 0.

Depending on the application, the final step is to separate the segmented lung tissue into left and right lungs. The thresholded lung regions are connected by the trachea and large airways and can be separated by region growing a trachea segmentation from the top of the segment [11, 39]. Further, the lungs often touch at the anterior and posterior junctions and need to be separated using another post-process that uses a maximum cut path to split the single lung component into the individual lungs [4, 11, 26].

The simple thresholding scheme gives a good gross estimate to the lung volume but often excludes small airways and vessels that a clinician would include with the lung annotation. These small regions can be filled through the use of morphological operations [11, 36], or by performing connected component analysis on the image slices [39] (see Fig. 8.3).

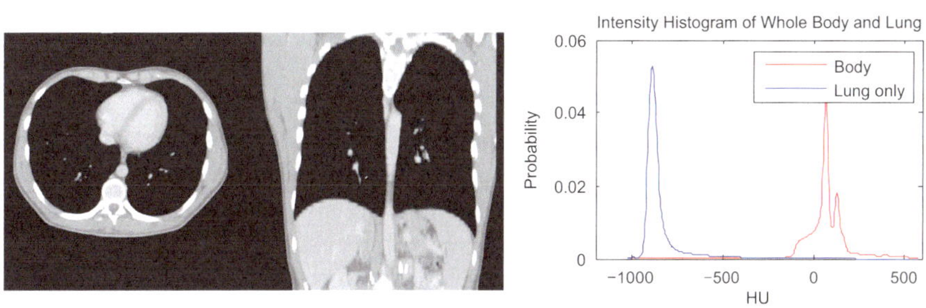

Fig. 8.2 Healthy lung tissue is easily separable from body tissue with a single threshold

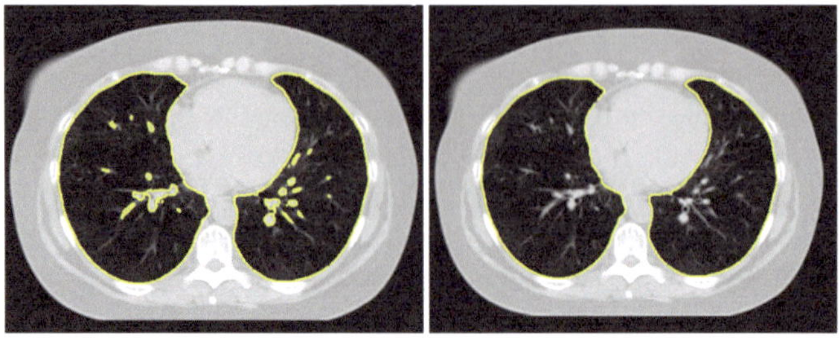

Fig. 8.3 Segmentation by simple thresholding often excludes airways and vessels (*left*). These vessels are easily removed by morphological operations or by removing small connected components on 2D slices (*right*)

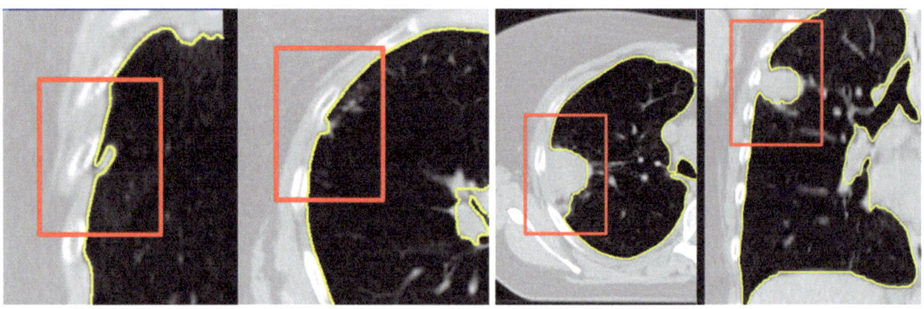

Fig. 8.4 Small juxtapleural nodules like those in the *left figure* can be included in the final segmentation through the use of morphological operations, but finding a set of parameters to include all possible tumors, such as those in the cases on the *right*, is challenging

Another subtle problem comes with nodules that lie on the boundary of the lung [27]. A complete segmentation of the lung is essential for cancer screening applications [3], and studies on computer aided diagnosis have found the exclusion of such nodules to be a limitation of automated segmentation and nodule detection methods [1]. These nodules can be included in the segmentation through the use of special post-processing steps, such as the adaptive border marching algorithm [23], which tries to include small concave regions on the lung slices. However, such algorithmic approaches are bound to fail for larger tumors whose size and shape are unconstrained (Fig. 8.4).

Even more problematic is interstitial lung disease, which causes a dramatic change in the attenuation and local texture pattern of lung parenchyma. Unlike the clearly separated histograms of healthy lung (Fig. 8.3), such diseased tissue will often have attenuation values that overlap with the surrounding body tissue (Fig. 8.5). Although higher thresholds, such as – 300 HU [39], can be used to include more lung tissue, simple thresholding methods are incapable of robustly segmenting these challenging pathologies.

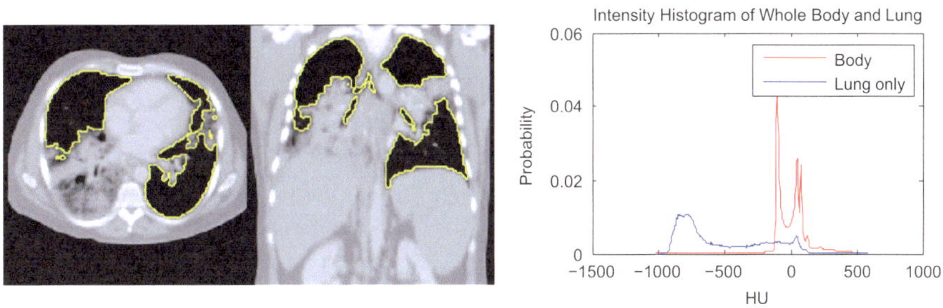

Fig. 8.5 Lungs with diffuse pulmonary disease has higher density tissue and is difficult to separate with a simple thresholding

Cues for Segmenting Pathological Lung

Intensity alone is the single strongest cue for segmenting healthy lung tissue, but in order to address the high density lung tissue associated with interstitial lung disease, and the different shapes associated with varying tumors, cues based on texture, anatomy, or shape priors must be exploited.

Texture Cues

Diseased parenchyma has a different texture pattern which can often be extracted through the use of texture features [20, 37, 39]. Texture, the local structural pattern of intensities, is commonly characterized by measurements obtained from a co-occurrence matrix [9], which records the joint frequency of intensity values between two pixels separated by a fixed offset computed over small volumes of interest around each image voxel. Quantities derived from this co-occurrence matrix, such as entropy, can be used to directly identify diseased tissue [39], or statistical classifiers can be trained to distinguish healthy from pathological tissue using features derived from this matrix [37].

Anatomical Cues

As the appearance of the pathological lung parenchyma can vary dramatically, texture and intensity cues are incapable of capturing all pathologies. These quantities, which are internal to the lung, can be combined with neighboring anatomical context, such as distance and curvature of the ribs. For example, Prasad et al. use the curvature of the ribs in order to adaptively choose a threshold for the lung segmentation [22]. As the lung border should also lie close to the ribcage and spine, distance to these anatomical structures can be combined with intensity features in classification of the lung border [12].

Shape Modeling

In order to avoid segmentations with unlikely shapes, such as the one in Fig. 8.5, a shape prior can be used as an additional cue for segmenting challenging cases. Although some inconsistencies in the shape can be removed, for example, by post-processing operations [11] or through ensuring smoothness in the resulting segmentations [12], the result should be constrained to be lung-like. Explicit statistical models of shape variability, such as a point distribution model that models the shape variability with a low-dimensional linear subspace can be used to constrain the resulting segmentation [6]. These models have been effectively used to overcome pathologies [30, 32].

Segmentation-by-registration are another class of methods that enforce a prior constraint on the resulting segmentations. In such approaches, a reference image complete with annotations is aligned to the target image through the process of image alignment. The target segmentation is then derived from the aligned reference image. To increase generality, multiple reference images can be aligned to the target image and the final segmentation can be taken as the fused result. Depending on the matching score used in the registration, such methods have shown to be effective for pathological lungs [28].

Multi-stage Learning for Lung Segmentation

To ensure robustness, a complete solution to the segmentation of pathological lung in CT has to include components that address shape and appearance variability caused by both tumors and diffuse lung disease. In this section we introduce a robust machine learning method for segmenting challenging lung cases that uses external anatomical information to position a statistical mesh model on the image. A large database of annotated images is used to train discriminative classifiers to detect initial poses of the mesh models and to identify stable boundary landmarks [30]. The boundary of this initialization is then guided by texture and appearance patterns to identify the boundary of the lung. Finally, as pathologies often only occupy a small portion of the lung, a fine-scale level set surface refinement is used to ensure the final segmentation includes all healthy regions as well as preserving the segmentation in the pathological regions [18]. The elements of the system are illustrated in Fig. 8.6.

Learning-Based Robust Initialization

For the initialization phase, the carina of the trachea is detected in the input volume. Given the carina location, a Hierachical Detection Network (HDN) [31] is used to detect an initial set of pose parameters of statistical shape models of each lung

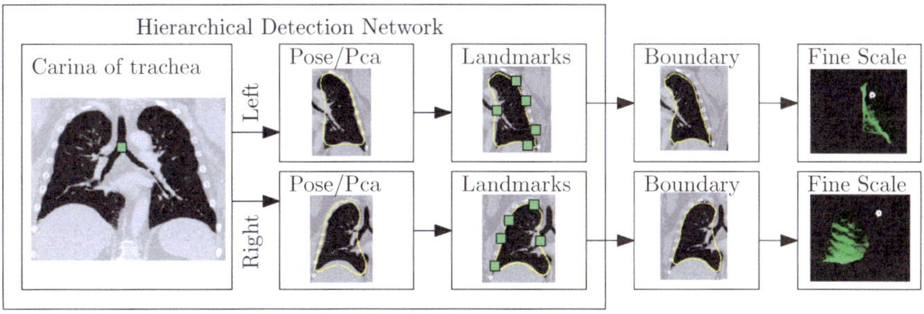

Fig. 8.6 A hierarchical detection network is used to initialize the lung segmentations from a set of stable landmarks. These segmentations are further refined by trained boundary detectors and finally by a fine-scale level set refinement

(Sections "Hierarchical Detection Network" and "Pose Detection"). In the next level of the hierarchy, stable landmark points on the mesh surface are refined to get an improved lung segmentation that is less sensitive to appearance changes within pathologies (Section "Refinement Using Stable Landmarks"). As we will see, these landmark points tend to use nearby anatomical context, e.g., ribs, to improve the segmentation. A further refinement comes by displacing the mesh surface so as to maximize the score of an appearance-based classifier (Section "Freeform Refinement").

Input Annotation Database

A set of CT images complete with manual annotation of the lungs is used as input to the algorithm. In an offline training step, statistical shape models of the shape variation within the database annotations are learned.

The input annotation meshes are first brought into correspondence and remeshed so that each annotation mesh has the same number of points and a consistent triangulation. Each annotation mesh, $\mathscr{M}_k = (\mathscr{P}_k, \mathscr{T})$, then consists of a set of points, $\mathscr{P}_k = \{\mathbf{v}_{ki} \in \mathbb{R}^3\}_{i=1}^{N}$, and a single set of triangle indices, $\mathscr{T} = \{\triangle_j \in \mathbb{Z}^3\}_{j=1}^{N_{tri}}$.

The variability in the point coordinates is modeled through a low-dimensional linear basis giving a statistical shape model,

$$\mathscr{S} = (\{\hat{\mathbf{v}}\}_{i=1}^{N}, \{U_j\}_{j=1}^{M}), \tag{8.1}$$

that consists of a mean shape, $\{\hat{\mathbf{v}}\}_{i=1}^{N}$, and the linear basis shapes, $U_j = \{u_{ij}\}_{i=1}^{N}$. The linear basis is empirically estimated by performing PCA on the aligned input annotation meshes. The alignment uses procrustes analysis to remove translation, orientation, and scale variation of the corresponding meshes.

A mesh in the *span* of the basis can be approximated by modulating the basis shape vectors and applying a similarity transform

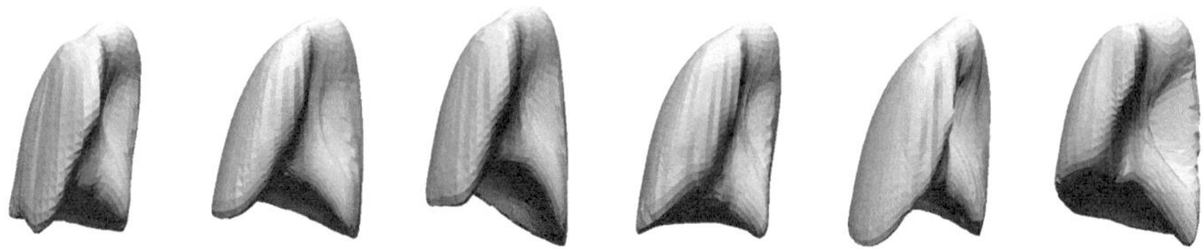

$\lambda_1 = -3$ $\lambda_1 = 3$ $\lambda_2 = -3$ $\lambda_2 = 3$ $\lambda_3 = -3$ $\lambda_3 = 3$

Fig. 8.7 The variability of right lung shape model by using one of the first three basis vectors to represent the shape

$$g(\mathbf{v}_i; \{\lambda_j\}, \mathbf{p}, \mathbf{r}, \mathbf{s}) = \mathbf{p} + \mathbf{M}(\mathbf{s}, \mathbf{r}) \sum_j \left(\hat{\mathbf{v}}_i + \mathbf{u}_{ij}\lambda_j\right), \tag{8.2}$$

where $\mathbf{M}(\mathbf{s}, \mathbf{r})$ is the rotation and scale matrix parameterized by rotation angles, $\mathbf{r}$, and anisotropic scale, $\mathbf{s}$. $\mathbf{p}$ is a translation vector, and $\{\lambda_j\}$ are the shape coefficients. Figure 8.7 illustrates the variability encoded by the first three basis vectors for a model of the right lung.

Each training shape can be approximated in the same manner, meaning each training shape has an associated pose and shape coefficient vector. In the following description of the image-based detection procedure, the relationship between these pose and shape coefficients and the image features is modeled with machine learning so that the parameters of the shape model can be inferred on unseen data.

Hierarchical Detection Network

The Hierarchical Detection Network (HDN) uses an efficient sequential decision process to estimate the unknown states (e.g., object poses or landmark positions) of a sequence of objects that depend on each other [31]. In the case of lung segmentation, the unknown states are the poses and shape coefficients that align a statistical model of the lung to the image, which depend on the detected trachea landmark point. The location of stable lung boundary points are dependent on the pose parameters of the lungs.

The HDN infers multiple dependent object states sequentially using a model of the prior relationship between these objects. Let $\boldsymbol{\theta}_t$ denote the unknown state of an object (e.g., the 9 parameters of a similarity transform or the 3D coordinates of a landmark), and let the complete state for $t + 1$ objects, $\boldsymbol{\theta}_0, \boldsymbol{\theta}_1, \ldots, \boldsymbol{\theta}_t$, be denoted as $\boldsymbol{\theta}_{0:t}$. Given a d-dimensional input volume, $V : \mathbb{R}^d \mapsto \mathbb{R}$, the estimation for each object, t, uses an observation region $V_t \subseteq V$. The complete state is inferred from the input volume by maximizing the posterior density, $f(\boldsymbol{\theta}_{0:t}|V_{0:t})$, which is recursively decomposed into a product of individual likelihoods, $f(V_t|\boldsymbol{\theta}_t)$, and the transition probability between the objects, $f(\boldsymbol{\theta}_t|\boldsymbol{\theta}_{0:t-1})$.

The recursive decomposition of the posterior is derived by applying a sequence of *prediction* and *update* steps. For object t, the *prediction* step ignores the observation region, V_t, and approximates the posterior, $f(\boldsymbol{\theta}_{0:t}|V_{0:t-1})$, using a product of the transition probability, $f(\boldsymbol{\theta}_t|\boldsymbol{\theta}_{0:t-1})$, and the posterior of the preceding objects:

$$f(\boldsymbol{\theta}_{0:t}|V_{0:t-1}) = f(\boldsymbol{\theta}_t|\boldsymbol{\theta}_{0:t-1}, V_{0:t-1})f(\boldsymbol{\theta}_{0:t-1}|V_{0:t-1}), \tag{8.3}$$

$$= f(\boldsymbol{\theta}_t|\boldsymbol{\theta}_{0:t-1})f(\boldsymbol{\theta}_{0:t-1}|V_{0:t-1}), \tag{8.4}$$

as $\boldsymbol{\theta}_t$ and $V_{0:\,t\,-\,1}$ are assumed to be conditionally independent given $\boldsymbol{\theta}_{0:t\,-\,1}$.

The observation region, V_t, is then combined with the prediction in the *update* step,

$$f(\boldsymbol{\theta}_{0:t}|V_{0:t}) = \frac{f(V_{0:t}|\boldsymbol{\theta}_{0:t})f(\boldsymbol{\theta}_{0:t})}{f(V_{0:t})} = \frac{f(V_t|V_{0:t-1}, \boldsymbol{\theta}_{0:t})f(V_{0:t-1}|\boldsymbol{\theta}_{0:t})f(\boldsymbol{\theta}_{0:t})}{f(V_t|V_{0:t-1})f(V_{0:t-1})} \tag{8.5}$$

$$= \frac{f(V_t|\boldsymbol{\theta}_t)f(\boldsymbol{\theta}_{0:t}|V_{0:t-1})}{f(V_t|V_{0:t-1})}, \tag{8.6}$$

where the denominator is a normalizing term, and the derivation assumes V_t and $(V_{0:t-1}, \boldsymbol{\theta}_{0:t-1})$ are conditionally independent given $\boldsymbol{\theta}_t$. The likelihood term, $f(V_t|\boldsymbol{\theta}_t)$, is modeled with a discriminative classifier,

$$f(V_t|\boldsymbol{\theta}_t) = f(y = +1|V_t, \boldsymbol{\theta}_t), \tag{8.7}$$

where the random variable $y \in \{-1, 1\}$ denotes the occurrence of the tth object at pose $\boldsymbol{\theta}_t$. The posterior, $f(y = +1|V_t, \boldsymbol{\theta}_t)$, is modeled with a powerful tree-based classifier, the Probabilistic Boosting Tree (PBT) [33], which is trained to predict the label, y, given the observation region, V_t and a state, $\boldsymbol{\theta}_t$.

The prediction step models the dependence between the objects with the transition prior. In the case of lung segmentation, each object is dependent on one of the previous objects, meaning

$$f(\boldsymbol{\theta}_t|\boldsymbol{\theta}_{0:t-1}) = f(\boldsymbol{\theta}_t|\boldsymbol{\theta}_j), \quad \exists j \in \{0, 1, 2, \ldots, t-1\}. \tag{8.8}$$

The relation between the objects, $f(\boldsymbol{\theta}_t \mid \boldsymbol{\theta}_j)$, is modeled using a Gaussian distribution whose parameters are learned from training data. In our application, the poses of each lung are dependent on the initial carina landmark point (Fig. 8.6). The stable landmarks, which are distributed on the boundary of the lungs, are then dependent on the pose of the lung.

The full posterior, $f(\boldsymbol{\theta}_{0:t} \mid V_{0:t})$, is approximated through sequential importance sampling, where a set of weighted particles (or samples), $\{\boldsymbol{\theta}_t^j, w_t^j\}P_{j=1}$, is used to approximate the posterior at state t, and these particles are propagated, in sequence, to the next object (see [31] for more details).

Pose Detection

The pose of each lung is represented with a 9-dimensional state vector, $\boldsymbol{\theta}_t = \{\mathbf{p}_t, \mathbf{r}_t, \mathbf{s}_t\}$, containing a translation vector $\mathbf{p} \in \mathbb{R}^3$, Euler angles for orientation $\mathbf{r}$, and an anisotropic scale, $\mathbf{s}$. The 9 pose parameters are decomposed into three sequential estimates of the respective 3-dimensional quantities [21, 42],

$$f(\boldsymbol{\theta}_t|V_t) = f(\mathbf{p}_t|V_t)f(\mathbf{r}_t|\mathbf{p}_t, V_t)f(\mathbf{s}_t|\mathbf{p}_t, \mathbf{r}_t, V_t), \quad (8.9)$$

allowing for efficient estimation by using fewer particles during inference. For position, the classifier in (8.7) is trained using 3D Haar features, whereas orientation and scale are estimated using steerable features [42].

The pose detection aligns the mean shape to the image, giving an initial segmentation. Additional detail is incorporated into the segmentation by then detecting the first three shape coefficients, $\boldsymbol{\theta}_t = \{\lambda_1, \lambda_2, \lambda_3\}$ from (8.2), using the HDN.

A uniform sampling of shape coefficients, $\lambda_k^{\min} \leq \lambda_k \leq \lambda_k^{\max}$, is used during detection. The bounds, $[\lambda_k^{\min}, \lambda_k^{\max}]$, are estimated from the shape coefficients of the training data. These uniformly sampled coefficients are augmented with the results of the pose estimation to get a candidate set of particles. Steerable features extracted from the image volume at vertices of the mesh are used to train the classifier in (8.7).

Refinement Using Stable Landmarks

The alignment of the shape models to the input volume through the above described detection process is still sensitive to the appearance and shape changes of pathologies. For this reason, we utilize a robust improvement of the shape alignment that detects a set of stable landmark points on the surface of the lung [30]. This subset of landmark points are chosen as a stable subset of mesh vertices by using the reliability of their corresponding detectors.

Training and Identifying Stable Landmarks. During training, all the input annotations are brought into correspondence using registration in order to build the statistical shape model (Section "Input Annotation Database"). Each one of the mesh vertices is then a potential landmark. Let $\mathbf{p}_{i\,j}$ denote the location of landmark, i, in training volume j. A position detector is trained for each landmark independently, and the detected result for each detector gives a predicted landmark location: $\mathbf{d}_{i\,j}$. The covariance of the error for each detector is then computed as $\mathbf{C}_i = \sum_j (\mathbf{d}_{ij} - \mathbf{p}_{ij})(\mathbf{d}_{ij} - \mathbf{p}_{ij})^\top$.

Landmarks that are stable should have low uncertainty, meaning that the score

$$s_i = \text{trace}(\mathbf{C}_i), \quad (8.10)$$

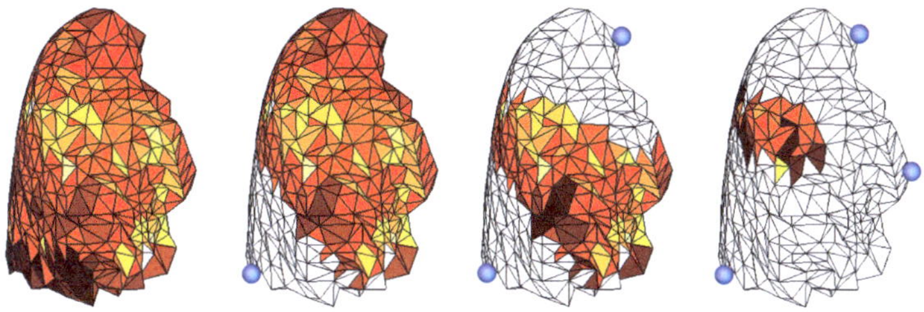

Fig. 8.8 An illustration showing the spatial filtering process used when selecting stable landmarks. The landmark with lowest error is selected on the *bottom left* of the lung, then a region within that landmark is ignored for future selection (*triangles marked white*). The process continues until no more vertices can be selected. Here we used a large filter parameter of $r = 100$ mm for illustration purposes

should be low. Further, the selected landmarks should be spatially distributed along the surface of the object. In order to select a subset of stable and well-distributed landmarks, a greedy selection scheme with a spatial filtering of radius r is used. First, the landmark with the lowest s_i is greedily chosen. Then the mesh vertices within radius r of this vertex on the mean mesh are no longer considered. The process then continues by iteratively choosing the next best landmark and removing nearby vertices from consideration (see Fig. 8.8). Let $L \subset \{1, 2, \ldots, N\}$ denote the mesh indices of the selected landmarks.

The parameter r gives a trade-off between the spatial distribution of the vertices and the stability of the chosen landmarks. In our experiments we found that a radius of $r = 20$ mm gives a good balance.

Alignment of Shape to Landmarks. During detection, in the HDN framework, the stable landmark positions are first predicted from the pose detection in section "Pose Detection". The resulting detected position of the landmark gives a constraint on where the corresponding vertex should move. As not all vertices have corresponding stable landmarks, the entire statistical mesh model must then be deformed to fit the detected landmark positions. This is accomplished by finding a smoothly varying nonrigid transformation using a thin-plate spline that transforms the input landmark vertices from their pose estimate $\mathbf{d}_i^0$ (Section "Pose Detection") to their detected positions, $\mathbf{d}_i$. The transform takes on the following form

$$f(\mathbf{x}) = \sum_{i \in L} \mathbf{a}_i r_i^2 \log(r_i) + \mathbf{A}\mathbf{x}, \tag{8.11}$$

where $r_i = |\mathbf{x} - \mathbf{d}_i^0|$ is the distance between a point $\mathbf{x} \in \mathbb{R}^3$ and the pre-image of the landmark point. $\mathbf{A}$ is a 3×4 affine transformation matrix, and $\mathbf{a}_i$ are 3×1 vector weights for each landmark point. The unknowns, $\mathbf{A}$ and $\mathbf{a}_i$, are obtained by solving the linear system that arises when constraining the transformation such that $f(\mathbf{d}_i^0) = \mathbf{d}_i$.

Freeform Refinement

The estimation of the stable landmarks in the previous section provides a robust initial estimate of the lung surfaces. Although the landmarks provide a more detailed initialization than the first three shape coefficients from the preceding stage, a more detailed estimate is obtained through the use of a freeform surface deformation approach [21] that is similar to the methods used in the active shape model [6].

Given the input volume, V, the freeform surface deformation finds the most likely mesh, $\mathcal{M}$, within the linear span of the statistical shape model:

$$\max f(\mathcal{M}|V) \quad \text{s.t.} \quad \mathcal{M} \in \text{span}(\mathcal{S}). \tag{8.12}$$

The above posterior is computed as an average on the surface of the mesh, and at each surface point, the posterior evaluates a discriminitive classifier:

$$f(\mathcal{M}|V) = \frac{1}{N}\sum_{v_i} f(\mathbf{v}_i|V) = \frac{1}{N}\sum_{v_i} f(y_i = 1|\mathbf{v}_i, \mathbf{n}_i, V), \tag{8.13}$$

where the random variable $y_i = \{-1, +1\}$ takes a value of + 1 if the surface boundary exists at point $\mathbf{v}_i$ with normal $\mathbf{n}_i$ in the input volume.

The statistical classifier for the boundary, $f(y_i = 1|\mathbf{v}_i, \mathbf{n}_i, V)$, can take into account such things as raw image intensity, spatial texture, or distance to anatomical structures in order to discriminate between surface points either on or off the lung boundary. We use a classifier that automatically selects the best set of features [33]. If only healthy cases exist, the classifier will pick features like image gradient or raw intensity. However, robustness to pathological cases can be obtained by ensuring pathological cases exist in training.

Instead of maximizing (8.12) directly using the shape coefficients and pose of the shape model, the freeform refinement performs a sequence of local per-vertex optimizations followed by a projection of the shape back into the span of the shape space. The local optimization for a vertex, $\mathbf{v}_i$, searches for the best displacement, $d_i \in [-\tau, \tau]$, along the normal, $\mathbf{n}_i$ by maximizing the score of the classifier:

$$d_i = \underset{-\tau \leq d \leq \tau}{\text{argmax}} \, f(\mathbf{v}_i + d\mathbf{n}_i|V), \tag{8.14}$$

where τ defines a local search range around the point. The vertex position is then updated with the best displacement, $\mathbf{v}_i \leftarrow \mathbf{v}_i + d_i\mathbf{n}_i$. As this process is done independently for each vertex, the resulting surface may be irregular. The projection of the displaced shape into the shape space regularizes the result and ensures a valid shape.

Several iterations of the above local optimization and regularization steps are performed, with the search range, τ, being reduced at each iteration. In the final iterations, when the search range is small, the projection of the mesh into the shape space is replaced with mesh smoothing [21]. This form of regularization gives a more detailed shape by allowing the surface to deviate from span($\mathscr{S}$).

Fine-Scale Refinement

The detection results from the previous section ensure the lung surface encompasses tumors and pathological regions, but the explicit mesh representation is ineffective to represent fine-scale detail. In the final phase, we use an energy-based level set refinement. In addition to the common data and regularization terms, our energy includes a term to remove overlap between lungs (e.g., at the anterior/posterior junctions), and another term to keep the refined solution close to the detection meshes that are output from the previous phase (Section "Freeform Refinement"). This energy framework can easily incorporate constraints from other adjacent structures such as the heart or liver to further improve the segmentation accuracy [18].

The detected lung surfaces, $\mathscr{C}_i$, are first converted to signed distance functions, $\Phi_i(\mathbf{x}) : \Omega \subset \mathbb{R}^3 \mapsto \mathbb{R}$ where $|\nabla \Phi_i(\mathbf{x})| = 1$ and $\mathscr{C}_i = \{\mathbf{x} | \Phi_i(\mathbf{x}) = 0\}$. Further, $\Phi_i(\mathbf{x}) > 0$ if $\mathbf{x}$ is inside $\mathscr{C}_i$, and $\Phi_i(\mathbf{x}) < 0$ outside $\mathscr{C}_i$ (see [5] and references within for more details). Then for each organ we minimize the energy proposed by Kohlberger et al. [18]:

$$E(\Phi_i; \{\Phi_j\}_{j \neq i}) := \underbrace{E_{\mathrm{d}}(\Phi_i)}_{\text{data}} + \underbrace{E_{\mathrm{s}}(\Phi_i)}_{\text{smooth}} + \underbrace{\sum_{j \in N_j^o} E_{\mathrm{o}}(\Phi_i, \Phi_j)}_{\text{overlap}} + \underbrace{E_{\mathrm{p}}(\Phi_i, \Phi_i^0)}_{\text{prior}}. \quad (8.15)$$

The standard region-based data energy, E_{d}, measures deviation of the appearance of the inside and outside regions from their respective distributions [5],

$$E_{\mathrm{d}}(\Phi_i) := -\alpha \int_{\Omega} H(\Phi_i) \log(p_i^{\mathrm{in}}(I(\mathbf{x})|\Phi_i)) + (1 - H(\Phi_i)) \log(p_i^{\mathrm{out}}(I(\mathbf{x})|\Phi_i)) d\mathbf{x}, \quad (8.16)$$

where H denotes the Heaviside function. Here, the probability of intensities belonging to the inside or outside of the object, $p_i^{\mathrm{in/out}}$, are modeled with non-parametric Parzen densities (see [7]). This data energy will push the segmentation surface to occupy regions that look similar to its intensity distribution. On the other hand, when the intensity distributions between foreground (lung) and background (body) overlap, this term will have less influence. This happens for diseased cases with large tumors or diffuse lung disease cause p_i^{in} to contain high density tissue.

The smoothness term in (8.15) penalizes surface area of the desired segmentation,

$$E_s(\Phi_i) := \gamma \int_\Omega |\nabla H(\Phi_i)| d\mathbf{x}, \tag{8.17}$$

and is balanced with the weight coefficient γ.

The overlap term, $E_o(\Phi_i, \Phi_j)$, penalizes overlap between organ i and a set of neighboring organs, N_i^o:

$$E_o(\Phi_i, \Phi_j) := \beta \int_\Omega H(\Phi_i) H(\Phi_j) \Phi_j d\mathbf{x}. \tag{8.18}$$

As intended, this term only affects regions that lie within the intersection of both surfaces, and the constraint is proportional to the depth of penetration into the surface Φ_j.

Finally, the prior shape term prefers the surface to be close to the detected shape, Φ_i^0:

$$E_p(\Phi_i, \Phi_i^0) := \int_\Omega \underbrace{\omega_{l(\mathbf{x})}^{\text{in}} H(\Phi_i^0(\mathbf{x}) - \Phi_i(\mathbf{x}))}_{\text{Inside deviations}} + \underbrace{\omega_{l(\mathbf{x})}^{\text{out}} H(\Phi_i(\mathbf{x}) - \Phi_i^0(\mathbf{x}))}_{\text{Outside deviations}} d\mathbf{x}. \tag{8.19}$$

The prior term utilizes a set of positive valued spatially varying surface weights $\omega_{l(\mathbf{x})}^{\text{in}}$ and $\omega_{l(\mathbf{x})}^{\text{out}}$ to control the penalization of the surface deviations occurring either inside or outside the detected shape. These surface weights are specified on the surface of the detected mesh, $\{\mathbf{p}_j\}$, which is pre-annotated with corresponding weights, $\{\omega_j^*\}$:

$$\omega_{l(\mathbf{x})}^* = \omega_j^* \qquad \text{where} \qquad j = \text{argmin}_j \|\mathbf{x} - \mathbf{p}_j\|^2. \tag{8.20}$$

To maintain a consistent weighting over the energy minimization, the points, $\mathbf{p}_j$, are also evolved during the minimization [19].

In practice, since our detection result is typically undersegmented, we use a large uniform penalization for the interior deviations, $\omega_{l(\mathbf{x})}{}^{\text{in}} = 10$. In order to allow the fine-scale refinement to fill in small details, we use a smaller weight for the exterior surface deviations and constrain the solution to not deviate much from the detection in the region of the airways. Figure 8.9 illustrates the spatially varying exterior weights, $\omega_{l(\mathbf{x})}^{\text{out}}$.

The contribution of the other terms are balanced by qualitative tuning on a few cases. Here we used a weight of $\alpha = 2$ for the data term, a smoothness weight of $\gamma = 15$, to keep the lung surface smooth, and a large weight on the overlap term, $\beta = 1,000$.

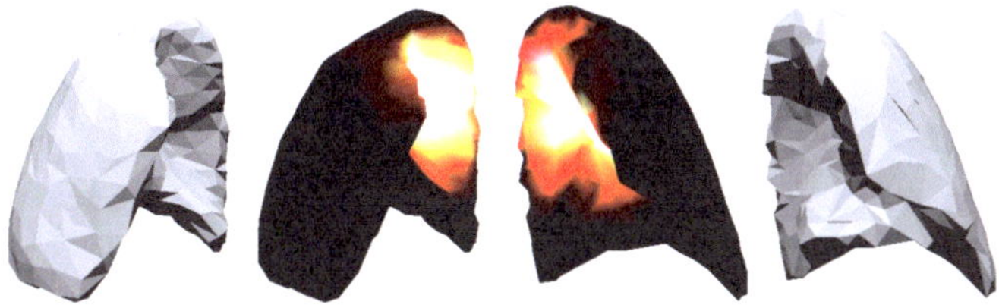

Fig. 8.9 An illustration of the spatially varying exterior surface constraint weights for the left and right lung on the surface of the detected points, $\{\mathbf{p}_j\}$. The *dark regions* map to $\omega^{\text{out}} = 0.1$ and the *white regions* map to $\omega^{\text{out}} = 5$. Larger weights are given in a region near the main bronchi

Optimization

Each of the lungs (and possibly other adjacent organs) has a corresponding energy in the form of (8.15), and the minimizers of these energies are coupled by the overlap penalization term (8.19). In practice, interleaving gradient descents for each of the organs is sufficient to get a desired solution [18].

Specifically, each lung is refined along the negative gradient of the energy term,

$$\frac{\partial \Phi_i}{\partial t} \frac{(\Phi_i^{t+1} - \Phi_i^t)}{\delta t} = -\frac{\partial E(\Phi_i; \{\Phi_j^t\}_{j \neq i})}{\partial \Phi_i}, \tag{8.21}$$

where the gradient for the coupled overlap term uses the solution from the previous time, Φ_j^t. Each organ is then evolved along (8.21) in lockstep using a discrete time step δt.

The gradient descent is terminated when either a fixed number of iterations is reached or if the movement of the surface in a given iteration falls below a predefined threshold. For an efficient solution, the level set surfaces are represented with a narrow-band scheme within $\pm$ 2 voxels of the zero crossing.

A Software Architecture for Detection and Segmentation

In order to implement our lung segmentation algorithm, we use an Integrated Detection Network (IDN) [29], which is a modular design that specifically caters to such detection networks. IDN promotes modularity and reusability through a basic abstraction that decomposes algorithms into the operations, which are called *Modules*, and the *Data* that these modules consume and produce. In contrast to a blackboard model, where information is globally shared through a blackboard, e.g., as done by Brown et al. for lung segmentation [4], the connections between modules illustrate the data flow of the entire algorithm. Data is only shared with a module if it is necessary.

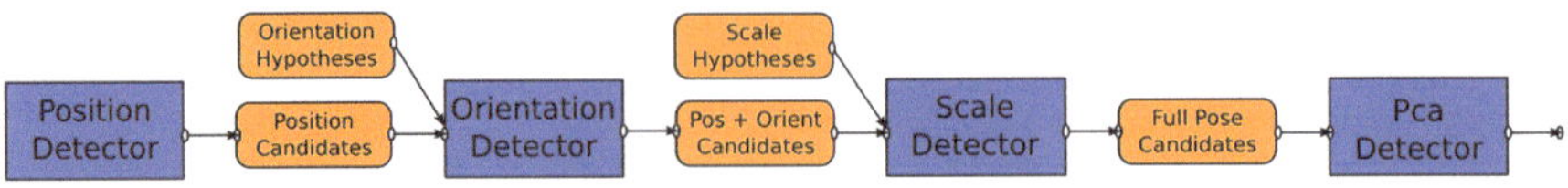

Fig. 8.10 Modules making up the pose estimation are connected by a set of pose candidates, with each detector augmenting more information to its output candidates. All *Modules* consume the CT volume as input

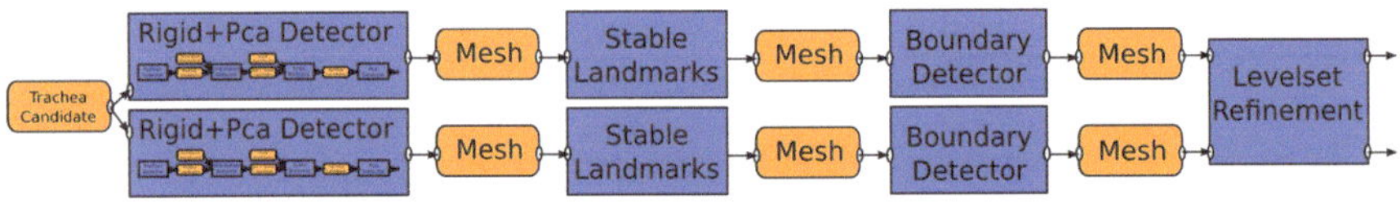

Fig. 8.11 The full pipeline uses the pose estimation, with the later modules performing consecutive refinements of the mesh

Each *Module* provides a set of input slots for incoming *Data* and owns a (possibly empty) set of output *Data* objects. Different *Module* operations may be connected as long as their connecting *Data* object type agrees with the respective input/output types of the *Module*. The connections between these *Modules* through their *Data* forms an acyclic graph.

Modules and *Data* carry all the necessary information to allow both training and detection. In this way, the spatial dependencies between objects in the HDN can be directly encoded with an IDN network, and this same network of *Modules* can be used to train the classifiers as well as to perform the detection and segmentation.

Pose Detection Modules

Pose detection *Modules* parallel their respective HDN detections and take as input a set of candidate poses and produce an augmented set of candidates, where, for example, the output of the orientation detector contains both position and orientation. Estimation of the object pose and the first few PCA coefficients is achieved by connecting the individual detectors, as illustrated in Fig. 8.10.

Segmentation Modules

The main components of the segmentation are also decomposed into independent modules. The stable landmark detector uses an input mesh to predict the locations of the stable landmarks and outputs a mesh deformed to fit these landmark positions. The learning-based boundary refinement refines a mesh, as does the level set refinement (Fig. 8.11). All of these elements can be interchanged provided the input/output types agree. Notice that the final IDN graph parallels the original flowchart of the algorithm in Fig. 8.6.

Experiments

In this section, we perform a qualitative and quantitative analysis at several stages of our algorithm.[1] We use a data set of 260 diagnostic CT scans, which has images of varying contrast and slice thickness (ranging from 0.5 to 5 mm). The lung surfaces have been manually annotated in each of these scans by an expert. This data was randomly partitioned into two sets: 192 volumes that were used to train our detectors, and another 68 volumes that were used for testing. The shape models (Section "Input Annotation Database") computed from the input annotations have a total of 614 vertices for each the left and right lung.

As the stable landmarks are selected by their error rates, we first illustrate the error rates for all the candidate landmarks by computing the accuracy on the training data. We then show how the automatic greedy selection of spatially varying landmarks tends to choose a set of well-distributed landmarks that are close to anatomical structures. We then demonstrate on testing data how this landmark-based initialization helps improve the results over the pose+PCA detector on challenging cases. Finally, we illustrate how the fine-scale refinement further improves the accuracy, even in the presence of pathologies.

Landmark Errors

Figure 8.12 illustrates the landmark scores (computed as the average distance between detected and ground truth) for all 614 landmarks computed on the training set for the right lung (as in section "Refinement Using Stable Landmarks").

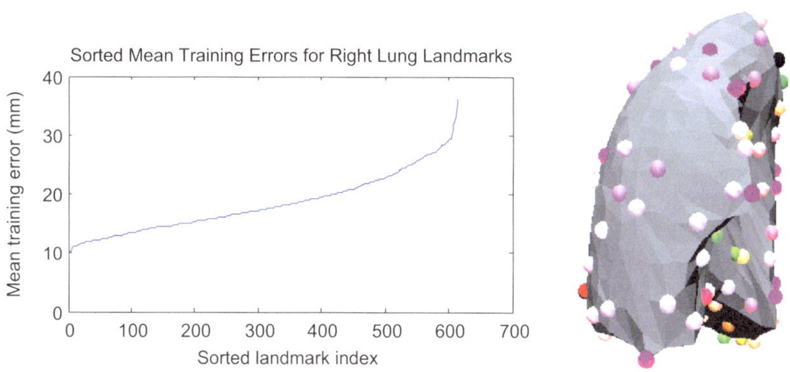

Fig. 8.12 Sorted mean errors of the 614 landmarks computed from all training volumes for the right lungs, and the 143 selected landmarks obtained using the spatial filtering with parameter of $r = 20$ mm visualized on the mesh

[1] The initial analysis and comparison of the performance of the boundary landmarks also appears in our earlier conference publication [30].

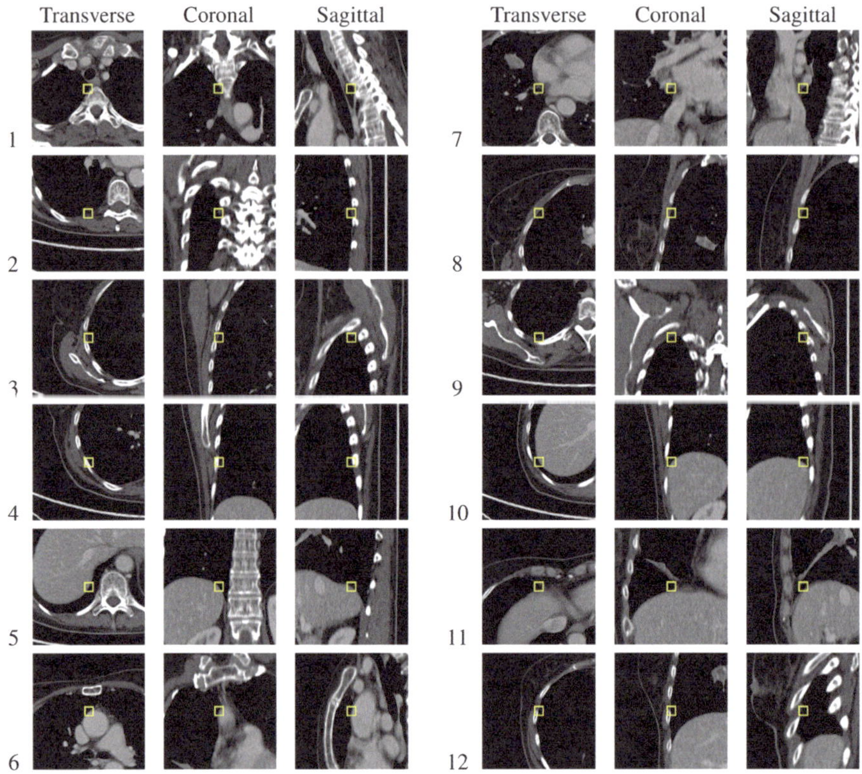

Fig. 8.13 Using a larger spatial filter radius (70 mm), the 12 strongest landmarks selected of the 614 mesh vertices are shown. These landmarks are selected near distinctive anatomical structures such as ribs (3, 4, 5, 12), vertebrae (1, 2) and top (5) and bottom of the lung (9, 10, 11). Reprinted from [30] with kind permission from Springer Science and Business Media

The larger errors on the right of the plot show that some of the landmarks are less reliable; these landmarks are less likely to be selected. For the landmarks with lower scores, some of the error is attributed to slight misalignments that occur during the correspondence establishment phase used to generate the ground truth landmark positions. When using a spatial radius of $r = 20$ mm, a total of 143 landmarks were chosen for the right lung and 133 for the left lung.

For illustration purposes, by increasing the spatial filtering radius to $r = 70$ mm, we show that the greedy selection is effective in choosing a distributed set of 12 stable landmarks (Fig. 8.13). The resulting landmarks are often chosen close to anatomical structures, such as ribs and vertebrae. The spatial filtering also ensures that some landmarks are also selected near the top and bottom of the lungs.

Table 8.1 Testing results of symmetrical point-to-mesh comparisons (in mm's) between the detected results and annotations for both lungs, with and without stable landmark detection [30], and also with the final level set refinement presented in section "Fine-scale Refinement"

Lung	Landmark	Level set	Mean (std.)	Med.	Min	Max	80 %
Right	No	No	2.35 ± 0.86	2.16	1.40	6.43	2.57
Right	Yes	No	1.98 ± 0.62	1.82	1.37	4.87	2.18
Right	Yes	Yes	1.30 ± 0.64	1.12	0.91	4.60	1.38
Left	No	No	2.31 ± 2.42	1.96	1.28	21.11	2.22
Left	Yes	No	1.92 ± 0.73	1.80	1.19	6.54	2.15
Left	Yes	Yes	1.34 ± 0.77	1.13	0.93	6.78	1.39

Segmentation Accuracy and Quality

In this next experiment, we analyze the improvement that is attained at several stages of the algorithm on our testing set. First, we ran the algorithm up to the freeform refinement without the use of the stable landmarks (i.e., skipping section "Refinement Using Stable Landmarks"). We then included the stable landmark stage of the algorithm. And finally, we then ran the full algorithm including the level set refinement. For comparison, the symmetric surface-to-surface distance was computed between the detected and ground truth segmentation.

The results in Table 8.1 show that the inclusion of the stable landmarks gave a significant ($p < 0.05$) decrease in the surface-to-surface distance for both the left and right lung [30]. In the case of the left lung, notice the decrease in the maximum error. This is caused by the stable landmarks correcting a failure case. Finally, notice that the fine-scale level set refinement further reduced this error by filling in the small scale details.

The main advantage of the stable landmarks is the ability to overcome a poor initialization that can occur due to appearance variability in pathologies. Figure 8.14 illustrates several qualitative examples of pathologies where the robust landmarks lead to an improved result of the free-form refinement.

As the fine-scale surface refinement is constrained by the initial surface estimate, a good initialization is important for final accuracy. Figure 8.15 illustrates that the final level set refinement fills in the small regions and that the segmentation still includes the large pathological regions due to the surface prior constraint.

In Fig. 8.16, we demonstrate that all the terms of the level set energy are necessary. When the *prior* and *overlap* terms are not used (only the data and regularization terms in (8.15)), the resulting segmentation excludes the pathological region even though the initialization includes this region. Further, without the *prior* term, the level set leaks into the airways and results in a non-smooth surface near the hilum. Enabling the *prior* term fixes these problems, but the segmentation still has overlap near the anterior junction (middle of Fig. 8.16). Only when both the *prior* and *overlap* terms are enabled is the desired segmentation achieved.

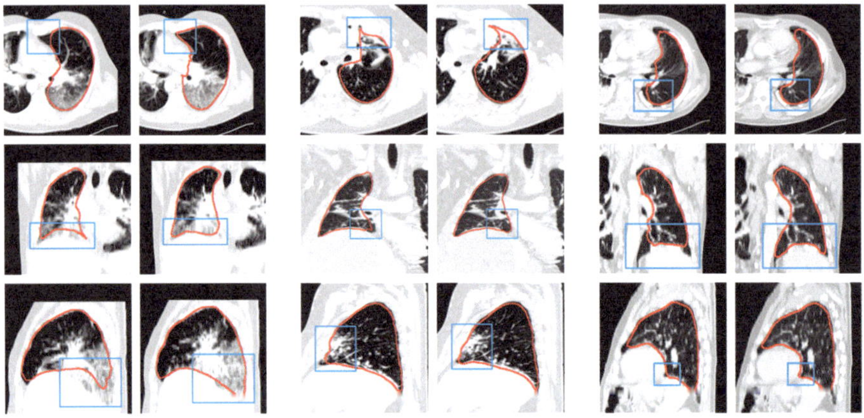

Fig. 8.14 Comparison of freeform boundary results without using the stable landmarks (*left column* of every set) and with stable landmark detection (*right column* of every set). Reprinted from [30] with kind permission from Springer Science and Business Media

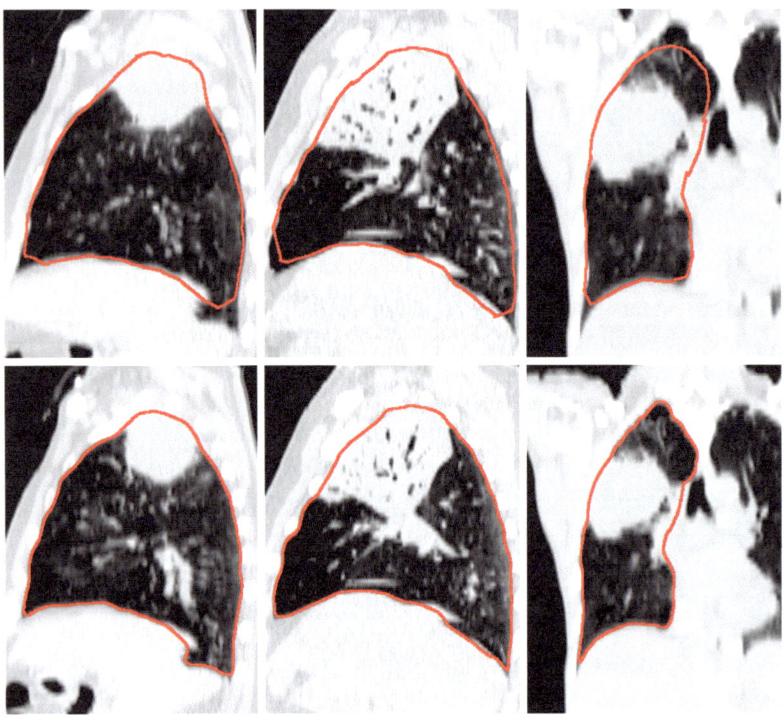

Fig. 8.15 Comparison of the basic boundary detection (*top*) and fine-scale level set refinement (*bottom*) on three example cases. The basic boundary detection gives a good coarse estimate that includes the high density tissue, and the fine-scale refinement not only remains close in these regions but also includes the fine-scale voxel-level details

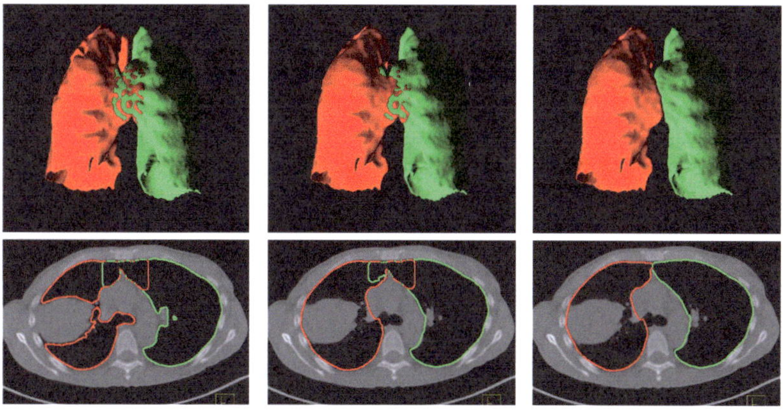

Fig. 8.16 In this example, the same data from the *right* of Fig. 8.15 is used to demonstrate that both the *overlap* and *prior* terms are necessary to obtain good segmentations in the level set refinement. Without the *prior* term, the segmentation doesn't include the tumor (*left*), and without the overlap term, the resulting segmentations may have overlap (*left* and *middle*). With both terms enabled, the desired segmentation, which includes the pathological region and removes overlap, is obtained (*right*)

Conclusion

In this article we presented a multi-stage learning method for segmenting challenging lung cases in thoracic CT. The algorithm overcomes the diversity of lung appearance in the presence of pathologies through the use of a statistical shape model and by detecting robust landmarks that use anatomical context outside the lung.

As pathologies may only affect a portion of the lung, it is important to also use a fine-scale refinement to obtain highly accurate segmentations in the healthy regions. Graph-based methods can be used for this refinement [12], but we propose to use a level set approach that uses adaptive region intensity constraints and enforces that the refined surface cannot deviate too far from the robustly initialized detected surfaces. We have illustrated that the resulting segmentation is robust to a variety of pathologies, including high density tissue associated with diffuse lung disease as well as tumors.

Intelligent editing may still be necessary to fix up failures in extreme cases [17]. However, the same principles used in our automatic algorithm, such as the use of machine learning to integrate shape, texture, and anatomical cues, can be used to guide the development of such interactive techniques.

References

1. Abe Y, Hanai K, Nakano M, Ohkubo Y, Hasizume T, Kakizaki T, Nakamura M, Niki N, Eguchi K, Fujino T, Moriyama N (2005) A computer-aided diagnosis (CAD) system in lung cancer screening with computed tomography. Anticancer Res 25:483–488
2. Adams H, Bernard M, McConnochie K (1991) An appraisal of CT pulmonary density mapping in normal subjects. Clin Radiol 43(4):238–42
3. Armato III S, Sensakovic W (2004) Automated lung segmentation for thoracic CT: Impact on computer-aided diagnosis. Acad Radiol 11(9):1011–1021
4. Brown MS, McNitt-Gray MF, Mankovich NJ, Goldin JG, Hiller J, Wilson LS, Aberle DR (1997) Method for segmenting chest CT image data using an anatomical model: preliminary results. IEEE Trans Med Imag 16(6):828–839
5. Chan T, Vese L (2001) Active contours without edges. IEEE Trans Image Process 10 (2):266–277
6. Cootes T, Hill A, Taylor C, Haslam J (1994) Use of active shape models for locating structures in medical images. Image Vis Comput 12(6):355–365
7. Cremers D, Rousson M, Deriche R (2007) A review of statistical approaches to level set segmentation: Integrating color, texture, motion and shape. Int J Comput Vis 72(2):195–215
8. Haider C, Bartholmai B, Holmes D, Camp J, Robb R (2005) Quantitative characterization of lung disease. Comput Med Imag Graph 29(7):555–563
9. Haralick RM, Shanmugam K, Dinstein I (1973) Textural features for image classification. IEEE Trans Syst Man Cybern 3(6):610–621
10. Hedlund L, Anderson R, Goulding P, Beck J, Effmann E, Putman C (1982) Two methods for isolating the lung area of a CT scan for density information. Radiology 144(2):353–357
11. Hu S, Hoffman E, Reinhardt J (2002) Automatic lung segmentation for accurate quantitation of volumetric X-ray CT images. IEEE Trans Med Imag 20(6):490–498
12. Hua P, Song Q, Sonka M, Hoffman E, Reinhardt J (2011) Segmentation of pathological and diseased lung tissue in CT images using a graph-search algorithm. International Symposium on Biomedical Imaging, Chicago, IL, March 2011
13. International Consensus Statement (2000) Idiopathic pulmonary fibrosis: diagnosis and treatment. American Thoracic Society (ATS) and the European Respiratory Society (ERS), vol 161, pp 646–664
14. International Consensus Statement (2002) American thoracic society/European respiratory society international multidisciplinary consensus classification of the idiopathic interstitial pneumonias. Am J Respir Crit Care Med 165:277–304
15. Kanazawa K, Kawata Y, Niki N, Satoh H, Ohmatsu H, Kakinuma R, Kaneko M, Moriyama N, Eguchi K (1998) Computer-aided diagnosis for pulmonary nodules based on helical CT images. Comput Med Imag Graph 22(2):157–167
16. King TE (2005) Clinical advances in the diagnosis and therapy of the interstitial lung diseases. Am J Respir Crit Care Med 172(3):268–279 (2005)
17. Kockelkorn T, van Rikxoort E, Grutters J, van Ginneken B (2010) Interactive lung segmentation in CT scans with severe abnormalities. In: International Symposium on Biomedical Imaging, Rotterdam, Netherlands, pp 564–567, 14–17 April 2010
18. Kohlberger T, Sofka M, Zhang J, Birkbeck N, Wetzl J, Kaftan J, Declerck J, Zhou S (2011) Automatic multi-organ segmentation using learning-based segmentation and level set optimization. In: Mediacl Image Computing and Computer-assisted Iintervention 2011
19. Kohlberger T, Uzunbaş MG, Alvino C, Kadir T, Slosman DO, Funka-Lea G (2009) Organ segmentation with level sets using local shape and appearance priors. In: Proceedings of MICCAI: Part II. pp 34–42. MICCAI '09
20. Korfiatis P, Kalogeropoulou C, Karahaliou A, Kazantzi A, Skiadopoulos S, Costaridou L (2008) Texture classification-based segmentation of lung affected by interstitial pneumonia in high-resolution CT. Med phys 35:5290

21. Ling H, Zhou SK, Zheng Y, Georgescu B, Suehling M, Comaniciu D (2008) Hierarchical, learning-based automatic liver segmentation. In: CVPR, pp 1–8, IEEE Computer Society, Los Alamitos, CA, USA, 2008
22. Prasad M, Brown M, Ahmad S, Abtin F, Allen J, da Costa I, Kim H, McNitt-Gray M, Goldin J (2008) Automatic segmentation of lung parenchyma in the presence of diseases based on curvature of ribs. Acad. Radiol. 15(9):1173–1180
23. Pu J, Roos J, Yi C, Napel S, Rubin G, Paik D (2008) Adaptive border marching algorithm: Automatic lung segmentation on chest CT images. Comput Med Imag Graph 32(6):452–462
24. Reeves AP, Kostis WJ (2000) Computer-aided diagnosis for lung cancer. Radiol Clin North Am. 38(3):497–509
25. Robinson P, Krell L (1979) Pulmonary tissue attenuation with computed tomography: comparison of inspiration and expiration scans. J Comput Assist Tomogr 3(6):740–748
26. Silva A, Silva JS, Santos BS, Ferreira C (2001) Fast pulmonary contour extraction in X-ray CT images: A methodology and quality assessment. In: SPIE Conf on Medical Imaging: Physiology and Function from Multidimensional Images. vol 4321, pp 216–224
27. Sluimer I, Schilham A, Prokop M, van Ginneken B (2006) Computer analysis of computed tomography scans of the lung: a survey. IEEE Trans Med Imag 25(4):385–405
28. Sluimer I, Prokop M, van Ginneken B (2005) Toward automated segmentation of the pathological lung in CT. IEEE Trans Med Imag 24(8):1025–1038
29. Sofka M, Ralovich K, Birkbeck N, Zhang J, Zhou S (2011) Integrated detection network (IDN) for pose and boundary estimation in medical images. In: Proceedings of the 8th International Symposium on Biomedical Imaging (ISBI 2011). Chicago, IL, 30 March–2 April 2011
30. Sofka M, Wetzl J, Birkbeck N, Zhang J, Kohlberger T, Kaftan J, Declerck J, Zhou S (2011) Multi-stage learning for robust lung segmentation in challenging CT volumes. In: Medical Image Computing and Computer-Assisted Intervention, MICCAI '11, Toronto, Canada, 18–22 September 2011
31. Sofka M, Zhang J, Zhou S, Comaniciu D: Multiple object detection by sequential Monte Carlo and hierarchical detection network. In: IEEE Conference on Computer Vision and Pattern Recognition, San Francisco, CA, 13–18 June 2010
32. Sun S, McLennan G, Hoffman EA, Beichel R (2010) Model-based segmentation of pathological lungs in volumetric ct data. In: The Third International Workshop on Pulmonary Image Analysis, Beijing, 20 September 2010
33. Tu Z (2005) Probabilistic boosting-tree: learning discriminative models for classification, recognition, and clustering. In: International Conference on Computer Vision, ICCV 2005, pp 1589–1596, vol 2,Beijing, 17–21 October 2005
34. Uchiyama Y, Katsuragawa S, Abe H, Shiraishi J, Li F, Li Q, Zhang CT, Suzuki K, Doi K (2003) Quantitative computerized analysis of diffuse lung disease in high-resolution computed tomography. Med Phys 30:2440–2454
35. Ukil S, Reinhardt J (2009) Anatomy-guided lung lobe segmentation in X-ray CT images. IEEE Trans Med Image 28(2):202–214
36. Ukil S, Reinhardt JM (2005) Smoothing lung segmentation surfaces in three-dimensional X-ray CT images using anatomic guidance. Acad. Radiol 12(12):1502–1511
37. Uppaluri R, Hoffman EA, Sonka M, Hartley PG, Hunninghake GW, McLennan G (1999) Computer recognition of regional lung disease patterns. Am J Respir Crit Care Med 160 (2):648–654
38. Uppaluri R, Mitsa T, Sonka M, Hoffman EA, Mclennan G (1997) Quantification of pulmonary emphysema from lung computed tomography images. Am J Respir Crit Care Med 156:248–254
39. Wang J, Li F, Li Q (2009) Automated segmentation of lungs with severe interstitial lung disease in CT. Med phys 36:4592
40. Wang J, Lib F, Doib K, Lia Q (2009) A novel scheme for detection of diffuse lung disease in MDCT by use of statistical texture features. In: SPIE 7260, 27 February 2009

41. Zhang L, Hoffman E, Reinhardt J (2005) Atlas-driven lung lobe segmentation in volumetric X-ray CT images. IEEE Trans Med Image 25(1):1–16
42. Zheng Y, Barbu A, Georgescu B, Scheuering M, Comaniciu D (2007) Fast automatic heart chamber segmentation from 3D CT data using marginal space learning and steerable features. In: IEEE International Conference on Computer Vision, ICCV 2007, pp 1–8, Rio de Janeiro, 14–21 October 2007

Part III
Image Processing and Analysis

Chapter 9
Bone Suppression in Chest Radiographs by Means of Anatomically Specific Multiple Massive-Training ANNs Combined with Total Variation Minimization Smoothing and Consistency Processing

Sheng Chen and Kenji Suzuki

Abstract Most lung nodules that are missed by radiologists as well as computer-aided detection (CADe) schemes overlap with ribs or clavicles in chest radiographs (CXRs). The purpose of this study was to separate bony structures such as ribs and clavicles from soft tissue in CXRs. To achieve this, we developed anatomically (location-) specific multiple massive-training artificial neural networks (MTANNs) which is a class of pixel-based machine learning combined with total variation (TV) minimization smoothing and a histogram-matching-based consistency processing technique. Multi-resolution MTANNs have previously been developed for rib suppression by use of input CXRs and the corresponding "teaching" images for training. Although they were able to suppress ribs, they did not suppress rib edges, ribs close to the lung wall, and the clavicles very well because the orientation, width, contrast, and density of bones are different from location to location and the capability of a single set of multi-resolution MTANNs is limited. To address this issue, the anatomically specific multiple MTANNs developed in this work were designed to separate bones from soft tissue in different anatomic segments of the lungs. Each of multiple anatomically specific MTANNs was trained with the corresponding anatomic segment in the teaching bone images. The output segmental images from the multiple MTANNs were merged to produce a whole bone image. Total variation minimization smoothing was applied to the bone image for reduction of noise while edges were preserved.

S. Chen (✉)
University of Shanghai for Science and Technology, Room 402, Building of Optical and Electrical Engineering School, 516 Jungong Road, Shanghai 200093, China

Department of Radiology, University of Chicago, 5841 South Maryland Avenue, MC 2026, Chicago, IL 60637, USA
e-mail: chnshn@hotmail.com

K. Suzuki
Department of Radiology, University of Chicago, 5841 South Maryland Avenue, MC 2026, Chicago, IL 60637, USA
e-mail: k-suzuki@aoi.bsd.uchicago.edu.

K. Suzuki (ed.), *Computational Intelligence in Biomedical Imaging*,
DOI 10.1007/978-1-4614-7245-2_9, © Springer Science+Business Media New York 2014

This bone image was then subtracted from the original CXR to produce a soft-tissue image where the bones were separated out. In order to ensure the contrast and density in different segments were consistent, a histogram-matching technique was applied to the input segmental images. This new method was compared with the conventional MTANNs by using a database of 110 CXRs with pulmonary nodules. Our new anatomically (location-) specific MTANNs separated rib edges, ribs close to the lung wall, and the clavicles from soft tissue in CXRs to a substantially higher level than the conventional MTANNs did, while the visibility of lung nodules and vessels was maintained. Thus, our image-processing technique for bone-soft-tissue separation by means of our new anatomically specific multiple MTANNs would be potentially useful for radiologists as well as for CAD schemes in detection of lung nodules on CXRs.

Introduction

The prevalence of chest diseases has been increasing over a long period of time. Every year, more than nine million people worldwide die from chest diseases [1]. Chest radiography (chest X-ray: CXR) is by far the most commonly used diagnostic imaging technique for identifying chest diseases such as lung cancer, tuberculosis, pneumonia, pneumoconioses, and pulmonary emphysema. This is because CXR is the most cost-effective, routinely available, and dose-effective diagnostic tool and has the ability to reveal certain unsuspected pathologic alterations [2]. Among different chest diseases, lung cancer is responsible for more than 900,000 deaths each year, making it the leading cause of cancer-related deaths in the world. CXRs are regularly used for detecting lung cancer [3–5] as there is evidence that early detection of the tumor can result in a more favorable prognosis [6–8].

Although CXR is widely used for the detection of pulmonary nodules, the occurrence of false-negatives for nodules on CXRs is relatively high, and CXR is inferior to CT with respect to the detection of small nodules. This failure to detect nodules has been attributed to their size and density and to obscuring by structures such as ribs, clavicles, mediastinum, and pulmonary blood vessels. It has been well demonstrated that the detection of lung cancer at an early stage using CXRs is a very difficult task for radiologists. Studies have shown that up to 30 % of nodules in CXRs could be missed by radiologists, and that 82–95 % of the missed nodules were partly obscured by overlying bones such as ribs and clavicles [9, 10]. However they would be relatively obvious on soft-tissue images if the dual-energy subtraction technique was used [11]. Therefore, a computer-aided detection (CADe) scheme [12, 13] for nodule detection on CXRs has been investigated because the computer prompts indicating nodules could improve radiologists' detection accuracy [14–16]. A major challenge for current CADe schemes is the detection of nodules overlapping with ribs, rib crossings, and clavicles, because the majority of false positives (FPs) are caused by these structures [17, 18]. This leads to a lower sensitivity as well as specificity of a CADe scheme. In order to overcome these challenges, Kido et al. [19, 20] developed a CADe scheme based on single-exposure dual-energy

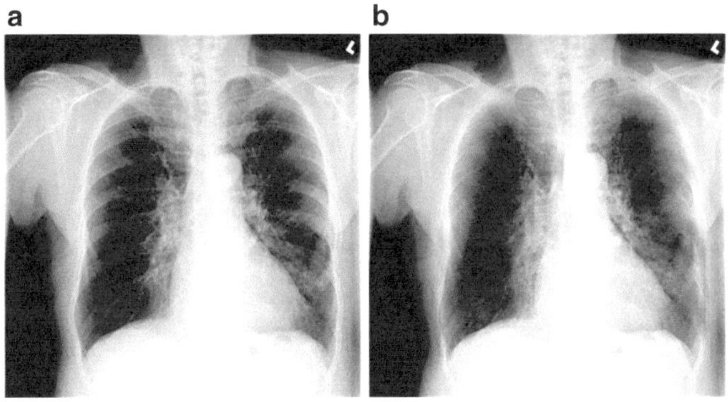

Fig. 9.1 Illustration of (**a**) an original standard chest radiograph and (**b**) the corresponding VDE soft-tissue image by use of our original MTANN method

computed radiography. A dual-energy subtraction technique [21, 22] was used for separating soft tissue from bones in CXRs by use of two X-ray exposures at two different energy levels. The technique produces soft-tissue images from which bones are extracted. By using these images, the performance of their CADe scheme was improved. In spite of its great advantages, a limited number of hospitals use the dual-energy radiography system because specialized equipment is required. In addition, the radiation dose can, in theory, be double compared to that for standard CXR.

Suzuki et al. first developed a supervised image-processing technique for separating ribs from soft tissue in CXRs by means of a multi-resolution massive-training artificial neural network (MTANN) [23, 24] which is a class of pixel-based machine learning [25] and is considered a supervised highly nonlinear filter based on artificial neural network regression. Real dual-energy images were used as teaching images for training of the multi-resolution MTANN. Once the multi-resolution MTANN was trained, real dual-energy images were no longer necessary. An observer performance study with 12 radiologists demonstrated that the suppression of bony structures in CXRs improved the diagnostic performance of radiologists in their detection of lung nodules substantially [26]. Ahmed and Rasheed [27] presented a technique based on independent component analysis for the suppression of posterior ribs and clavicles in order to enhance the visibility of nodules and to aid radiologists during the diagnosis process. Loog et al. [28] proposed a supervised filter learning technique for the suppression of ribs. The procedure is based on K-nearest neighbor regression, which incorporates knowledge obtained from a training set of dual-energy radiographs with their corresponding subtraction images for the construction of a soft-tissue image from a previously unseen single standard chest image. The MTANN [23, 24] was able to separate ribs from soft tissue in CXRs; however, rib edges, ribs close to the lung wall, and clavicles were not completely suppressed (Fig. 9.1). The reason for this is that the orientation, width, contrast, and density of bones are different from location to location in the CXR, and the capability of a single set of multi-resolution MTANNs is limited.

The purpose of this study was to separate rib edges, ribs close to the lung wall, and clavicles from soft tissue in CXRs. To achieve this goal, we newly developed anatomically (location-) specific multiple MTANNs, each of which was designed to process the corresponding anatomic segment in the lungs. A composite VDE bone image was formed from multiple output images of the anatomically specific multiple MTANNs by using anatomic segment masks, which were automatically segmented. In order to make the contrast and density of the output image of each set of MTANNs consistent, histogram matching was applied to process the training images. Before a VDE bone image was subtracted from the corresponding CXR to produce a VDE soft image, a total variation (TV) minimization smoothing method was applied to maintain rib edges. Our newly developed MTANNs were compared with our conventional MTANNs.

Methods

Database

The database used in this study consisted of 119 posterior–anterior CXRs acquired with a computed radiography (CR) system with a dual-energy subtraction unit (FCR 9501 ES; Fujifilm Medical Systems, Stamford, CT) at The University of Chicago Medical Center. The dual-energy subtraction unit employed a single-shot dual-energy subtraction technique, where image acquisition is performed with a single exposure that is detected by two receptor plates separated by a filter for obtaining images at two different energy levels [29–31]. The CXRs included 118 abnormal cases with pulmonary nodules and a "normal" case (i.e., a nodule-free case). Among them, eight nodule cases and the normal case were used as a training set, and the rest were used as a test set. The matrix size of the chest images was 1,760 $\times$ 1,760 pixels (pixel size, 0.2 mm; grayscale, 10 bits). The absence and presence of nodules in the CXRs were confirmed through CT examinations. Most nodules overlapped with ribs and/or clavicles in CXRs.

Multi-Resolution MTANNs for Bone Suppression

For bone suppression, the MTANN [32] consisted of a machine-learning regression model such as a linear-output multilayer ANN regression model [33], which is capable of operating directly on pixel data. This model employs a linear function instead of a sigmoid function as the activation function of the unit in the output layer. This was used because the characteristics of an ANN have been shown to be significantly improved with a linear function when applied to the continuous mapping of values in image processing [33, 34]. Other machine-learning regression models can be used in the MTANN framework (a.k.a., pixel-based machine learning [25]) such as support vector regression and nonlinear Gaussian process regression models [35]. The output is a continuous value.

The MTANN involves training with massive subregion-pixel pairs which we call a massive-subregions training scheme. For bone suppression, CXRs are divided pixel by pixel into a large number of overlapping subregions (or image patches). Single pixels corresponding to the input subregions are extracted from the teaching images as teaching values. The MTANN is massively trained by using each of a large number of the input subregions (or patches) together with each of the corresponding teaching single pixels. The inputs to the MTANN are pixel values in a subregion (or an image patch), R, extracted from an input image. The output of the MTANN is a continuous scalar value, which is associated with the center pixel in the subregion, represented by

$$O(x,y) = ML\{I(x-i,y-j)|(i,j) \in R\}, \tag{9.1}$$

where $ML(\cdot)$ is the output of the machine-learning regression model, and $I(x,y)$ is a pixel value of the input image. The error to be minimized by training of the MTANN is represented by

$$E = \frac{1}{P}\sum_{c}\sum_{(x,y)\in R_T}\{T_c(x,y) - O_c(x,y)\}^2, \tag{9.2}$$

where c is the training case number, O_c is the output of the MTANN for the cth case, T_c is the teaching value for the MTANN for the cth case, and P is the number of total training pixels in the training region for the MTANN, R_T.

Bones such as ribs and clavicles in CXRs include various spatial-frequency components. For a single MTANN, suppression of ribs containing such variations is difficult, because the capability of a single MTANN is limited, i.e., the capability depends on the size of the subregion of the MTANN. In order to overcome this issue, multi-resolution decomposition/composition techniques were applied.

First, input CXRs and the corresponding teaching bone images were decomposed into sets of images of different resolution and these were then used for training three MTANNs in the multi-resolution MTANN. Each MTANN is an expert for a certain resolution, i.e., a low-resolution MTANN is responsible for low-frequency components of ribs, a medium-resolution MTANN is for medium-frequency components, and a high-resolution MTANN for high-frequency components. Each resolution MTANN is trained independently with the corresponding resolution images. After training, the MTANNs produce images of different resolution, and then these images are combined to provide a complete high-resolution image by use of the multi-resolution composition technique. The complete high-resolution image is expected to be similar to the teaching bone image; therefore, the multi-resolution MTANN would provide a VDE bone image in which ribs are separated from soft tissues.

Anatomically (Location-) Specific Multiple MTANNs

Although an MTANN was able to suppress ribs in CXRs [23], the single MTANN did not efficiently suppress rib edges, ribs close to the lung wall, and the clavicles, because the orientation, width, contrast, and density of bones are different from location to location, and because the capability of a single MTANN is limited. To improve the suppression of bones at different locations, we extended the capability of a single MTANN and developed an anatomically specific multiple-MTANN scheme that consisted of eight MTANNs arranged in parallel, as shown in Fig. 9.2a. Each anatomically specific MTANN was trained independently by use of normal cases and nodule cases in which nodules were located in the corresponding anatomic segment. The lung field was divided into eight anatomic segments; a left-upper segment for suppression of left clavicles and ribs, a left hilar segment for suppression of bone in the hilar area, a left middle segment for suppression of ribs in the middle of the lung field, a left lower segment for suppression of ribs in the left lower lobe, a right upper segment, a right hilar segment, a right middle segment, and a right lower segment. For each anatomically specific MTANN, the training samples were extracted specifically from the corresponding anatomic segment mask (the training region in Eq. 9.2).

After training, each of the segments in a non-training CXR was inputted into the corresponding trained anatomically specific MTANN for processing of the anatomic segment in the lung field, e.g., MTANNs No. 1 was trained to process the left-upper segment in the lung field in which the clavicle lies; MTANNs No. 2 was trained to process the left hilar segment, etc., as illustrated in Fig. 9.2b. The eight segmental output sub-images from the anatomically specific multiple MTANNs were then composited to an entire VDE bone image by use of the eight anatomic segment masks. To blend the sub-images smoothly near their boundaries, anatomic segmentation masks smoothed by a Gaussian filter were used to composite the output sub-images, represented by

$$f_b(x,y) = \sum_{i=1}^{8} O_i(x,y) \times f_G[M_i(x,y)], \tag{9.3}$$

where $f_b(x,y)$ is the composite bone image, O_i is the ith trained anatomically specific MTANN, $f_G(\cdot)$ is a Gaussian filtering operator, and M_i is the ith anatomic segmentation mask.

Training Method

In order to make the output image of each set of anatomical segment MTANNs consistent in density and contrast, it is preferable to use similar CXRs to train each anatomical segment. A normal case was therefore selected for training the eight

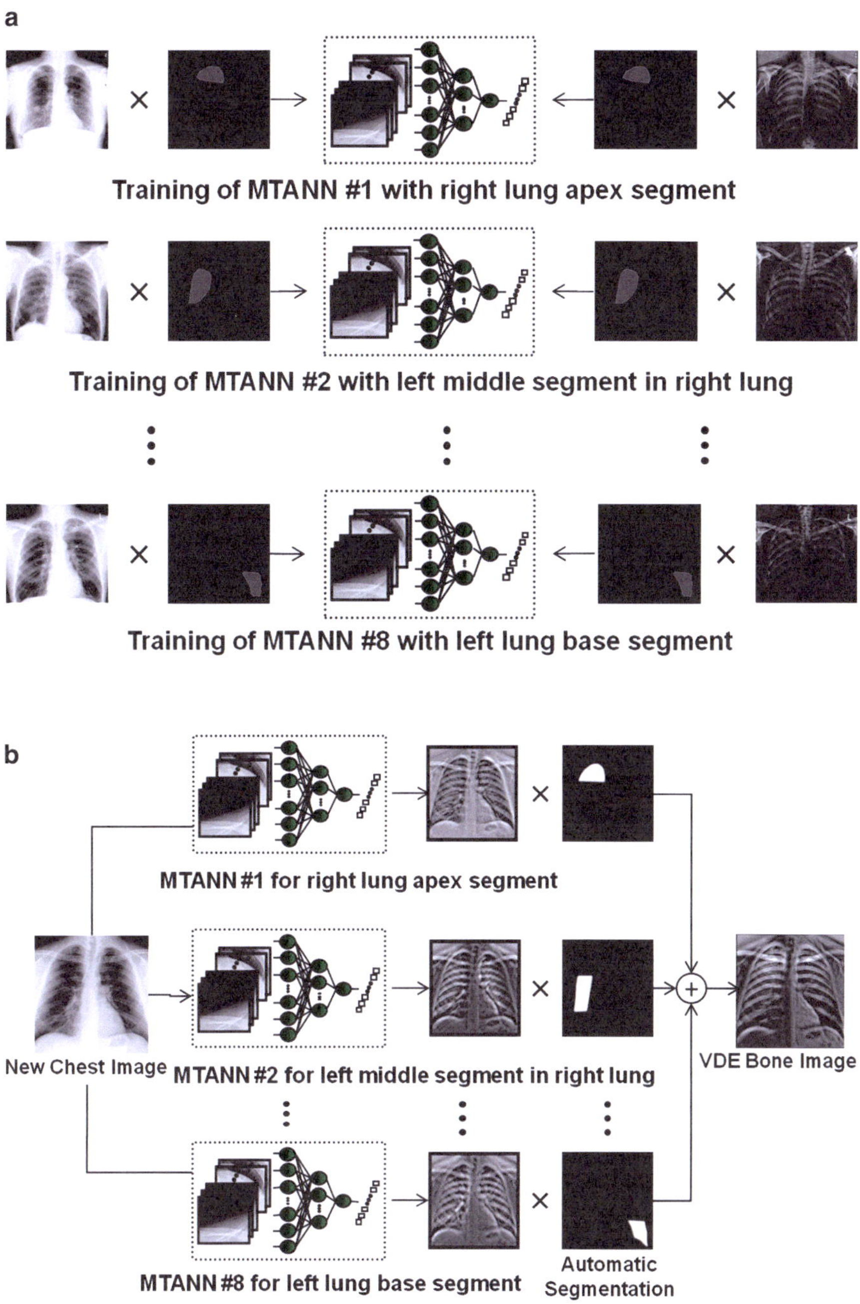

Fig. 9.2 Architecture and training of our new anatomically specific MTANNs. (**a**) Training phase. (**b**) Execution phase

MTANNs with different segments of the lung field. In order to maintain nodule contrast while suppressing bone structures, nodule cases were used to train the anatomical segment-specific multiple MTANNs as well. As it is impossible to find an abnormal case where each of eight typical nodules is located in each of the eight anatomical segments in the lung field, eight different nodule cases were required for training eight anatomical MTANNs. For each nodule case, a nodule was located in the anatomical segment that was used to train the corresponding MTANN. As a result, nine CXRs were used, i.e., one normal case and eight nodule cases, along with the corresponding dual-energy bone images for training the eight sets of multi-resolution MTANNs.

For training of overall features in each anatomic segment in the lung field, 10,000 pairs of training samples were extracted randomly from the anatomic segment for each anatomically specific MTANN: 5,000 samples from the normal case; and 5,000 samples from the corresponding nodule case. A three-layered MTANN was used, where the numbers of input, hidden, and output units were 81, 20, and 1, respectively. Once the MTANNs are trained, the dual-energy imaging system is no longer necessary. The trained MTANNs can be applied to standard CXRs for suppression of bones; thus, the term "virtual dual-energy" (VDE) technology. The advantages of this technology over real dual-energy imaging are that there is no need for special equipment to produce dual-energy images, or no additional radiation dose to patients.

Because of differences in acquisition conditions and patients among different CXRs, the density and contrast vary within the different training images. This makes the training of the eight anatomically specific MTANNs inconsistent. To address this issue, a histogram-matching technique was applied to training images to equalize the density and contrast. Histogram matching is a technique for matching the histogram of a given image with that of a reference images. We used a normal case as the reference image to adjust the nodule cases. First the cumulative histogram F_1 of the given image and that F_2 of the reference image were calculated. Then, the histogram transfer function $M(G_1) = G_2$ was calculated so that $F_1(G_1) = F_2(G_2)$. Finally, the histogram transfer function M was applied to each pixel in the given image.

The proportion of background also varies among different CXRs. The histogram matching of an image with a larger proportion of the background to another with a small proportion may cause the density of the lung field in the matched image to appear darker than the target image. For this reason, only the histogram of the body without the background was matched in the target image. The background was first segmented, which typically corresponds to the highest signal levels in the image where the unobstructed radiation hits the imaging plate. Several factors make the detection of these regions a challenging task. First, the radiation field across the image may be nonuniform due to the orientation of the X-ray source relative to the imaging plate, and the effect of scatter in thicker anatomical regions compounds this problem. Further, for some examinations, multiple exposures may be carried out on a single plate, resulting in multiple background levels. The noise attributes of the imaging system were used to determine if the variation around a candidate background pixel is a typical range of direct exposure pixel values. The corresponding values of candidate background pixels were accumulated in a histogram, and the resulting distribution of background pixel values invariably contained well-defined peaks, which served as markers for selecting the background threshold. After analyzing the histogram, the intensity values to the left of the background peak clearly represented the background, while those to the right represented, to a progressively greater extent, the intensity values of image information. The portion of the histogram to the right of the background peak was processed to find the point at which the histogram first exhibited a change in its curvature from negative to positive. For an increase in intensity, a negative curvature corresponds to a decreasing rate of occurrence of background pixels, while a positive curvature corresponds to an increasing rate of occurrence. In this manner, it was possible to create a difference histogram to obtain a positive slope at the intensity position to the right of the background peak. At this position, we could determine the counts for the least intense pixels, whose intensities are mostly due to the signal. After finding the intensity level representative of the minimum signal intensity level, this level was applied as a signal threshold for segmenting the background. This approach successfully dealt with the problems of non-uniform backgrounds. Figure 9.3 illustrates our background segmentation. A background peak is seen in the histogram illustrated in Fig. 9.3a. Figure 9.3c illustrates a segmentation threshold determined by finding the right bin to the background peak in the difference histogram. Figure 9.3d shows the background segmentation result by using the threshold value.

Automated Anatomic Segmentation

To train and process anatomically specific MTANNs, a given CXR was divided into anatomic segments. Each segment was inputted into each of anatomically specific MTANNs simultaneously. Each MTANN provided the corresponding segment of a VDE bone image where bones were extracted. Because each MTANN is an expert for a specific anatomic segment, the signal-to-noise ratio is highest in the corresponding anatomic segment among all segments, as illustrated in Fig. 9.4. Merging all anatomic segments provided a complete single VDE bone image where the signal-to-noise ratio is high in all segments.

To determine eight anatomic segments, an automated anatomic segmentation method was developed based on active shape models (ASMs) [36]. First, the lung fields were segmented automatically by using a multi-segment ASM (M-ASM) scheme [37], which can be adapted to each of the segments of the lung boundaries (which we call a multi-segment adaptation approach), as illustrated in Fig. 9.5. As the nodes in the conventional ASM are equally spaced along the entire lung shape, they do not fit parts with high curvatures. In our developed method, the model was improved by the fixation of selected nodes at specific structural boundaries that we call transitional landmarks. Transitional landmarks identified the change from one boundary type (e.g., a boundary between the lung field and the heart) to another

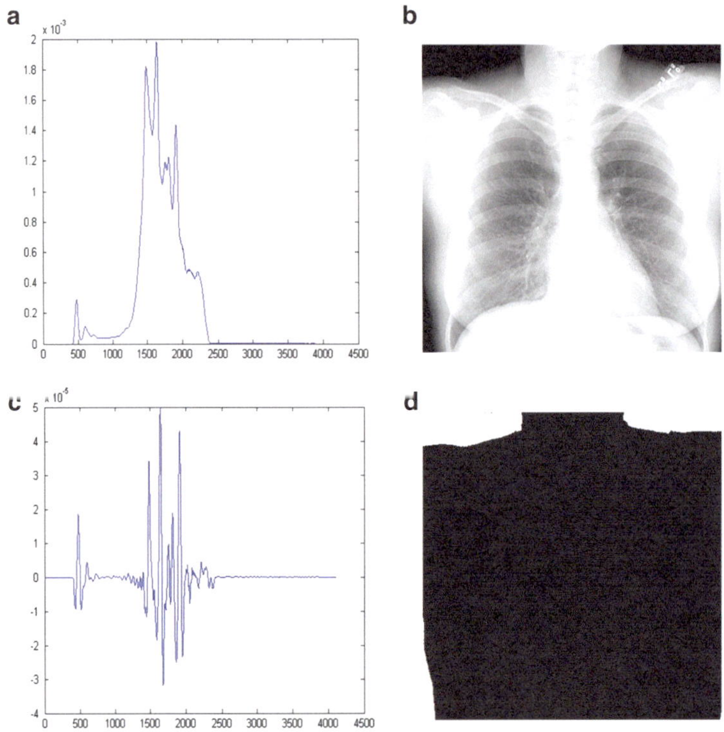

Fig. 9.3 Background segmentation. (**a**) Histogram of pixel values in CXR (**b**). (**b**) Original CXR. (**c**) Differences between two neighboring bins in histogram (**a**). (**d**) Background segmentation result

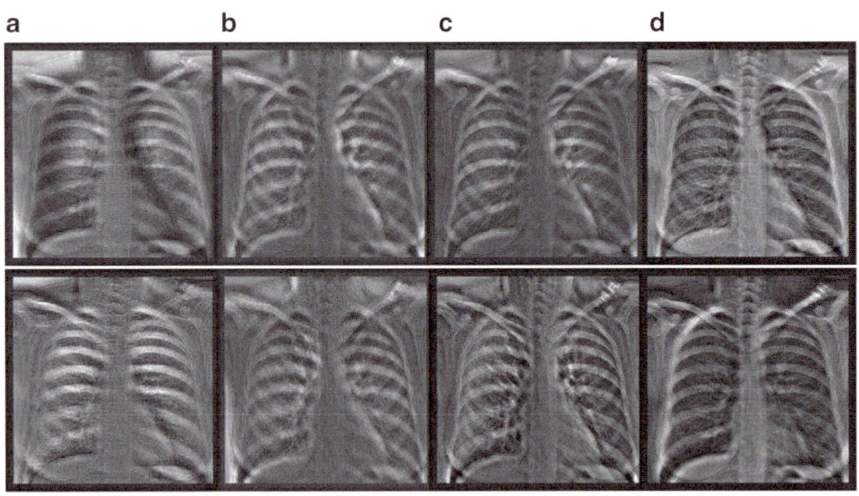

Fig. 9.4 Eight output bone images of the trained anatomically specific multiple MTANNs. (**a**) Output from the segment MTANNs trained for the hilar region, (**b**) Output from the MTANNs trained for the lower region of the lung, (**c**) Output from the MTANNs trained for the middle region of the lung, (**d**) Output from the MTANNs trained for the upper region of the lung

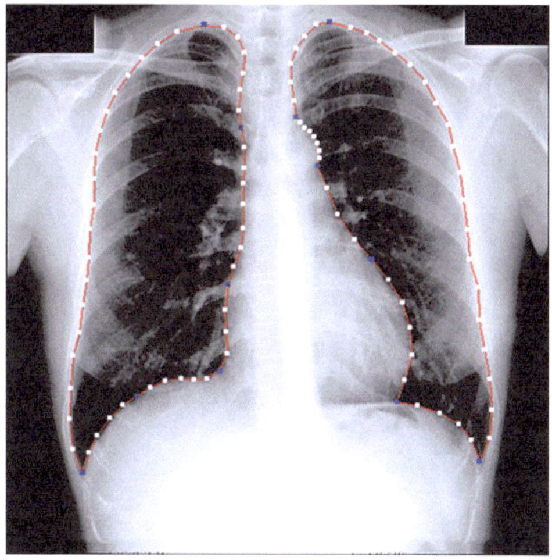

Fig. 9.5 Lung segmentation using our M-ASM. *Blue points* represent the transitional landmarks of two boundary types

(e.g., a boundary between the lung field and the diaphragm). This resulted in multiple segmented lung field boundaries where each segment is correlated with a specific boundary type (heart, aorta, rib cage, diaphragm, etc.). The node-specific ASM was built by using a fixed set of equally spaced nodes for each boundary segment. Our lung M-ASM consisted of a total of 50 nodes for each lung boundary that were not equally spaced along the entire contour. A fixed number of nodes were assigned to each boundary segment, and they were equally spaced along each boundary (as shown in Fig. 9.5). For example, the boundary between the left lung field and the heart consisted of 11 points in every image, regardless of the actual extent of this boundary in the image (see Fig. 9.5). This allowed the local features of nodes to fit a specific boundary segment rather than the whole lung, resulting in a marked improvement in the accuracy of boundary segmentation. From the training images, the relative spatial relationships among the nodes in each boundary segment were learned in order to form the shape model. The nodes were arranged into a vector x and projected into the principal component shape space, represented by the following equation:

$$b = V^T(x - \overline{x}), \tag{9.4}$$

where $V = (V_1 V_2 \ldots V_M)$ is the matrix of the first M eigenvectors for the shape covariance matrix, and $b = (b_1 b_2 \ldots b_M)^T$ is a vector of shape coefficients for the primary axes. The shape coefficients were constrained to lie in a range $\pm m\sqrt{\lambda_i}$ to generate only a plausible shape and projected back to node coordinates, represented by:

$$x = \overline{x} + Vb, \tag{9.5}$$

where m usually has a value between 2 and 3 [38], and was 2.5 in our experiment.

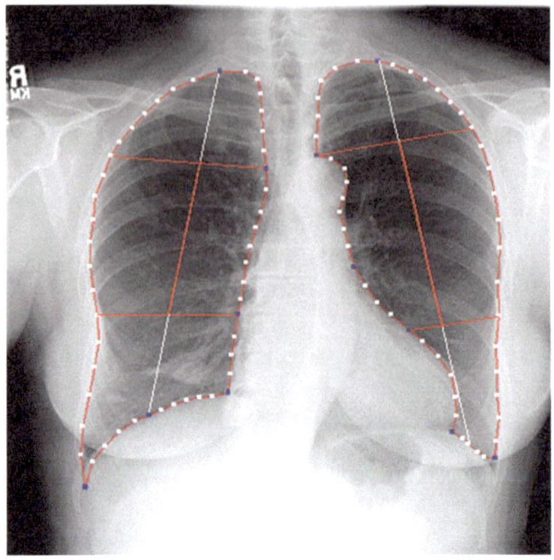

Fig. 9.6 Result of automated anatomic segmentation based on our M-ASM

After the lungs were segmented, they were automatically divided into eight anatomic segments by using the boundary types and the transitional landmarks. By using the landmark points, we obtained the upper region, lower region, and hilar region in each lung, as illustrated in Fig. 9.6. The eight output segmental images from the multiple MTANNs were merged into a single VDE bone image:

$$f_b(x,y) = \sum_{i=1}^{8} f^i{}_b(x,y)^* m^i{}_b(x,y), \tag{9.6}$$

where $f^i{}_b(x,y)$ is the output image from the *i-th* MTANN and $m^i{}_b(x,y)$ is the anatomic segment mask for the *i-th* MTANN. The anatomic segment masks were smoothed by a Gaussian filter so that an unnatural discontinuity between anatomical segments in the merged image was eliminated.

Creation of Soft-Tissue Images

After the VDE bone image was obtained, the VDE soft image could be acquired by use of the subtraction technique. In this study, we focused on the suppression of ribs and clavicles in the lung regions, because this is where most nodules overlap with bony structures. For processing only in the lungs, lung segmentation was used, and suppression was done only in the segmented lungs in the subtraction technique. After the segmentation, a Gaussian filter was applied for smoothing the edges of the segmented lung regions to create an image $m(x,y)$ for masking the outside of the lung regions. The masking image was normalized to have values from 0 to 1. For suppression of ribs in an original CXR, the VDE bone image $f_b(x,y)$ produced by

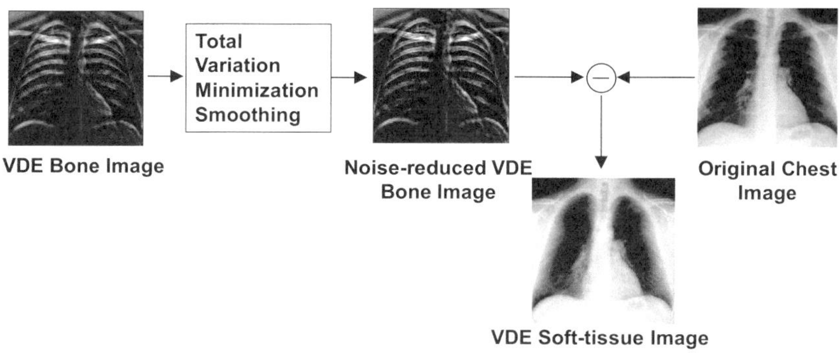

Fig. 9.7 Method for obtaining a soft-tissue image from a bone image

the anatomically specific multiple MTANN was subtracted from the original CXR $g(x,y)$ with the masking image $m(x,y)$ as follows:

$$f_S(x,y) = g(x,y) - w_C \times f_b(x,y) \times m(x,y), \tag{9.7}$$

where w_C is a weighting parameter for determining the contrast of ribs. By changing the weighting parameter w_C, one can obtain processed CXR with different contrast of ribs and clavicles.

As mentioned above, owing to noise in a VDE bone image, the Gaussian smoothing method was applied. Although it smooths the noise in the VDE bone image, it can also smooth bone edges. As a result, the bone edges remain in the VDE soft-tissue image when subtracting the VDE bone image from the corresponding original CXR. In this paper, we propose a TV minimization noise smoothing method which can smooth the noise in the VDE bone image while preserving the edge information of bones (Fig. 9.7). TV minimization problems were first introduced in the context of image smoothing by Rudin et al. [39]. The main advantage of the TV formulation is the ability to preserve edges in the images. This is because of the piecewise smooth regularization property of the TV norm. We assume the noise in the VDE bone image is white Gaussian noise:

$$z(x,y) = u(x,y) + \eta(x,y), \tag{9.8}$$

where $u(x,y)$ is an unknown piecewise constant two-dimensional function representing the noise-free original image, $z(x,y)$ is the noisy observation of $u(x,y)$, and $\eta(x,y)$ is white Gaussian noise. A conventional additive noise suppression technique such as Wiener filtering is applied in order to find $u(x,y)$ which minimizes the functional:

$$T(u) = \frac{1}{2}\|u - z\|^2 + \alpha J(u), \tag{9.9}$$

Common choices for J are

$$J(u) = \int u^2 dx, \tag{9.10}$$

Equation (9.9) often induces blur in images and spurious oscillations when u is discontinuous.

Therefore, we consider the nonlinear TV functional:

$$J_{TV}(u) = \int_\Omega |\nabla u| dx, \tag{9.11}$$

where ∇u denotes the gradient of u:

$$\nabla u = \left(\frac{\partial u}{\partial x}, \frac{\partial u}{\partial y}\right)$$

Here, u is not required to be continuous.

However, the Euclidean norm is not differentiable at zero. To avoid difficulties associated with the non-differentiability, the modification

$$J_\beta(u) = \int_\Omega \sqrt{|\nabla u|^2 + \beta^2} dx$$

is utilized here. The functional to be minimized is

$$T(u) = \frac{1}{2}\|u - z\|^2 + \alpha \int_\Omega \sqrt{|\nabla u|^2 + \beta^2} dx, \tag{9.12}$$

The Eular–Lagrange equation associated with Eq. (9.12) is

$$\begin{aligned} u + \alpha L(u) u &= z, \ x \in \Omega \\ \frac{\partial u}{\partial n} &= 0, \ x \in \partial\, \Omega , \end{aligned} \tag{9.13}$$

where $L(u)$ is a differential operator whose action on u is given by

$$L(u)u = -\nabla \cdot \left(\frac{1}{\sqrt{|\nabla u|^2 + \beta^2}} \nabla u\right), \tag{9.14}$$

It is an elliptic nonlinear partial differential equation (PDE). From Eq. (9.14), we can see that the smoothing decreases as the gradient strength increases; and thus, the smoothing stops across edges.

There are many standard numerical optimization techniques such as conjugate gradient method. However, these standard methods tend to perform poorly on TV minimization problems. In this paper we adopt the nonlinear multi-grid method to deal with this problem. Unlike the conventional methods, the multi-grid algorithm can solve nonlinear elliptic PDE with non-constant coefficients with hardly any loss in efficiency. In addition, no nonlinear equations need to be solved, except on the coarsest grid.

Suppose we discrete the nonlinear elliptic PDE of Eq. (9.13) on a uniform grid with mesh size h:

$$T_h(u_h) = z_h, \tag{9.15}$$

where: $T_h(u_h)$ denote $u_h + \alpha L_h(u_h)u_h$.

Let $\widetilde{u_h}$ denote some approximate solution and u_h denote the exact solution to Eq. (9.15). Then the correction is:

$$v_h = u_h - \widetilde{u}_h,$$

The residual is:

$$T_h(\widetilde{u_h} + v_h) - T_h(\widetilde{u}_h) = f_h - T_h(\widetilde{u}_h) = -d_h, \tag{9.16}$$

Now, we form the appropriate approximation T_H of T_h on a coarser grid with mesh size H (we will always take $H = 2\,h$). The residual equation is now approximated by:

$$T_H(u_H) - T_H(\widetilde{u}_H) = -d_H, \tag{9.17}$$

Since T_H has a smaller dimension, this equation will be easier to be solved. To define $\widetilde{u}_H$ and d_H on the coarse grid, we need a restriction operator R that restricts $\widetilde{u_h}$ and d_h to the coarse grid. That is, we solve:

$$T_H(u_H) = T_H(R\widetilde{u_h}) - Rd_h, \tag{9.18}$$

on the coarse gird. Then the coarse-grid correction is:

$$\widetilde{v}_H = u_H - R\widetilde{u_h},$$

Once we have a solution $\widetilde{v}_H$ on the coarse gird, we need a prolongation operator P that interpolates the correction to the fine gird:

$$\widetilde{v_h} = P\widetilde{v}_H,$$

So we have:

$$\widetilde{u}_{h\,new} = \widetilde{u_h} + P\widetilde{v}_H, \tag{9.19}$$

It is the two-grid algorithm and can be easily extended to a multi-grid.

The symbol of P is found by considering v_H to be 1 at some mesh point (x, y), zero elsewhere, and then asking for the values of Pv_H. The most popular prolongation operator is simple bilinear interpolation. It gives nonzero values at the nine points (x,y), $(x + h, y)$, …, $(x - h, y - h)$ and its symbol is:

$$\begin{bmatrix} 1/4 & 1/2 & 1/4 \\ 1/2 & 1 & 1/2 \\ 1/4 & 1/2 & 1/4 \end{bmatrix}, \tag{9.20}$$

The symbol of R is defined by considering v_h to be defined everywhere on the fine grid, and then asking what is Rv_h at (x,y) as a linear combination of these values. The choice for R is the adjoint operator to P. So that the symbol of R is:

$$\begin{bmatrix} 1/16 & 1/8 & 1/16 \\ 1/8 & 1/4 & 1/8 \\ 1/16 & 1/8 & 1/16 \end{bmatrix}, \tag{9.21}$$

At the coarsest-grid, we have one remaining task before implementing our nonlinear multi-grid algorithm: choosing a nonlinear relaxation scheme. Our first choice is the nonlinear Gauss–Seidel scheme. If the discretized Eq. (9.15) is written with some choice of ordering as:

$$T_i(u_1, \ldots, u_N) = z_i, i = 1, \ldots, N, \tag{9.22}$$

Then the nonlinear Gauss–Seidel scheme solves:

$$T_i\left(u_1, \ldots, u_{i-1}, u_i^{new}, u_{i+1}, \ldots, u_N\right) = z_i, \tag{9.23}$$

Often equation is linear in u_i^{new}, since the nonlinear terms are discretized by means of its neighbors. If this is not the case, we replace Eq. (9.19) by one step of a Newton iteration:

$$u_i^{new} = u_i^{old} - \frac{T_i\left(u_i^{old}\right) - z_i}{\partial T_i(u_i^{old})/\partial u_i}, \tag{9.24}$$

Results

Lung Field and Anatomic Segment

Lung segmentation plays an important role in the bone suppression in this study. Inaccurate segmentation means that the anatomical segment mask will not correspond to the region mask trained in the anatomically specific multiple MTANNs. As a result, the bone structures will not be suppressed in the VDE soft image very well. Figure 9.8 shows a failed case due to inaccurate segmentation of the lung field. Although some bones are suppressed, the clavicles are not suppressed. When the lung field was manually segmented into the eight anatomical segments, the clavicles were suppressed much more successfully.

In this study, 93 normal images from the public Japanese Society of Radiological Technology (JSRT) database were used for training of the M-ASM. The segmentation accuracy was computed by use of the overlap measure Ω:

$$\Omega = \frac{TP_{seg}}{TP_{seg} + FP_{seg} + FN_{seg}}, \tag{9.25}$$

where TP_{seg} is the area correctly classified as a lung field, FP_{seg} is the area incorrectly classified as a lung field, and FN_{seg} is the area incorrectly classified as the background. The mean and standard deviation of the overlap measure for all the 154 nodule images in the JSRT database were 0.913 and 0.023, respectively. For the 118 testing cases in the U of C database, because we did not have the lung field truth with which we compare our M-ASM segmentation results, we only evaluated segmentation results visually. Based on our visual evaluation, segmentation failed in ten cases. This may be because the M-ASM was trained with JSRT normal cases that were digitized from files, whereas the U of C database consists of digital radiographs with nodules from a CR system. We would like to leave the improvement in the performance of lung segmentation as our future work.

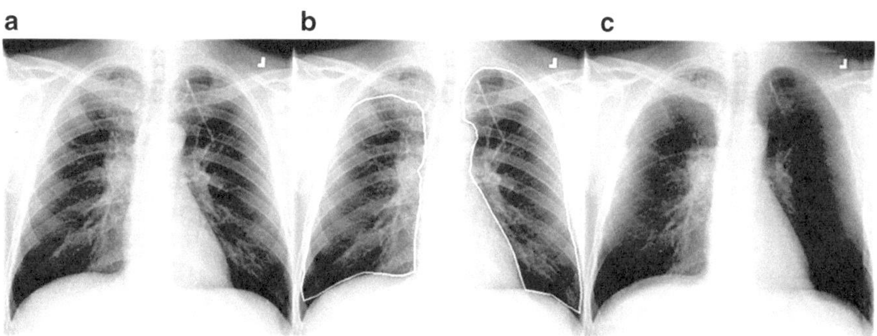

Fig. 9.8 Illustration of incomplete suppression caused by a lung segmentation failure. (**a**) an original image, (**b**) lung field segmentation, and (**c**) bone suppression within the segmented lung fields. The right clavicles in (**c**) are not suppressed

In these experiments, 50 points were used for each M-ASM for each lung, and the relative position of each point in the segmentation results is known. As shown in Fig. 9.5, the seventh point in the segment boundary between the lung field and the lung wall begins from the apex of the lung (the translating blue point), and the aortic arch blue point was used to achieve the upper lung segment. The sixth point begins from costophrenic angle (blue point in the lowest position) and the blue point in the ventricle border was used to segment the lower lung region. Finally, the apex point and the blue point in the hemidiaphragm were used to segment the middle region to obtain the hilar region.

As a result, we can automatically obtain anatomic segments based on the lung field segmentation results (Fig. 9.6).

Smoothing VDE Bone Images

In order to prove the effectiveness of the TV minimization smoothing method, we compared with the Gaussian smoothing method. As illustrated in Fig. 9.9, the edges of ribs remain in the soft-tissue image obtained by using the Gaussian smoothing method, whereas they disappear in the soft-tissue image obtained by using the TV minimization smoothing method.

In our experiment, the smoothing parameter used for the original VDE bone image was usually larger than that of the improved VDE bone image. The reason is that in our improved bone suppression method, each set of anatomic specific MTANNs only process patterns with less variation in a small, relatively uniform anatomic segment. The signal-to-noise ratio in the small anatomic segment is higher than that in the entire lung field.

The processing time for the Gaussian smoothing method was 0.2 s per case, whereas that for the TV minimization was only 1 s per case because of the efficiency of the multi-grid algorithm that was implemented in the TV minimization.

Evaluation

The newly developed anatomically specific multiple MTANNs were subjected to a validation test that included 110 nodule cases. The bone suppression performance was quantitatively evaluated by using the absolute error [4], defined as:

$$E_N = \sum_{x,\,y \in R_L} |b(x,y) - f_b(x,y)| / N_L(b_{\max} - b_{\min}), \tag{9.26}$$

where $f_b(x,y)$ is the VDE bone image, $b(x,y)$ is the corresponding "gold-standard" dual-energy bone image, R_L indicates lung regions, N_L is the number of pixels in R_L, and b_{max} and b_{min} are the maximum value and the minimum value in R_L in the dual-energy bone image, respectively. The result for the 110 CXRs was an average E_N of

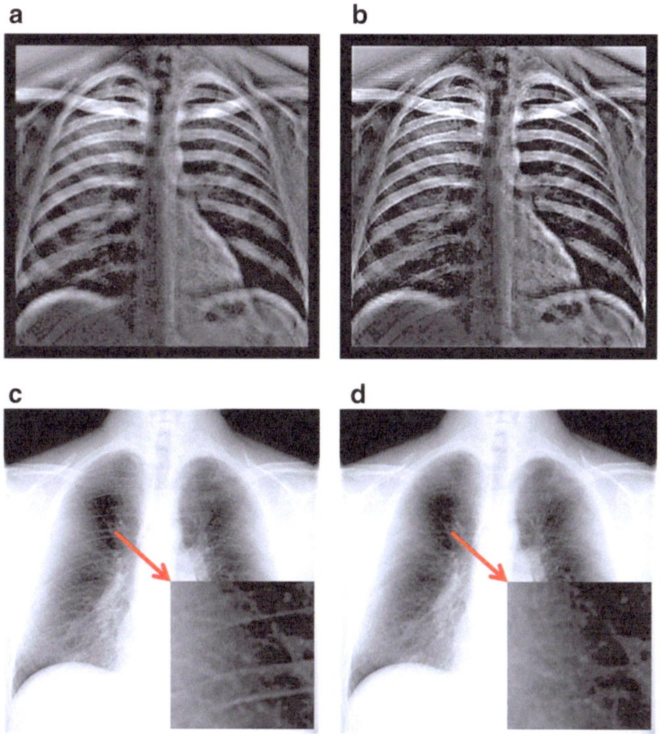

Fig. 9.9 Illustration of (**a**) a VDE bone image with Gaussian smoothing, (**b**) a VDE bone image with TV-minimization-based smoothing, (**c**) a VDE soft-tissue image corresponding to (**a**), and (**d**) a VDE soft-tissue image corresponding to (**b**), all by use of the anatomically specific multiple MTANNs

0.072 with a standard deviation of 0.012, which were lower than the result (E_N of 0.082 with a standard deviation of 0.014) for our previous method [4] at a statistically significant level ($P < 0.05$).

Figure 9.10 illustrates the results of bone suppression for a normal case. Compare to the old VDE soft-tissue images obtained by use of our previous technique, rib edges, the clavicles, and ribs close to the lung wall are suppressed better, while the visibility of soft tissue such as vessels is maintained. The quality of the VDE soft-tissue images is comparable to that of the "gold-standard" dual-energy soft-tissue images.

Figure 9.11 illustrates the results for a case where a nodule that not only overlaps with ribs but also is close to the lung wall. In our previous method, the ribs close to the lung wall were not successfully suppressed, and the contrast of the nodule in this area was similar to the original CXR. In the present improved method, the nodule was maintained while the surrounding ribs were suppressed, and the boundary of the nodule was clearer than that in the original CXR. Figure 9.12 illustrates a case

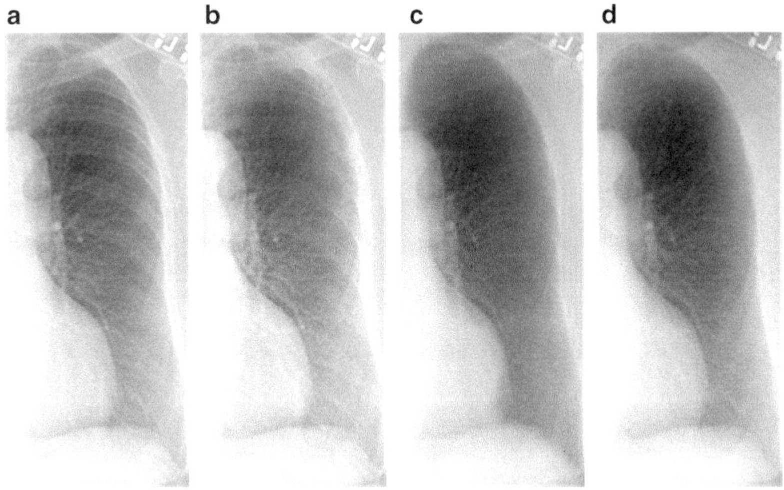

Fig. 9.10 Result for a non-training normal chest radiograph. (**a**) An original normal chest radiograph, (**b**) a VDE soft-tissue image obtained by use of our original MTANN technique, (**c**) a VDE soft-tissue image obtained by use of our new MTANN technique, and (**d**) the corresponding "gold-standard" dual-energy soft-tissue image

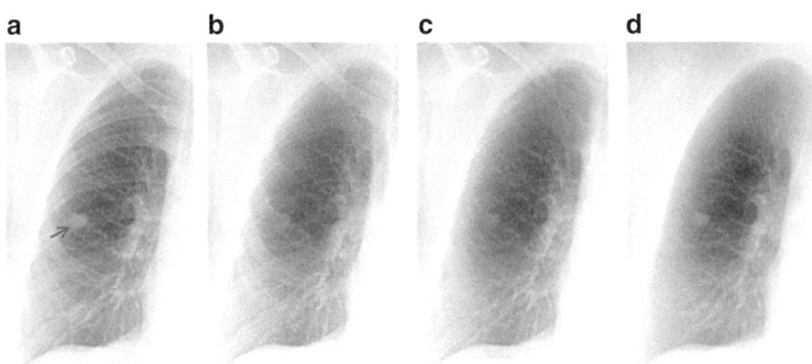

Fig. 9.11 Result for an abnormal chest radiograph with a nodule that overlaps with both anterior and posterior ribs. (**a**) An original abnormal chest radiograph with a nodule (indicated by a *red arrow*), (**b**) a VDE soft-tissue image obtained by use of our original MTANN technique, (**c**) a VDE soft-tissue image obtained by use of our new MTANN technique, and (**d**) the corresponding "gold-standard" dual-energy soft-tissue image

where the nodule that partly overlaps with bone. In our original results, the boundaries of the nodule were smoothed, and the contrast of the nodule was partly suppressed, whereas in the improved result, there were clear nodule boundaries and the contrast of the nodule was close to that of the soft-tissue image. Figure 9.13 illustrates a case of good preservation of nodules found in the left lung. Figure 9.14

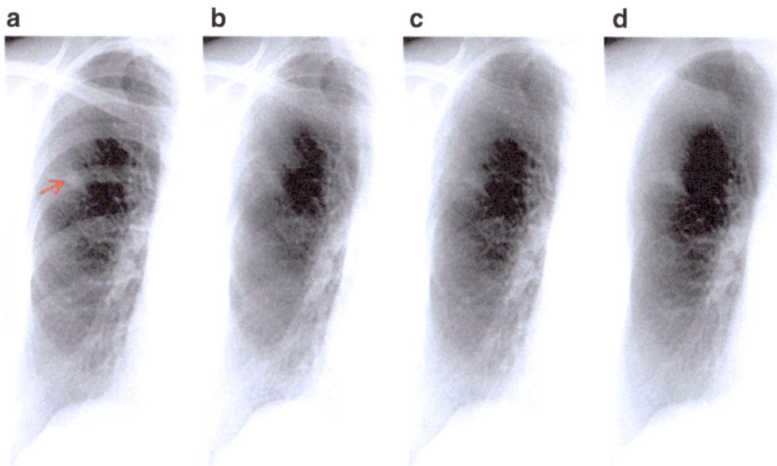

Fig. 9.12 Results for abnormal chest radiographs with a nodule that is mostly overlap with a rib. (**a**) An original abnormal chest radiograph with a nodule (indicated by a *red arrow*), (**b**) a VDE soft-tissue image obtained by use of our original MTANN technique, (**c**) a VDE soft-tissue image obtained by use of our new MTANN technique, and (**d**) the corresponding "gold-standard" dual-energy soft-tissue image

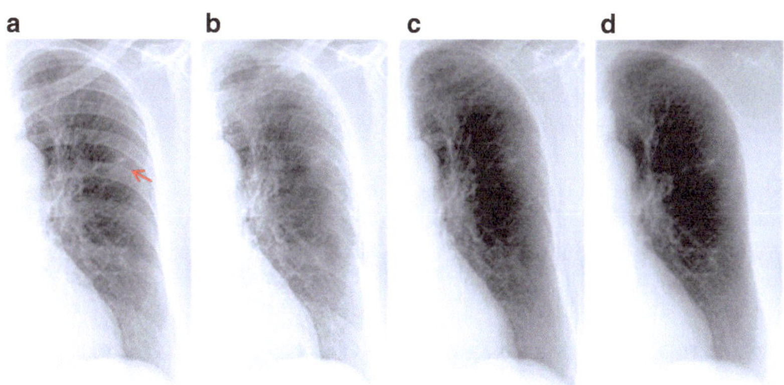

Fig. 9.13 Results for abnormal chest radiographs with a tiny nodule in the left lung. (**a**) An original abnormal chest radiograph with a nodule (indicated by a *red arrow*), (**b**) a VDE soft-tissue image obtained by use of our original MTANN technique, (**c**) a VDE soft-tissue image obtained by use of our new MTANN technique, and (**d**) the corresponding "gold-standard" dual-energy soft-tissue image

illustrates a case where the nodules were located in the hilar region. Both the contrast and shapes of the nodules were maintained very well in the images obtained with the present improved method, whereas in the images obtained with the original method, the nodules appeared diffused with smoothed boundaries.

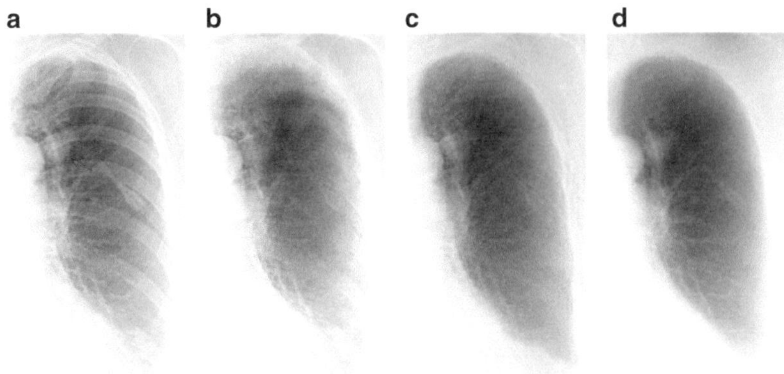

Fig. 9.14 Results for abnormal chest radiographs with a nodule in the hilar region of the lung. (**a**) An original abnormal chest radiograph with a nodule (indicated by a *red arrow*), (**b**) a VDE soft-tissue image obtained by use of our original MTANN technique, (**c**) a VDE soft-tissue image obtained by use of our new MTANN technique, and (**d**) the corresponding "gold-standard" dual-energy soft-tissue image

Discussion

In CXR, nodules generally overlap with ribs, which are often close to the lung wall. This causes a large number of FPs in the CADe scheme. In previously described method, the posterior ribs were suppressed well, but the anterior ribs were not suppressed sufficiently. In the VDE bone images, nodules still overlap with anterior ribs, which usually have a similar density to the nodules.

All the results in this paper were achieved by using a single set of same parameters. However, in order to obtain the best results, we can optimize the bone suppression amount for different CXRs acquired in different exposure settings.

Although the gray-level normalization for consistency improvement was used for training images to make the output images of each of the anatomically specific MTANNs in the bone suppression phase consistent, in some cases, there were still some differences between different anatomic segments in terms of the bone contrast and density. As a result, bones in some anatomical segments were not suppressed as much as were in other segments. This may be because variations in bone contrast and density in testing images were larger than those in the training images.

One of the advantages of the M-ASM segmentation method used in this work is that it is possible to know which point belongs to which type of anatomic boundary, and that which point is the transition point in the contour of the segmentation. Based on these points, the lung field can be automatically divided into segments based on the anatomy. It is helpful to suppress bones in different anatomical segments automatically.

In this study, we assume that the noise model in VDE bone images is Gaussian, and the TV-based models can answer fundamental questions arising in image restoration better than other models.

In our original method, only the posterior ribs were present in the VDE bone images. Owing to the anatomically specific multiple MTANNs used in this work, the anterior ribs were also present in the new VDE bone images. As the anterior ribs in a CXR are usually close to the lung wall, their suppression using this novel method was seen to be significantly better than that using the original method.

Although nine cases were used (one normal and eight abnormal cases) for training the anatomically specific multiple MTANNs, only one normal case and one nodule case were used for each anatomic segment. In spite of the small number of cases used, the MTANNs produced reliable results for non-training cases. However, the MTANN would be more robust against variations among cases if a larger number of cases were used for training.

As the use of the MTANN requires only software, this technique can be utilized on an existing viewing workstation. Although we applied a TV minimization-based smoothing method, the processing time for creating a VDE soft-tissue image and a VDE bone image from a CXR is very short, i.e., 1.63 s on a PC-based workstation (CPU: Intel Pentium IV, 3.2 GHz) because the efficient multi-grid solving method was used. Thus, the software can be applied prior to interpretation in every case without incurring any delay.

As the fine structures of soft tissues such as small vessels are mostly maintained in the VDE soft-tissue images, these images could potentially be used for quantitative assessment of interstitial lung diseases that are characterized by fine patterns. In addition, this technique can easily be applied to anatomic regions other than the lungs by training with dual-energy images of specific anatomic segments.

Conclusion

We have developed an anatomically (location-) specific multiple MTANN scheme to suppress bony structures in CXRs. With our new technique, rib edges, ribs close to the lung wall, and the clavicles were suppressed substantially better than was possible with our conventional technique, while soft tissue such as lung nodules and vessels was maintained. Thus, our technique would be useful for radiologists as well as for CADe schemes in the detection of lung nodules in CXRs.

Acknowledgments The authors are grateful to Heber MacMahon, MD, for his valuable clinical suggestions. Initial bone suppression technology and source code have been non-exclusively licensed to Riverain Medical (Riverain Technologies). It is the policy of University of Chicago that investigators disclose publicly actual or potential financial interests that may appear to be affected by research activities.

References

1. Murray CJ, Lopez AD (1997) Mortality by cause for eight regions of the world: global burden of disease study. Lancet 349:1269–1276
2. Murphy GP et al (1995) American Cancer Society textbook of clinical oncology, 2nd edn. The American Cancer Society, Atlanta
3. Frost JK et al (1984) Early lung cancer detection: results of the initial (prevalence) radiologic and cytologic screening in the Johns Hopkins study. Am Rev Respir Dis 130:549–554
4. Fontana RS et al (1984) Early lung cancer detection: results of the initial (prevalence) radiologic and cytologic screening in the Mayo Clinic study. Am Rev Respir Dis 130:561–565
5. Henschke CI et al (1994) Radiographic screening for cancer. Proposed paradigm for requisite research. Clin Imaging 18:16–20
6. Heelan RT et al (1984) Non-small-cell lung cancer: results of the New York screening program. Radiology 151:289–293
7. Sobue T et al (1992) Survival for clinical stage I lung cancer not surgically treated. Comparison between screen-detected and symptom-detected cases. The Japanese Lung Cancer Screening Research Group. Cancer 69:685–692
8. Flehinger BJ et al (1992) The effect of surgical treatment on survival from early lung cancer. Implications for screening. Chest 101:1013–1018
9. Austin JH et al (1992) Missed bronchogenic carcinoma: radiographic findings in 27 patients with a potentially resectable lesion evident in retrospect. Radiology 182:115–122
10. Shah PK et al (2003) Missed non-small cell lung cancer: radiographic findings of potentially resectable lesions evident only in retrospect. Radiology 226:235–241
11. Li F et al (2008) Improved detection of small lung cancers with dual-energy subtraction chest radiography. AJR Am J Roentgenol 190:886–891
12. Giger ML et al (1988) Image feature analysis and computer-aided diagnosis in digital radiography. 3. Automated detection of nodules in peripheral lung fields. Med Phys 15:158–166
13. van Ginneken B et al (2001) Computer-aided diagnosis in chest radiography: a survey. IEEE Trans Med Imaging 20:1228–1241
14. Abe K et al (1993) Computer-aided diagnosis in chest radiography. Preliminary experience. Invest Radiol 28:987–993
15. Kobayashi T et al (1996) Effect of a computer-aided diagnosis scheme on radiologists' performance in detection of lung nodules on radiographs. Radiology 199:843–848
16. Kakeda S et al (2004) Improved detection of lung nodules on chest radiographs using a commercial computer-aided diagnosis system. AJR Am J Roentgenol 182:505–510
17. Matsumoto T et al (1992) Image feature analysis of false-positive diagnoses produced by automated detection of lung nodules. Invest Radiol 27:587–597
18. Xu XW et al (1997) Development of an improved CAD scheme for automated detection of lung nodules in digital chest images. Med Phys 24:1395–1403
19. Kido S et al (2002) Detection of simulated pulmonary nodules by single-exposure dual-energy computed radiography of the chest: effect of a computer-aided diagnosis system (part 2). Eur J Radiol 44:205–209
20. Kido S et al (2002) Computerized detection of pulmonary nodules by single-exposure dual-energy computed radiography of the chest (part 1). Eur J Radiol 44:198–204
21. Glocker R, Frohnmayer W (1925) Uber die rontgenspektroskopische Bestimmung des Gewichtsanteiles eines Elementes in Gememgen und Verbindungen. Ann Phys 76:369–395
22. Jacobson B, Mackay RS (1958) Radiological contrast enhancing methods. Adv Biol Med Phys 6:201–261
23. Suzuki K et al (2006) Image-processing technique for suppressing ribs in chest radiographs by means of massive training artificial neural network (MTANN). IEEE Trans Med Imaging 25:406–416

24. Suzuki K et al (2004) Suppression of the contrast of ribs in chest radiographs by means of massive training artificial neural network. In: Proceedings of SPIE medical imaging (SPIE MI), San Diego, pp 1109–1119
25. Suzuki K (2012) Pixel-based machine learning in medical imaging. Int J Biomed Imaging 2012:18
26. Oda S et al (2009) Performance of radiologists in detection of small pulmonary nodules on chest radiographs: effect of rib suppression with a massive-training artificial neural network. AJR Am J Roentgenol 193:W397–W402
27. Ahmed B, Rasheed T (2007) Rib suppression for enhancing frontal chest radiographs using independent component analysis. In: Adaptive and natural computing algorithms. Lecture notes in computer science, vol 4432. Springer, New York, pp 300–308
28. Loog M et al (2006) Filter learning: application to suppression of bony structures from chest radiographs. Med Image Anal 10:826–840
29. Ishigaki T et al (1986) One-shot dual-energy subtraction imaging. Radiology 161:271–273
30. Ishigaki T et al (1988) One-shot dual-energy subtraction chest imaging with computed radiography: clinical evaluation of film images. Radiology 168:67–72
31. Stewart BK, Huang HK (1990) Single-exposure dual-energy computed radiography. Med Phys 17:866–875
32. Suzuki K et al (2003) Massive training artificial neural network (MTANN) for reduction of false positives in computerized detection of lung nodules in low-dose CT. Med Phys 30:15
33. Suzuki K et al (1995) Recognition of coronary arterial stenosis using neural network on DSA system. Syst Comput Jpn 26:66–74
34. Suzuki K et al (2003) Neural edge enhancer for supervised edge enhancement from noisy images. IEEE Trans Pattern Anal Mach Intell 25:1582–1596
35. Xu J, Suzuki K (2011) Massive-training support vector regression and Gaussian process for false-positive reduction in computer-aided detection of polyps in CT colonography. Med Phys 38:14
36. van Ginneken B et al (2006) Segmentation of anatomical structures in chest radiographs using supervised methods: a comparative study on a public database. Med Image Anal 10:19–40
37. Chen S et al (2011) Development and evaluation of a computer-aided diagnostic scheme for lung nodule detection in chest radiographs by means of two-stage nodule enhancement with support vector classification. Med Phys 38:15
38. van Ginneken B et al (2002) Active shape model segmentation with optimal features. IEEE Trans Med Imaging 21:924–933
39. Rudin LI et al (1992) Nonlinear total variation based noise removal algorithms. Physica D 60:259–268

Chapter 10
Image Segmentation for Connectomics Using Machine Learning

T. Tasdizen, M. Seyedhosseini, T. Liu, C. Jones, and E. Jurrus

Abstract Reconstruction of neural circuits at the microscopic scale of individual neurons and synapses, also known as connectomics, is an important challenge for neuroscience. While an important motivation of connectomics is providing anatomical ground truth for neural circuit models, the ability to decipher neural wiring maps at the individual cell level is also important in studies of many neurodegenerative diseases. Reconstruction of a neural circuit at the individual neuron level requires the use of electron microscopy images due to their extremely high resolution. Computational challenges include pixel-by-pixel annotation of these images into classes such as cell membrane, mitochondria and synaptic vesicles and the segmentation of individual neurons. State-of-the-art image analysis solutions are still far from the accuracy and robustness of human vision and biologists are still limited to studying small neural circuits using mostly manual analysis. In this chapter, we describe our image analysis pipeline that makes use of novel supervised machine learning techniques to tackle this problem.

Introduction

Supervised machine learning techniques have shown great potential and have become important tools of choice in many problems. This is particularly true for image analysis [1, 2]. Image analysis approaches with hand designed, deterministic filters are being replaced with approaches that use filters and operations learned

T. Tasdizen (✉) • M. Seyedhosseini • C. Jones
Electrical and Computer Engineering Department, Scientific Computing and Imaging Institute, University of Utah, Lake City, UT 84112, USA
e-mail: tolga@sci.utah.edu

T. Liu • E. Jurrus
School of Computing, Scientific Computing and Imaging Institute, University of Utah, Lake City, UT 84112, USA

K. Suzuki (ed.), *Computational Intelligence in Biomedical Imaging*,
DOI 10.1007/978-1-4614-7245-2_10,

from human generated ground truth. This supervised learning strategy has been shown to outperform traditional methods in many image analysis applications. In this chapter, we will focus on one such application: neural circuit reconstruction from electron microscopy (EM) images at the scale of individual neurons and synapses. We will refer to this problem as connectomics [3–10].

An important motivation for connectomics is providing anatomical ground truth for neural circuit models. Connectomics is also important in studies of many neurodegenerative diseases. For instance, a loss of photoreceptors in the retina can cause neurons to rewire [11, 12] and neural circuits undergo remodeling in response to seizures in epilepsy [13, 14]. Serial section EM, where a block of tissue is cut into sections and imaged, has sufficient detail for identification of individual neurons and their synaptic connections in a three-dimensional (3D) volume; however, this is a difficult and time-consuming image analysis task for humans. Furthermore, state-of-the-art automated image analysis solutions are still far from the accuracy and robustness of human vision. Therefore, biologists are still limited to studying small neural circuits using mostly manual analysis. Reconstruction of a neural circuit from an electron microscopy volume requires segmentation of individual neurons in three dimensions and the detection of synapses between them. Supervised learning approaches to this problem typically involve pixel-by-pixel annotation of these images into classes such as cell membrane, mitochondria, and synaptic vesicles with a classifier learned from training data. We will refer to this step as the pixel classifier. This is generally followed by another step which segments individual neurons based on the cell membrane pixels detected by the classifier in the initial step. This second step can be as simple as a flood fill operation on the thresholded output of the pixel classifier from the first step or as complex as a second classifier which learns to merge/split regions obtained from the pixel classifier's output as in our approach. This two-step strategy is taken because cell membranes are similar in local appearance to many other intracellular structures (see Fig. 10.1) which makes their detection with deterministic filter banks or segmentation with techniques such as active contours very difficult.

The supervised learning strategy for connectomics has its own challenges that need to be addressed. First, generating training data from electron microscopy images can be a cumbersome task for humans. On the other hand, no training data is needed for deterministic approaches. Second, the training set can be extremely large since each pixel in the training image becomes a training example. This requires a lengthy training stage. In comparison, no training time is spent in deterministic approaches. Third, overfitting is a possibility as in any machine learning application. Finally, the cell membrane classification step demands extremely high accuracy. Even with high pixel accuracy rates such as 95 %, which is acceptable in many other applications, it is virtually certain that almost every neuron in a volume will be incorrectly segmented due to their global, tree-like structure, and correspondingly large surface area. The lack of reliable automated solutions to these problems is the current bottleneck in the field of connectomics. In this chapter, we will describe our approach to deal with each of these problems.

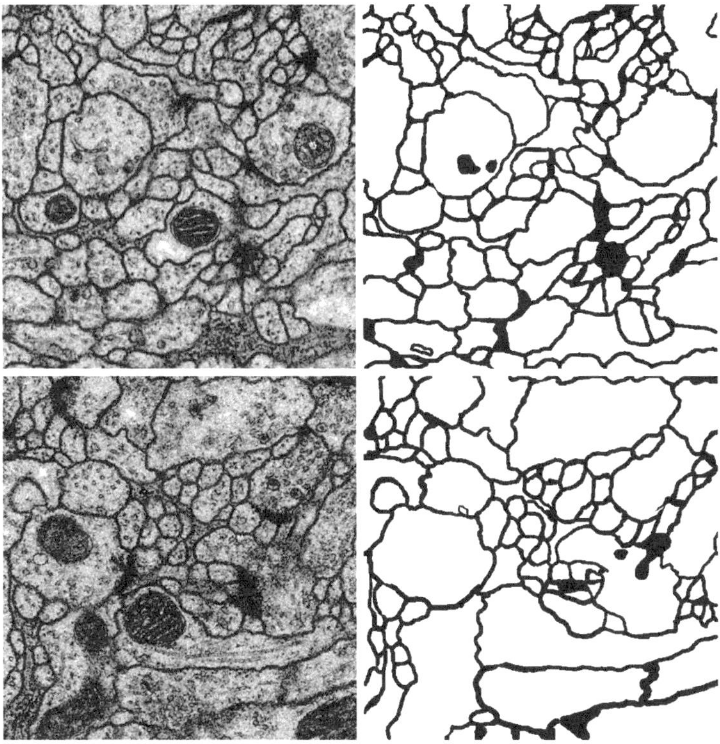

Fig. 10.1 *Left*: Two ssTEM sections from the Drosophila first instar larva VNC [8]. *Right*: Corresponding ground truth maps for cell membranes (*black*). *Data: Cardona Lab, ETH*

Background

Connectomics from Electron Microscopy

Compared with other imaging techniques, such as MRI [15] and scanning confocal light microscopy [16–20], electron microscopy provides much higher resolution and remains the primary tool for connectomics. The only complete reconstruction of a nervous system to date has been performed for the nematode *Caenorhabditis elegans* (*C. elegans*) which has 302 neurons and just over 6,000 synapses [21–23]. This reconstruction, performed manually, is reported to have taken more than a decade [4]. Recently, high throughput serial section transmission electron microscopy (ssTEM) [5, 6, 9, 24–26] and serial block-face scanning electron microscopy (SBFSEM) [4, 10, 27] have emerged as automated acquisition strategies for connectomics. Automatic Tape-Collecting Lathe Ultramicrotome (ATLUM) [28] is another promising technology for speeding up data collection for connectomics.

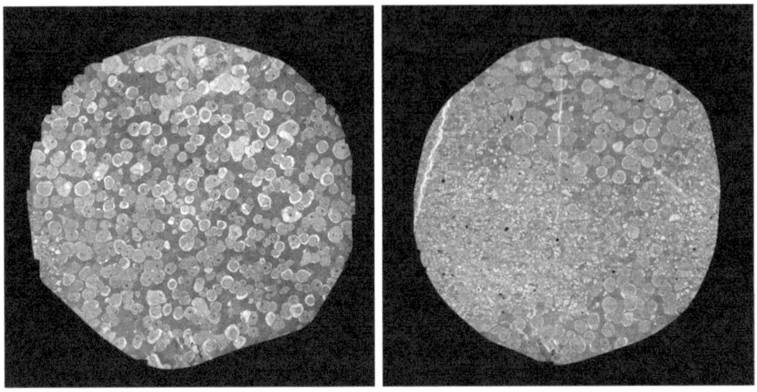

Fig. 10.2 Two sections from the retinal connectome [32] which comprises 341 sections. Each section is $\sim$ 32 GB and comprises 1,000 image tiles, each 4, 096 $\times$4, 096 pixels. The circular area with data is approximately 132, 000 pixels in diameter. The complete dataset is $\sim$ 16 TB. *Data: Marc Lab, University of Utah*

In the ssTEM technique, sections are cut from a specimen block and suspended so that an electron beam can pass through it, creating a projection which can be captured digitally or on film with 2 nm in-plane resolution. This extremely high resolution is sufficient for identifying synapses visually. An important trade-off occurs with respect to the section thickness: thinner sections, e.g. 30 nm, are easier to analyze because structures are crisper due to less averaging whereas thicker sections, e.g. 90 nm, are easier to handle physically without loss. Through mosaicking of many individual images [29, 30], ssTEM offers a relatively wide field of view to identify large sets of cells as they progress through the sections. Image registration techniques are necessary to align the sections into a 3D volume [6, 31].

In the SBFSEM technique, sections are cut away, and the electron beam is scanned over the remaining block face to produce electron backscatter images. Since the dimensions of the solid block remain relatively stable after sectioning, there is no need for image registration between sections. However, the in-plane resolution is closer to 10 nm which is a disadvantage compared to ssTEM. Typical section thicknesses for SBFSEM are 30–50 nm.

New projects using the techniques described above capture very large volumes containing several orders of magnitude more neurons than the *C. elegans*. As an example, Fig. 10.2 shows two mosaic sections from a *16 TB* ssTEM retina volume [32] that was assembled with our algorithms [6, 31]. It is not feasible to reconstruct complete neural circuits in these datasets with manual methods. Moreover, population or screening studies are unfeasible since fully manual segmentation and analysis would require years of manual effort per specimen. As a result, automation of the computational reconstruction process is critical for the study of these systems.

Finally, as an alternative to SBFSEM and ssTEM, fully 3D approaches such as focused ion-beam scanning electron microscopy (FIBSEM) [33] and electron tomography [34–36] produce nearly isotropic datasets. Both techniques are limited to studying small volumes which is a disadvantage for their use for connectomics. FIBSEM uses a focused-ion beam to mill away sections instead of cutting sections with a knife. While it is clear that these datasets are easier to analyze accurately, the amount of data and the time it would take to acquire and analyze them is prohibitive for large-scale circuit reconstruction applications for the time being.

Neuron Segmentation

Figure 10.2b shows the complexity of the problem. This image which is 132, 000 pixels in diameter contains thousands of neuronal processes. The larger structures seen in Fig. 10.2a are the cell bodies of these processes. Reconstructing neural circuits from EM datasets involves segmenting individual neurons in 3D and finding the synapses between them. Neuron segmentation is the immediate challenge and thus has gathered significantly more attention than synapse detection. The only successful automatic synapse detection approaches so far have been limited to FIBSEM data which offers almost isotropic resolution [37]. In this chapter, we limit our attention to neuron segmentation. There are two general strategies for neuron segmentation. One strategy is to directly segment neurons in 3D [38, 39]. However, this can be difficult in many datasets due to the anisotropic nature of the data. The large section thickness often causes features to shift significantly between sequential images both in ssTEM and SBFSEM, decreasing the potential advantages of a direct 3D approach. The other strategy first segments neurons in two-dimensional (2D) images followed by linking them across sections to form a complete neuron [40–43]. Our approach fits in this second category. In this chapter, we focus on the 2D neuron segmentation problem. For linking 2D neuron regions across sections we refer the reader to [41, 44–46].

Image Processing Methods

Neuron segmentation has been studied mostly using semi-automated methods [8, 24, 40, 43, 47]. Fully automatic segmentation is complicated by two main challenges: complex intracellular structures such as vesicles and mitochondria that are present in the ssTEM images and the extremely anisotropic resolution of the data, e.g. 2 nm in-plane vs. 40 nm out-of-plane. Previous automatic EM segmentation methods include active contours which rely on an gradient term to drive the segmentation [42, 48–53]. This gradient/edge term can be ambiguous because of the locally similar appearance of neuron and intracellular membranes. Figure 10.1 shows two ssTEM sections from the Drosophila first instar larva ventral nerve cord (VNC) [8] and their corresponding cell membrane ground truth maps drawn by a human expert. Notice that the intensity profile of cell membranes completely overlaps with many other intracellular structures such as mitochondria (large, dark round structures) and synapses (elongated, dark structures). Furthermore, notice that when the cell membranes are parallel to the cutting plane in 3D they appear fuzzy and of lighter intensity. In our earlier work, we used directional diffusion to attempt to remove intracellular structures from similar images [54]. Other researchers have used Radon-like features [55] to try to isolate cell membranes without using supervised learning. These deterministic methods have had limited success.

Furthermore, due to the very anisotropic resolution, a typical approach is to segment neurons in 2D sections followed by a separate stage to link the segments in 3D as mentioned earlier. Active contours can be propagated through the sections with the help of Kalman filtering [50]; however, this propagation can be inaccurate because of the large changes in shape and position of neurons from one section to the next. The large shape change stems from the anisotropy of the volume while the position change problem stems from the anisotropy as well as the fact that each section is cut and imaged independently resulting in nonrigid deformations. While our and other registration methods [31, 56, 57] can be used to fix the position change problem to a large extent, the shape change problem remains. Consequently, due to this poor initialization, active contours can get stuck on edges of intracellular structures and fail to segment neurons properly. Hence, active contours have been most successful in earlier SBFSEM images which only highlight extracellular spaces removing almost all contrast from intracellular structures. While this simplifies segmentation, it also removes important information such as synapses that are critical to identifying functional properties of neurons [7]. The other drawback is that active contours typically segment one neuron at a time whereas a typical volume has tens of thousands of neurons. While graph-cut methods [58–60] can simultaneously segment a large number of neurons, they still have the intracellular membrane problem. Combined with machine learning methods [61], they have an improved detection accuracy and can be used more reliably.

Machine Learning Methods

As discussed, intracellular structures are present in images which can be a source of confusion for neuron segmentation. Supervised lassifiers have been applied to the problem of neuron membrane detection as a precursor to segmentation and have proven more successful [5, 38, 39, 62, 63]. Membrane detection results can be with a method as simple as flood-filling for segmentation or as an edge term in active contour or graph-cut methods to overcome the problem due to intracellular structures. Jain et al. [39] use a convolutional network for restoring membranes in SBFSEM images. Similar to Markov random field (MRF) [64, 65] and conditional random fields (CRF) [66, 67] models, convolutional networks impose a spatial coherency on the membrane detection results. However, convolutional nets define a less rigid framework where the spatial structure is learned and they can make use of context from larger regions, but typically need many hidden layers. The large number of hidden layers can become problematic in training with backpropagation and simplifications such as layer-by-layer training are often needed [68]. The series neural network architecture [63] used here also takes advantage of context and samples image pixels directly to learn membrane boundaries.

While supervised learning for cell membrane detection has met moderate success, all methods require substantial user interaction for initialization and correcting errors in the subsequent segmentation step [40]. As discussed in section "Introduction", the cell membrane classification step demands extremely high accuracy. Neurons have a global tree-like geometry with a correspondingly large surface area between neighboring neurons (cell membranes). A single local area of false negatives on this cell membrane leads to under-segmentation. Therefore, even with high pixel accuracy rates such as 95 % it is virtually certain that almost every neuron in a volume will be incorrectly under-segmented. Furthermore, neurons have very narrow cross-sections in many places which create many possibilities for over-segmentation when intracellular structures with similar local appearance to cell membranes are co-located with these constrictions. Researchers have investigated approaches to improve the accuracy of such classifiers. A 2-step classification where a membrane detection classifier is followed by a higher-level classifier that learns to remove spurious boundary segments causing over-segmentation was proposed [38]. Funke et al. [46] proposed a tree structure for simultaneous intra-section and inter-section segmentation. However, their model can only segment a 3D volume of consecutive sections and cannot segment a single section. Moreover, the final optimization problem in their model can be complicated given a set of complete trees of an image stack. Another promising direction is to optimize segmentation error rather than pixel-wise classification error, focusing learning on critical pixels where a mistake in classification results in a segmentation error [69, 70]. Topological constraints have also been proposed as an alternative to the pixel-wise classification error metric [71]. A recent study proposed to combine tomographic reconstruction with ssTEM to achieve a virtual resolution of 5 nm out-of-plane [72]. Finally, perceptual grouping applied to membrane detection classifier results was used in [61].

Another approach to improving the accuracy of cell membrane detection is to use multi-scale methods. In early computer vision work, the neocognitron [73], which is a network composed of alternating layers of simple cells for filtering and complex cells for pooling and downsampling inspired by Hubel and Wiesel [74], was proposed for object recognition. Learning in the neocognitron is unsupervised. Convolutional nets in their original form are similar to the neocognitron in terms of their architecture; however, learning is supervised [75]. Convolutional nets have been applied to face detection [76, 77], face recognition [78], and general object recognition [79, 80]. However, the convolutional nets applied to connectomics [39, 69–71] have not taken advantage of the multi-scale nature of the neocognitron. In a different microscopy imaging application, Ning et al. have applied multi-scale convolutional nets to the problem of segmentation of subcellular structures in Differential Interference Contrast microscopy [81]. We proposed a multi-scale version of our series neural network architecture [82] that we also employ here. Recently, deep convolutional nets have been proposed for learning hierarchical image features [83, 84]. While these deep convolutional nets are trained in an unsupervised manner by presenting a set of training images containing the object of interest [85], their outputs can also be used as features in an object recognition application. This approach was recently used in the winning entry of the ISBI EM image segmentation challenge [86].

Methods

In this section, we will describe our algorithms for segmenting EM images. Section "Convolutional Networks and Auto-context Overview" discusses convolutional networks and auto-context methods which motivate our method. Section "Series of Artificial Neural Networks Pixel Classifier" introduced our series of artificial neural networks (ANN) framework. Section "Multi-scale Series of ANN Pixel Classifier" generalizes this framework to a multi-scale model. Section "Partial Differential Equation Based Post Processing" discusses a partial differential processing-based post-processing step to close gaps in the membrane detection results from the multi-scale series of artificial neural networks. This step typically results in a slight over-segmentation of the images. Therefore, section "Watershed Merge Tree Classifier" describes a watershed transform and supervised learning-based method for merging regions in the segmentation as necessary.

Convolutional Networks and Auto-Context Overview

As discussed in section "Machine Learning Methods", supervised machine learning methods have proven useful for detecting membranes in EM images. To address the challenges presented, we developed a machine learning method that combines two bodies of related work. The first by Jain et al. use a multilayer convolutional ANN to classify pixels as membrane or nonmembrane in specimens prepared with an extracellular stain [39]. The convolutional ANN has two important characteristics: it learns the filters for classification directly from data, and the multiple sequential convolutions throughout the layers of the network account for an increasing (indirect) filter support region. This method will work well for different types of image data, since it uses, as input, raw pixel data. In addition, the multiple convolutions enable the classifier to learn nonlocal structures that extend across the image without using large areas of the image as input. However, this method requires learning a very large number of parameters using backpropagation through many layers. Therefore, it is computationally intensive and requires very large training sets. Also of particular relevance is Tu's auto-context framework [87] from the computer vision literature, which uses a series of classifiers with contextual inputs to classify pixels in images. In Tu's method, the "continuous" output of a classifier, considered as a probability map, and the original set of features, are used as inputs to the next classifier. The probability map values from the previous classifiers provide context for the current classifier, by using a feature set that consists of samples of the probability map at a large neighborhood around each pixel. Theoretically, the series of classifiers improves an approximation of an a posteriori distribution [87]. Hence, each subsequent classifier extends the support of the probability map, improving the decision boundary in feature space, and thus the system can learn the context, or shapes, associated with a pixel classification problem. Similar to the convolutional network, this means that a classifier can make use of information relayed by previous classifiers from pixel values beyond the scope of its neighborhood. However, the particular implementation demonstrated by Tu uses 8,000 nonspecific, spatially dispersed, image features, and a sampling of probability maps in very large neighborhoods. This is appropriate for smaller scale problems. On the other hand, for large connectomics datasets, it can be impractical to calculate thousands of features in order to train the classifier. Similar to Jain et al. we choose to learn the image features directly from the data and use the image intensities as input to our architecture, rather than preprocessing the data and computing thousands of image features. This provides us with a much smaller set of features and allows for flexibility and training of large datasets. Also, the use of the series ANNs and increasing context allows us to focus on small sets of image features to detect membranes, while also eliminating pixels that represent vesicles or other internal structures.

Series of Artificial Neural Networks Pixel Classifier

Problem Formulation

Let $X = (x(i, j))$ be a 2D input image that comes with a ground truth $Y = (y(i, j))$ where $y(i, j) \in \{-1, 1\}$ is the class label for pixel (i, j). The training set is $T = \{(X_k, Y_k); k = 1, \ldots, M\}$ where M denotes the number of training images. Given an input image X, the maximum a posteriori (MAP) estimation of Y for each pixel is given by

$$\hat{y}_{MAP}(i,j) = \operatorname{argmax} p(y(i,j)|X). \tag{10.1}$$

It is not practical to solve (10.1) for large real-world problems. Instead of the exact equation an approximation can be obtained by using the Markov assumption

$$\hat{y}_{MAP}(i,j) = \operatorname{argmax} p(y(i,j)|X_{N(i,j)}), \tag{10.2}$$

where $N(i, j)$ denotes all the pixels in the neighborhood of pixel (i, j). In practice, instead of using the entire input image, the classifier has access to a limited number of neighborhood pixels at each input pixel (i, j). This approximation decreases the computational complexity and makes the training tractable on large datasets.

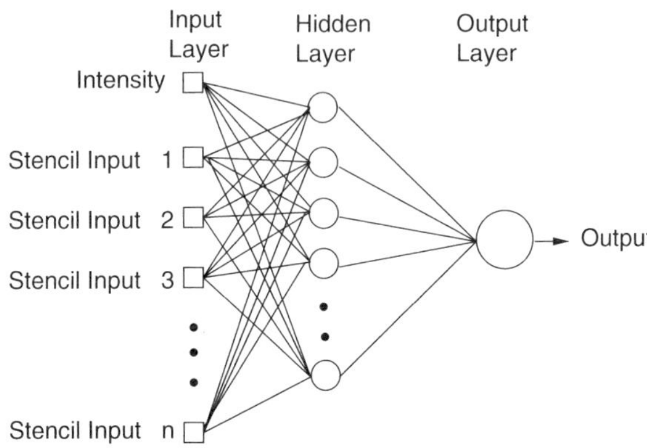

Fig. 10.3 Artificial neural network diagram with one hidden layer. Inputs to the network, in this framework, include the image intensity and the values of the image at stencil locations

Lets call the output image of this classifier $C = (c(i, j))$. In our series ANN, the next classifier is trained both on the neighborhood features of X and on the neighborhood features of C. The MAP estimation equation for this classifier can be written as

$$\hat{y}_{MAP}(i,j) = \operatorname{argmax} p(y(i,j)|X_{N(i,j)}, C_{N'(i,j)}), \tag{10.3}$$

where $N^{'}(i, j)$ denotes the neighborhood lattice of pixel (i, j) in the context image. Note that N and N' can represent different neighborhoods. The same procedure is repeated through the different stages of the series classifier until convergence. It is worth noting that (10.3) is closely related to the CRF model [66]; however, multiple models in series are learned which is an important difference from standard CRF approaches. It has been shown that this approach outperforms iterations with the same model [88].

Artificial Neural Network

Given the success of ANNs for membrane detection [5, 39], a multilayer perceptron (MLP) ANN is implemented as the classifier. An MLP is a feed-forward neural network which approximates a classification boundary with the use of nonlinearly weighted inputs. The architecture of the network is depicted schematically in Fig. 10.3. The output of each processing element (PE) (each node of the ANN) is given as [89, 90]

$$y = f(\mathbf{w}^T\mathbf{x} + b), \tag{10.4}$$

where f is, in this case, the *tanh* nonlinearity, $\mathbf{w}$ is the weight vector, and b is the bias. The input vector $\mathbf{x}$ to PEs in the hidden layer is the input feature vector discussed in more detail in section "Image Stencil Neighborhood". For the output PEs, $\mathbf{x}$ contains the outputs of the PEs in the hidden layer.

ANNs are a method for learning general functions from examples. They are well suited for problems without prior knowledge of the function to be approximated. They have been successfully applied to robotics [91, 92] and face and speech recognition [93, 94] and are robust to noise. Training uses gradient descent to solve for a solution which is guaranteed to find a local minimum. However, several trade-offs occur in training ANNs regarding the size of the network and the number of inputs. An ANN with too many hidden nodes can lead to overfitting of the network [89], resulting in a set of weights that fits well to the training data, but may not generalize well to test data. At the other extreme, if the number of hidden nodes is insufficient, the ANN does not have enough degrees of freedom to accurately approximate the decision boundary. The number of features should also be kept small to mitigate the problem of high dimensional spaces. Generally speaking, as the dimensionality of the input space increases, the number of observations becomes increasingly sparse which makes it difficult to accurately learn a decision boundary. Additionally, the training time tends to scale with the amount of training data and size of the network, and therefore training smaller networks with fewer features is generally preferable. Hence, the number of inputs to each ANN should be large enough to describe the data, but small enough for manageable training times.

Image Stencil Neighborhood

Good feature selection in any classification problem is critical. In this application, one possible approach uses large sets of statistical features as the input to a learning algorithm. These features can include simple local and nonlocal properties, including the pixel values, mean, gradient magnitude, standard deviation, and Hessian eigenvalues [38, 87, 95]. These attempt to present the learning algorithm with a large variety of mathematical descriptors to train on and are designed to work on a variety of data types. To achieve this generality, however, large numbers of these features are required to train a classifier. Another approach is to design a set of matched filters and apply them to an image to approximate a pixel's similarity to a membrane. This works well if the membranes in the image are uniform and respond well using cross correlation [96, 97]. Moreover, the design of the filter bank requires significant a priori knowledge of the problem. Yet, the fixed design may not be optimal for the dataset. Most importantly, the match filters have to be redesigned for datasets with different characteristics. On the other hand, learning these filters from training data, as in the case of convolutional networks [39], has the advantage that no a priori knowledge is required. A similar idea has been used in texture classification where it was shown that direct sampling of the image with a patch is actually a simpler and more universal approach for training a classifier compared to the use of filter banks [98]. Image patches have also been used successfully for texture segmentation [99] and image filtering [100–102]. Similarly, using image neighborhoods as in (10.2) allows the ANNs to learn directly on the input intensity data, giving the classifier more flexibility in finding the correct

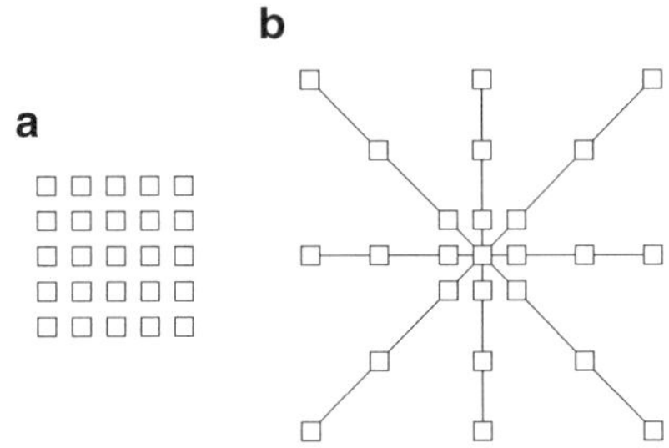

Fig. 10.4 Two image neighborhood sampling techniques: image pixels sampled using (**a**) a patch and (**b**) a stencil. For this example, the stencil contains the same number of samples, yet covers a larger area of the data. This is a more efficient representation for sampling the image space.

decision boundary. A square image neighborhood can be defined as an image patch, shown in Fig. 10.4a, centered at pixel k, l,

$$N(i,j) = \left\{ I_{k+i,l+j} : k,l = -\frac{R-1}{2}, \ldots, \frac{R-1}{2} \right\}. \tag{10.5}$$

R is the width of the square image patch. Unfortunately, the size of the image patches required to capture sufficient context can be quite large. For this reason, we propose using as input to the ANNs the values from the image and probability map of the previous classifier sampled through a stencil neighborhood, shown in Fig. 10.4b. A stencil is also centered at pixel k, l and defined as,

$$N(i,j) = \cup_{a=1}^{n} B(i,j,a) \tag{10.6}$$

where

$$B(i,j,a) = \left\{ I_{i+ak,j+al} : k,l = -1,0,1 \right\}, \tag{10.7}$$

and n is the number of rows the stencil spans in the image. The stencil in Figs. 10.4 and 10.5 cover large areas representing the desired feature space, but samples it in a spatially adaptive resolution strategy. For large image features, stencils such as the one in Fig. 10.5 are required. In this way, an ANN can be trained using a low-dimensional feature vector from image data, without having to use the whole image patch. Since the number of weights to be computed in an ANN is dominated by the connection between the input and the hidden layers, reducing the number of inputs reduces the number of weights and helps regularize the learned network. Moreover, using fewer inputs generally allows for faster training. With this, one aims to provide the classifier with sparse, but sufficient context information and achieve faster training, while obtaining a larger context which can lead to improvements in membrane detection. This strategy combined with the serial use of ANNs grows the region of interest for classification within a smaller number of stages and without long training times.

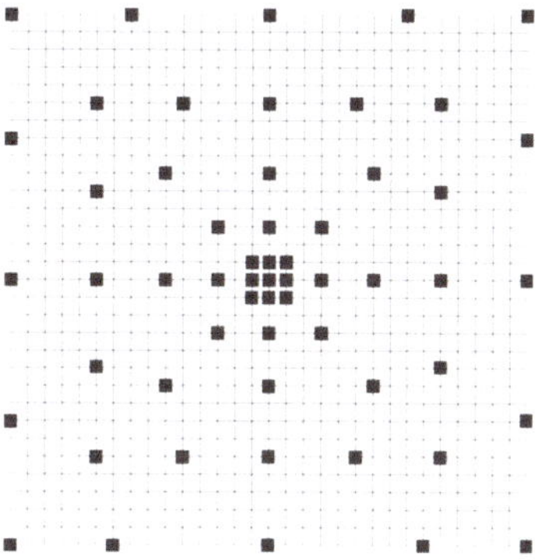

Fig. 10.5 Example of a larger image neighborhood sampling technique, covering a 31 ×31 patch of image pixels

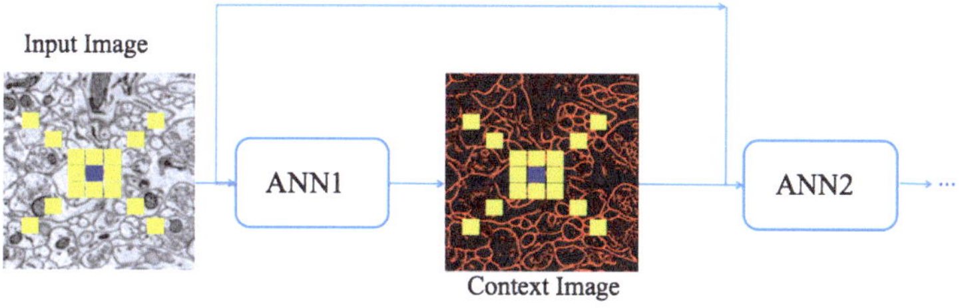

Fig. 10.6 Series neural network diagram demonstrating the flow of data between ANNs. The *blue* and *yellow squares* symbolize the center pixel and its neighborhood pixels in the stencil structure, respectively

Series Artificial Neural Networks

From the principles from auto-context, we architect a series of classifiers that leverage the output from previous networks to gain knowledge of a large neighborhood. The input to the first classifier is the image intensities around a pixel sampled using a stencil as described in section "Image Stencil Neighborhood". For the ANNs in the remaining series, the input vector contains the samples from the original image, used as input to the first ANN, appended with the values from the output of the previous classifier which was also sampled through the stencil neighborhood, yielding a larger feature vector. This second classifier is described mathematically with (10.3). While the desired output labels remain the same, each ANN is dependent on the information from the previous network and therefore must be trained sequentially, rather than in parallel. Figure 10.6 demonstrates this flow of data between classifiers. The lattice of squares represent the sampling stencil (shown more precisely in Fig. 10.5).

In summary, the series structure allows the classifiers to gather, with each step, context information from a progressively larger image neighborhood to the pixel being classified, as occurs with a convolutional ANN. The pixel values are sampled with a stencil neighborhood over each pixel, containing the pixels within the stencil (Fig. 10.5). The probability map feature vector is also obtained with a stencil

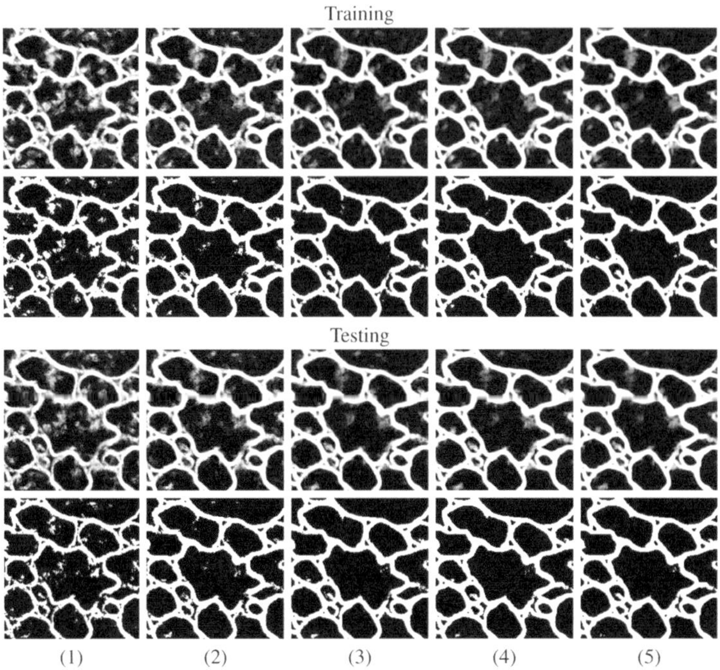

Fig. 10.7 Example output using the same image, first as part of a training set (*top two rows*), and then separately, as part of a testing set (*bottom two rows*), at each stage (1–5) of the network series. The output from each network is shown in rows 1 and 3. Rows 2 and 4 demonstrate the actual membrane detection when that output is thresholded. The network quickly learns which pixels belong to the membranes within the first 2–3 stages and then closes gaps in the last couple of stages

neighborhood placed over each pixel containing information about the classes, as determined by the previous classifier. Indirectly, the classification from the previous ANN contains information about features in surrounding pixels, that is not represented in the original feature set. This allows the subsequent networks in the series (Fig. 10.6) to make decisions about the membrane classification utilizing nonlocal information. Put differently, each stage in the series accounts for larger structures in the data, taking advantage of results from all the previous networks. This results in membrane detection that improves after each network in the series. Figure 10.7 visually demonstrates the classification improving between ANNs in the series as gaps in weak membranes are closed and intracellular structures are removed with each iteration in the series. The receiver operating characteristic (ROC) curves in Fig. 10.8 also demonstrate the increase in detection accuracy after each ANN in the series. Notice that the results converge after a few stages.

Combining the original image features with features sampled from the output of the previous classifier is important because, in this way, the membrane structure relevant for detection is enforced locally and then again at a higher level with each step in the series of classifiers. One of the advantages of this approach is that it

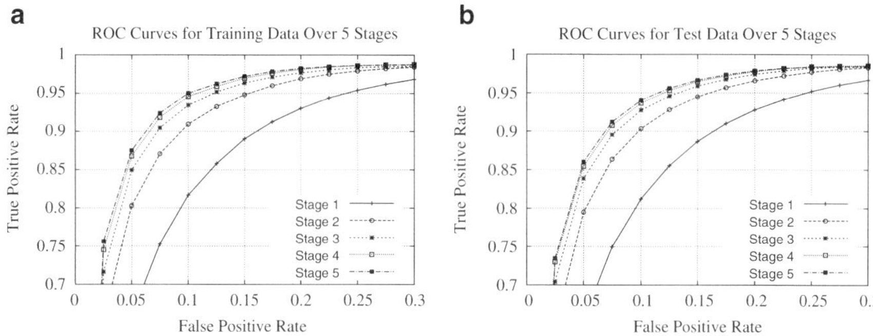

Fig. 10.8 ROC curves for the (**a**) training data and (**b**) testing data for each stage of the network on the *C. elegans* dataset

provides better control of the training, allowing the network to learn in steps, refining the classification at each step as the context information it needs to correctly segment the image increases. Again, note that the membrane structure is learned directly from the data. Compared to a single large network with many hidden layers and nodes, such as the convolutional ANN of Jain et al. [39], the proposed classifier is easier to train. This is mainly because each of the ANNs has a relatively small number of parameters. For example, for a single ANN, the number of parameters needed is approximately 500 for the first ANN and 1,100 for the remaining ANNs in the series. The number of weights in an ANN with a single-hidden layer is given by $(n + 1)h + (h + 1)$, where n is the number of inputs and h is the number of nodes in the hidden layer. For the first ANN in the series, $n = s$, where s is the number of points in the stencil. For the remaining ANNs in the series, $n = 2s$, since the original image and the output from the previous classifier are each sampled once. The total number of parameters across the whole series totals to approximately 5,000. In contrast, a convolutional ANN needs $(n + 1)h$ for the first layer, and $(n\,h + 1)h$ for the remaining layers, an h^2 dependence [39]. Hence, much less training data is needed in this approach, which is hard to obtain, since the ground truth must be hand labeled.[1] Furthermore, the training is simpler since backpropagation is less likely to get stuck on local minima of the performance surface [89, 90], and the network will train much faster. Moreover, this accounts for a smaller and simpler network which can be trained from smaller numbers of features in the input vector. The series of ANNs is much more attractive to train, as opposed to using a single large network with many hidden layers and nodes. A single large network would be time consuming and difficult to train due to the many local minima in the performance surface.

[1] According to the "rule-of-thumb" in [90], one needs at least 10 $\times$training samples of the total number of parameters. Thus, compared to Jain et al. [39] convolutional ANN, the approach presented here needs about 27 $\times$less training samples, for the values given.

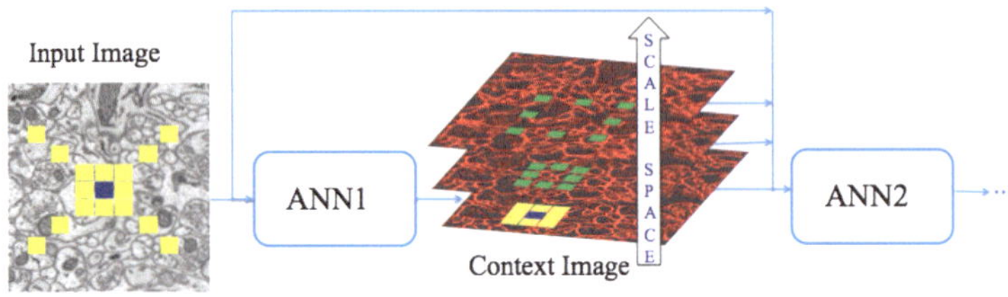

Fig. 10.9 Illustration of the multi-scale contextual model. Each context image is sampled at different scales (*green squares*). The *blue squares* represent the center pixel and the *yellow squares* show the selected input/context image locations at original scale

Multi-scale Series of ANN Pixel Classifier

In this section, we discuss how more information can be obtained by using a scale-space representation of the context and allowing the classifier access to samples of context at different scales. It can be seen from (10.3) that context image provides prior information to solve the MAP problem. Although the Markov assumption is reasonable and makes the problem tractable, it still results in a significant loss of information from global context because it only uses local information obtained from the neighborhood area. However, it is not practical to sample every pixel in a very large neighborhood area of the context due to computational complexity problem and overfitting. The series classifiers exploit a sparse sampling approach to cover large context areas as shown in Fig. 10.5. However, single pixel contextual information in the finest scale conveys only partial information about its neighborhood pixels in a sparse sampling strategy while each pixel in the coarser scales contains more information about its neighborhood area due to the use of averaging filters. Furthermore, single pixel context can be noisy whereas context at coarser scales is more robust against noise due to the averaging effect. In other words, while it is reasonable to sample context at the finest level a few pixels away, sampling context at the finest scale tens to hundreds of pixels away is error prone and results in a non-optimal summary of its local area. We will show how more information can be obtained by creating a scale space representation of the context and allowing the classifier access to samples of small patches at each scale. Conceptually, sampling from the scale space representation increases the effective size of the neighborhood while keeping the number of samples small.

Multi-scale Contextual Model

The multi-scale contextual model is shown in Fig. 10.9. In the conventional series structure, the classifiers simply take sparsely sampled context together with input image as input. In the multi-scale contextual model, each context image is treated as an image and a scale-space representation of context image is created by applying a

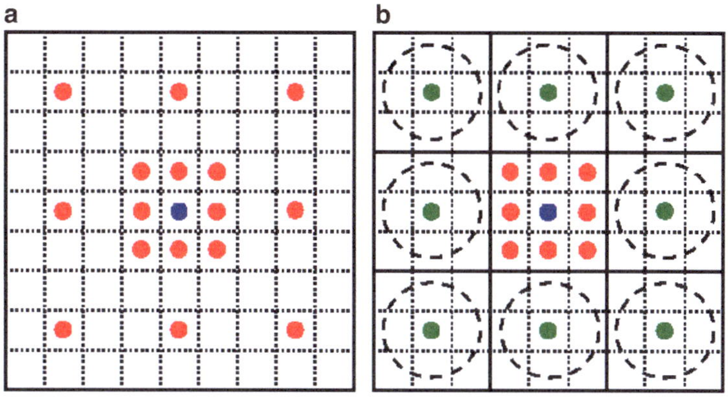

Fig. 10.10 Sampling strategy of context: (**a**) Sampling at a single scale (**b**) sampling at multi-scale. *Green circles* illustrate the summary of pixels in *dashed circles*. We use linear averaging to create the summary

set of averaging filters. This results in a feature map with lower resolution that is robust against the small variations in the location of features as well as noise. Figure 10.10 shows the multi-scale sampling strategy versus the single-scale sampling strategy. In Fig. 10.10b the classifier can have as an input the center 3×3 patch at the original scale and a summary of eight surrounding 3×3 patches at a coarser scale (The green circles denote the summaries of dashed circles). The green circles in Fig. 10.10b are more informative and less noisy compared to their equivalent red circles in Fig. 10.10a. The summaries become more informative as the number of scales increases. For example, in the first scale the summary is computed over 9 pixels (3×3 neighborhood) while it is computed over 25 pixels (5×5 neighborhood) in the second scale. Different methods such as Gaussian filtering, maximum pooling, etc. can be used to create the summary (green dots in Fig. 10.9) . From a mathematical point of view, (10.3) can be rewritten as:

$$\hat{y}_{MAP}(i,j) = \operatorname{argmax} p(y(i,j)|X_{N(i,j)}, C_{N'_0(i,j)}(0), C_{N'_1(i,j)}(1), \ldots, C_{N'_l(i,j)}(l)) \quad (10.8)$$

where $C(0), C(1), \ldots, C(l)$ denote the scale space representation of the context and $N'_0(i,j), N'_1(i,j), \ldots, N'_l(i,j)$ are corresponding neighborhood structures. Unlike (10.3) that uses the context in a single-scale architecture, (10.8) takes advantage of multi-scale contextual information. Even though the Markov assumption is still used in (10.8), the size of the neighborhood is larger and thus less information is lost compared to (10.3).

The series multi-scale contextual model updates the (10.8) iteratively:

$$\hat{y}^{k+1}_{MAP}(i,j) = \operatorname{argmax} p(y(i,j)|X_{N(i,j)}, C^k_{N'_0(i,j)}(0), C^k_{N'_1(i,j)}(1), \ldots, C^k_{N'_l(i,j)}(l)) \quad (10.9)$$

where $C^k(0), C^k(1), \ldots, C^k(l)$ are the scale space representation of the output of classifier at stage k, $k = 1, \ldots, K - 1$ and $\hat{y}^{k+1}_{MAP}(i,j)$ denotes the output of the stage $k + 1$. In turn, the $k + 1$'th classifier output as defined in (10.9) creates the context for the $k + 2$'th classifier. The model repeats (10.9) until the performance improvement between two consecutive stages becomes small. Because context is being used more effectively, the performance improvement through the stages is larger compared to the conventional series-ANN algorithm.

The overall performance of the multi-scale contextual model can be improved by extracting powerful features from the input image in addition to pixel intensities. It has been shown empirically that trying to segment the structures in connectome images using only geometric or textural features is not very effective [55]. Radon-like features (RLF) were proposed as a remedy to this problem as they are designed to leverage both the texture and the geometric information present in the connectome images to segment structures of interest. We refer the reader to [55] for further details of the RLF method. RLF method is an unsupervised method by itself but it can be integrated into supervised models as a feature extraction step. Furthermore, more powerful features can be obtained by computing RLF at multiple scales and for different edge threshold settings [82]. This richer set of features allow for correct detection of cell boundaries in the regions that cannot be detected by the original RLF as proposed in [55] and avoids the need for extensive parameter tuning.

Partial Differential Equation-Based Post-Processing

The partial differential equation (PDE) post-processing step is an entirely unsupervised process that improves the probability map by closing small to medium sized gaps in the membrane detection results. Typically the PDE post processing will generate an over-segmented image. Our motivation is that we can learn to fix over-segmentation errors with the watershed merge tree classifier as will be discussed in section "Watershed Merge Tree Classifier" whereas this is not possible for under-segmentation errors. In this section, we discuss how the probability map is updated at each iteration and the influence each term in the update equation has on the result.

Let f be an probability map where 1 represents locations with a low probability of being cell membrane and 0 represents locations with a high probability of being cell membrane. F is updated according to the rule $f_{k+1} = f_k + \Delta t(\Delta f)$, where

$$\Delta f = \alpha \Delta A + \beta \Delta B + \eta \Delta C \qquad (10.10)$$

and each term ΔA, ΔB, and ΔC represents a different characteristic of the probability map or underlying image that is to be optimized. The $\Delta\ t$ term is a parameter that can be adjusted to improve the stability of the update rule and the α, β, and η terms are parameters that can be used to control how much weight each different term in the PDE has relative to the other terms.

The first term in (10.10), ΔA, is defined as:

$$\Delta A = |\nabla f| \nabla \cdot \frac{\nabla f}{|\nabla f|} \tag{10.11}$$

where ∇ is the gradient operator and $\nabla\cdot$ is the divergence operator. The $\nabla \cdot \frac{\nabla f}{|\nabla f|}$ term in (10.11) computes the mean curvature at each pixel location in f and multiplying by $|\nabla f|$ ensures the stability. The effect of using the curvature is to force some smoothness along the boundaries between the membrane and non-membrane regions. Because the cells are generally large rounded structures with few sharp corners, high curvature areas are uncommon resulting in the curvature minimization term having the effect of favoring objects shaped like the interior of a typical cell. Without any other terms however, this would eventually reduce the areas with values close to 1 to shrink down to a small circle and eventually a single point. The other terms will counteract this behavior to give the desired result. In the discrete implementation of this curvature term, finite central difference is used to compute ∇f.

The second term in (10.10), ΔB, is defined as:

$$\Delta B = \nabla f \cdot \nabla G \tag{10.12}$$

where $\nabla G = \exp(-\frac{|\nabla I|^2}{\sigma})$ and I is a version of the original image filtered with the nonlocal means algorithm [101] to reduce the effects of noise. We chose the nonlocal means algorithm due to its success with textured images. The intent of this term is to push the edges of the probability map f to be along the edges of the original image. We assume that there is a strong edge between membrane and non-membrane regions. By itself this would produce a very jagged edge because of the noisy nature of the image. Combined with the curvature term, the edges of the probability map f will produce a clean edge that closely follows the edges in the original image. In the discrete implementation of this gradient term, an upwind scheme is used to compute ∇f and finite central difference is used to compute the ∇G and ∇I.

The final term in (10.10), ΔC, is defined as:

$$\Delta C = -.5\lambda_1 + .5\lambda_2 \tag{10.13}$$

where λ_1, λ_2 are the eigenvalues of the Hessian matrix of f, and $\lambda_1 > \lambda_2$. The larger eigenvalue of the Hessian of f represents the change across the gradient of f. By subtracting this term, it has the effect of inverse diffusion which tends to sharpen image features. This will effectively bring together areas of wide gray into a narrow dark region. Without the curvature term and gradient term this will cause some spurious detail to form, so a balance between this term and the other two terms is

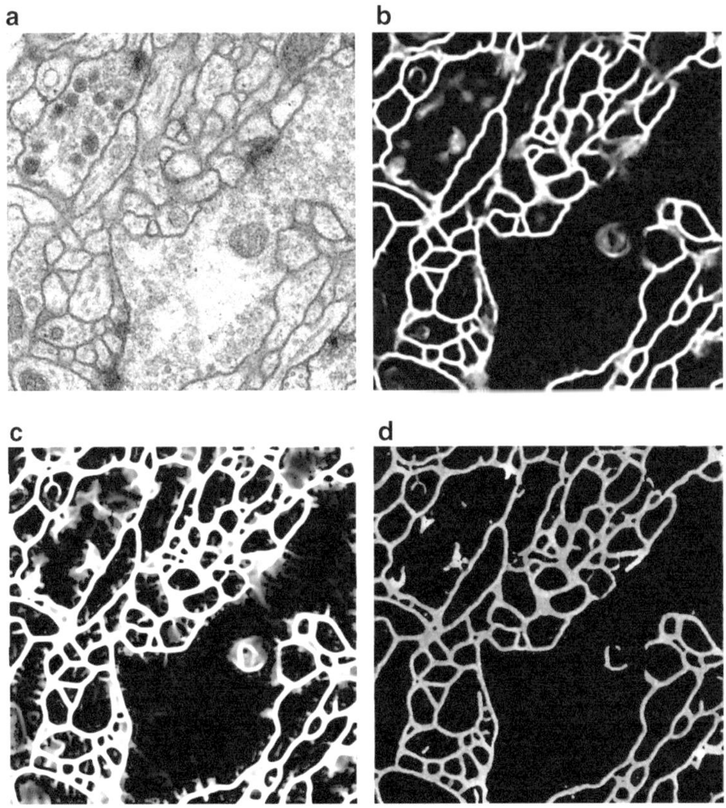

Fig. 10.11 Example of (**a**) original EM image, (**b**) multi-scale contextual membrane detection, (**c**) initial PDE result prior to thresholding , and (**d**) PDE result with replacement

necessary to ensure stability. The smaller eigenvalue of the Hessian of *f* represents the change in the direction perpendicular to the direction of the maximum gradient. Adding this term in allows growth extending the membranes at terminal points and connecting across regions that were missed in the initial probability map. In the discrete implementation of the Hessian, central differences are used to compute each of the 2nd derivatives. The number of iterations for the PDE is determined empirically according to the number of iterations that give the minimum rand error on the training data used in previous stages.

The result of running this algorithm is that the threshold giving the best result is at 1 resulting in everything less than 1 being considered non-membrane and everything equal to 1 being considered as membrane as seen in Fig. 10.11c. On some datasets this still offers significant improvement over just using the multi-scale series ANN; however, on other datasets the improvement is minimal. To be able to improve the thresholding and to be able to run the watershedding method described in the next section, we threshold the results of this PDE at the optimal

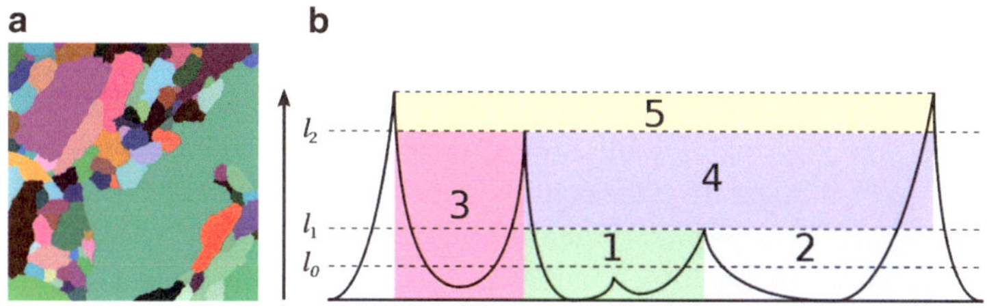

Fig. 10.12 Example of (**a**) initial watershed segmentation and (**b**) region merging with water level rising

threshold as determined on the training data and replace the areas classified as membrane with the intensity values from the original image. The result is an image where everything considered to be non-membrane has a value of 0 and everything considered to be membrane has the values from the original image as seen in Fig. 10.11d. Using the ISBI dataset, this algorithm improved both the training and the testing rand error as compared to the multi-scale series ANN by over 7 %.

Watershed Merge Tree Classifier

With the membrane detection and the PDE-based post-processing, we have a probability map for each image section indicating how probable every pixel can be membrane, as shown in Fig. 10.11. By simply applying thresholding on this map, we are able to get a segmentation. With this method, however, small mispredictions in pixels about membrane could lead to undesirable region merging and thus significant under-segmentation errors. With the watershed algorithm, we can also obtain a set of different segmentations by varying the water level. Yet a fixed global water level that works well through the entire image is difficult or even impossible to find due to various local terrains. On the contrary, we expect better results if we make specific local decisions according to different local situations, which motivates our watershed merge tree-based method.

Watershed Merge Tree

Consider a probability map as a three-dimensional terrain map with pixel probability as ridge height. Water rains into catchment basins, and regions with lower heights are flooded. An initial water level forms an initial segmentation as shown in Fig. 10.12a. With more water falling in and the water level rising over ridges, small regions merge into larger ones, and finally into one large region once the water level rises above the highest ridge in the map. Figure 10.12b gives a one-dimensional case for illustration: with initial water level l_0, we have regions 1, 2, and 3; when the water level rises to l_1, regions 1 and 2 merge to 4; region 3 merges with 4 and 5 at water level l_2. This technique produces a hierarchy of region merging that can be represented by a tree structure, which we call a watershed merge tree.

Here we give a formal definition of a watershed merge tree. A watershed tree $T = (\{N\}, \{E\})$, derived from the concept of a tree in the graph theory, consists of a set of nodes and edges between them. At depth d, a node N_i^d corresponds to an image region R_i^d; an edge from a parent node N_i^d to its child node $N_{i'}^{d+1}$ indicates region $R_{i'}^{d+1}$ is a subregion of region R_i^d; a local tree structure $(N_i^d, N_{i'_1}^{d+1}, N_{i'_2}^{d+1}, \ldots)$ represents region R_i^d can be the merging result of all of its subregion $\{R_{i'_1}^{d+1}, R_{i'_2}^{d+1}, \ldots\}$. For simplicity, we here consider the merge tree as a binary tree, which means only two regions merge each time. If several regions merge at the same water level, we merge two regions at a time and the merging order can be arbitrary.

As we use nonlocal features for the boundary classifier, which will be described in detail in the next section, it is difficult to extract some meaningful features from regions that are too small. Therefore, we use an initial water level l_0 to merge some very small regions beforehand in the initial segmentation, and further conduct a preprocessing step to get rid of regions smaller than n_r pixels by merging them with their neighbor regions with the lowest probability barrier.

Boundary Classifier

In order to decide which regions we should preserve as the final segmentation in the merge tree, we need information about how probable each potential merge could happen. Thus, we learn a boundary classifier from training data. For a pair of regions, we consider the set of pixels that are adjacent to the other region as a boundary. The output of the classifier is a probability that the boundary between the two regions is false, or in other words, the two regions should merge. The input of the classifier is a set of 141 features extracted from the two merging regions, including geometric features (region area, boundary lengths, region contour lengths, etc.), intensity statistics features of boundary pixels from both original EM images and membrane detection probability maps, and regional features (texton histogram difference and watershed region merging saliency). Here the watershed region merging saliency is defined as the difference between the minimum water level to merge the two regions and the minimum value in the membrane detection probability map.

We obtain the label that indicates whether a region pair (R_i^d, R_j^d) should merge or not by measuring the Rand error over the ground truth segmentation, which is defined as

$$E_k = \frac{1}{|R_i^d| \cdot |R_j^d|} \sum_{x_p, x_q \in R_i^d \cup R_j^d} \left| \sigma_{pq} - \beta_{pq}^k \right|, \tag{10.14}$$

where (x_p, x_q) represents any pixel pair from the union of the two merging regions, and

$$\sigma_{pq} = \begin{cases} 1 & \text{if } xp \text{ and } xq \text{ are in the same truth region} \\ 0 & \text{otherwise} \end{cases}$$
$$\beta^1_{pq} = \begin{cases} 1 & \text{always} \\ 0 & \text{never} \end{cases} \qquad (10.15)$$
$$\beta^2_{pq} = \begin{cases} 1 & \text{if } xp \text{ and } xq \text{ are in the same merging region} \\ 0 & \textit{otherwise.} \end{cases}$$

Here the Rand error E_1 measures the portion of pixel pairs that are misclassified against the ground truth segmentation if the two regions merge, and E_2 is that portion if the two regions keep split. Thus, we can decide the label by simply comparing the Rand errors as

$$l^d_{ij} = \begin{cases} +1(merge) & \text{if } E^1_R < E^2_R \\ -1(split) & \text{otherwise.} \end{cases} \qquad (10.16)$$

To balance the contributions of positive and negative examples, different weights are assigned to each type of examples. A random forest classifier [103] is trained with the weighted training examples and applied to make predictions about how likely a pair of regions should merge for the testing data.

Resolving the Merge Tree

The boundary classifier predicts the probability for every potential merge in a merge tree. We seek to take advantage of this information and obtain a consistent segmentation of the whole image in a sense of optimization. We define the consistency as that in the final segmentation any pixel should be labeled exactly once. In the context of our tree structure, if a node is selected, all of its ancestor and descendants cannot be selected, and its immediate sibling or a set of the descendants of its immediate sibling must be selected; if a node is not selected, one of its ancestors or a set of its descendants must be selected. In other words, exactly one node should be picked on each path from any leaf to the root. Figure 10.13 shows an artificial example. We have an initial over-segmentation shown in Fig. 10.13a, from which a merge tree is built as shown in Fig. 10.13c. Nodes 3, 6, 9, and 12 are picked for a consistent final segmentation shown in Fig. 10.13b. Consequently, the other nodes cannot be selected. Because we cannot have both purple region (node 9) and region 1 (or 2) exist, otherwise region 1 (or 2) would be labeled more than once as 1 (or 2) and 9, which is inconsistent by our definition. Meanwhile, if we select node 3, node 9 or nodes 1 and 2 together then must be picked in this case, otherwise

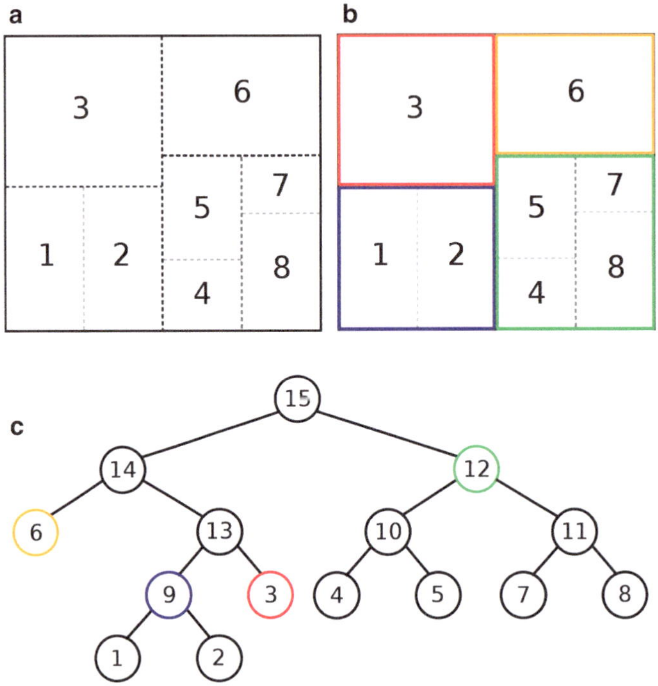

Fig. 10.13 Example of (**a**) initial over-segmentation, (**b**) consistent final segmentation, and (**c**) corresponding merge tree

region 1 or region 2 is not labeled in the final segmentation, which is also inconsistent.

In order to resolve the merge tree, we transform the probabilities of region pair merging into the form of potentials for each node in the tree. A region exists in the final segmentation because it neither splits into smaller regions nor merges with others into a larger region. Since each prediction that the classifier makes depends only on the two merging regions, we compute the potential that a node N_i^d is picked as the probability that its two child nodes $N_{i'_1}^{d+1}$ and $N_{i'_2}^{d+1}$ merge and at the same time N_i^d does not merge with its immediate sibling node N_j^d at the next higher water level to their parent node N_k^{d-1}. Thus, we define the potential for N_i^d as

$$P_i^d = p_{i'_1,i'_2}^{d+1} \cdot (1 - p_{i,j}^d), \tag{10.17}$$

where $p_{i'_1,i'_2}^{d+1}$ is the predicted probability that the two child nodes $N_{i'_1}^{d+1}$ and $N_{i'_2}^{d+1}$ merge, and $p_{i,j}^d$ is the probability that node N_i^d merge with its immediate sibling node N_j^d. In the example shown in Fig. 10.13c, the potential of node 9 is $P_9 = p_{1,2}(1 - p_{3,9})$. Since leaf nodes have no children, their potentials are defined as the probability that they do not merge penalized into half. Similarly, the root node has no parent, so its potential is half of the probability that its children merge.

Given the potentials of each node, we seek to locally optimize the node selection to form a complete consistent final segmentation. Here we apply a greedy approach. The node with the highest potential in the merge tree is picked. Then all of its ancestors and descendants are regarded as inconsistent options and removed from the tree. This procedure is repeated until there are no nodes left in the tree. All the picked nodes together make up a complete consistent final segmentation.

Results

In this section, we will demonstrate the results of our algorithms on two ssTEM and one SBFSEM dataset. In addition to visual results, quantitative results are provided using the pixel error and rand error metrics on the training and testing datasets.

C. elegans *Ventral Nerve Cord ssTEM*

Dataset

The nematode *C. elegans* is an important dataset for neural circuit reconstruction. Despite being a well-studied organism [21], there are still numerous open questions such as how genes regulate wiring [104] or how connectivity is altered to mediate different behaviors, for example between males and females [105]. Reconstructions of the full nervous system reveal topological characteristics important for researchers studying neuron wiring. The particular ssTEM dataset used here is from the VNC of the *C. elegans* and is important for studying the topological structure resulting from neurons making connections to local targets.

Series-ANN Pixel Classifier

In this experiment, a series classifier with 5 stages was trained. Additional networks could be included; however, for these datasets, the performance converges to a limit (Fig. 10.8) and improvement in membrane detection is minimal. Each ANN used in the experiments contained one hidden layer with 20 nodes. We experimented with more layers and different numbers of nodes but did not find significant advantages. It is important that the number of nodes be large enough to approximate a nonlinear boundary and small enough that the ANN does not overfit to the training data [106, 107]. Results using 10, 20, and 30 nodes turned out to be somewhat similar. Given the time versus performance trade-off, we chose 20 nodes. The networks were trained using backpropagation with a step size of 0. 0001 and momentum term of 0.5. We used early stopping as the criterion to determine when to terminate training [89, 90]. This means that a small portion of the training data (20 % in our case), called the validation set, is used only to test the classifier generalization performance. The training terminates when the lowest error on the validation set is attained. To mitigate problems with local minima, each network is trained for 5 Monte Carlo simulations using randomly initialized weights.

Post-processing and Segmentation

For this dataset the parameters were optimized empirically on the 15 images used as training images. The PDE ran for 288 iterations with δt equal to 0. 1875, α equal to 0. 1, β equal to 0. 6, and η equal to 1. This places the most weight on the inverse diffusion-based growth term, significant weight on the gradient term, and minimal weight on the curvature term. Following 288 iterations of the pde, the result was thresholded with a threshold of 0. 4 and all of the membrane areas were replaced with their values from a denoised version of the original image. The denoising was done using a nonlocal means denoising algorithm. Following this replacement the watershed process was started using the resultant image. For the watershed merge tree classification, the initial water level was 5 % of the maximum value in each probability map. Due to large section size, we merged regions smaller than $n_r = 300$ pixels with their neighbors in the preprocessing step; 7×7 texture patches were extracted from the original EM images for generating the texton dictionary and building texton histograms as boundary classifier features. A random forest with 500 trees was trained for boundary classification. Figure 10.14 shows the results of the ANN series and post-processing methods for four different test images. Table 10.1 shows the pixel and Rand error of the series ANN model alone and ANN series model followed by PDE post-processing and watershed merge tree segmentation. Notice that while the post-processing worsens the pixel accuracy slightly, it significantly improves the Rand error. Since Rand error is a measure of segmentation errors, this particular trade-off between the pixel accuracy and Rand error is desirable.

Drosophila Ventral Nerve Cord ssTEM

Dataset

The second dataset we experimented with is a stack of 60 images from an ssTEM dataset of the Drosophila first instar larva VNC [8, 108]. It has a resolution of $4 \times 4 \times 50$ nm/pixel and each 2D section is 512×512 pixels. The corresponding binary labels were annotated by an expert neuroanatomist. During the International Symposium on Biomedical Imaging (ISBI) Electron Microscopy Image Segmentation Challenge 30 images were used for training and the remaining images were used for testing.

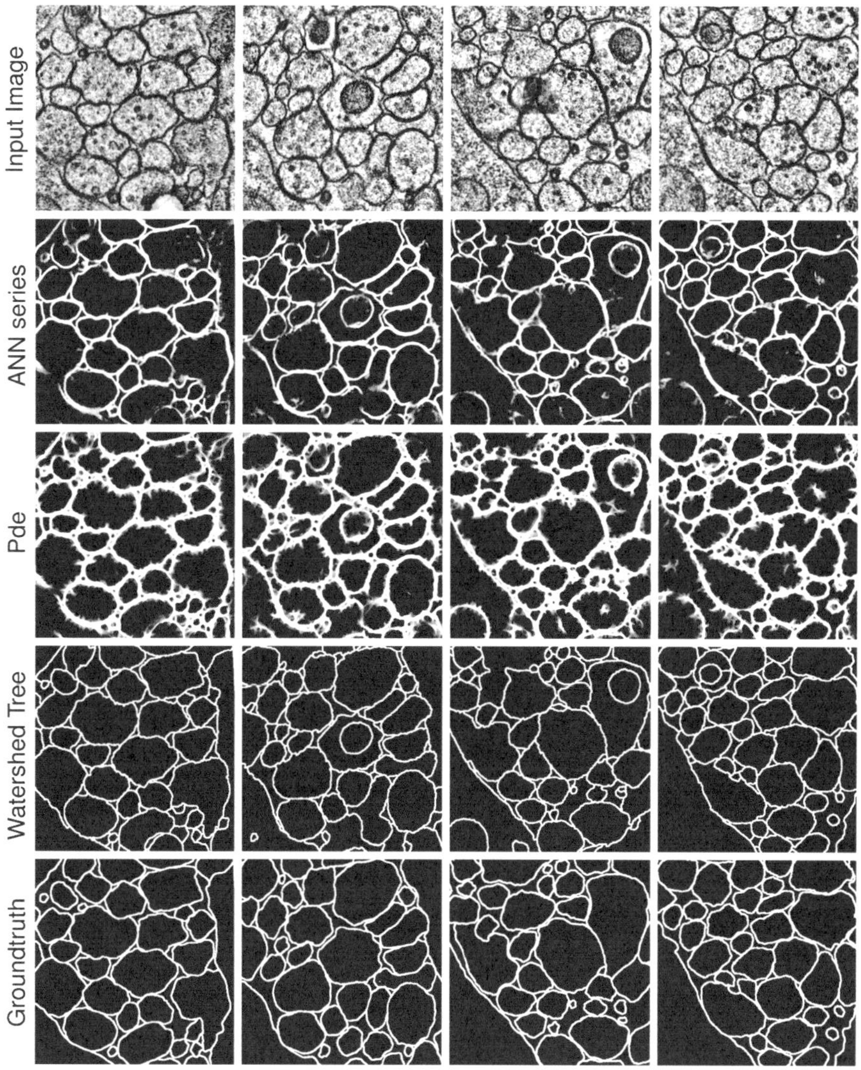

Fig. 10.14 Test results for membrane detection for four different input images from *C. elegans* VNC. The first row shows the input images, row 2 shows the conventional ANN series results, row 3 shows the PDE post-processing results (applied on the results in row 2), and row 4 shows the watershed merge tree results (applied on the results in row 3), and the last row shows the corresponding groundtruth images. All the images in this figure are zoomed in for the sake of better visualization of the details

Table 10.1 Testing performance of the ANN series model and post-processing methods (pde + watershed merge tree) for the *C. elegans* ssTEM dataset

	Training		Testing	
Method	Rand error	Pixel error	Rand error	Pixel error
Series ANN	0.2113	0.0327	0.2285	0.0324
Post-processing	0.0986	0.0431	0.1498	0.0432

Multi-scale Series-ANN Pixel Classifier

In this experiment, a series classifier with five stages was trained using multi-scale contextual method. Each MLP-ANN in the series had one hidden layer with ten nodes. To optimize the network performance, five million samples were randomly selected from the training images such that the training set contained twice the number of negative samples, i.e., the non-membrane samples, than positive samples, i.e., membrane samples. To compute the feature vector for the input image pixels, an 11 by 11 stencil was used to sample the input image and the RLF maps for cell boundaries (at two scales) and mitochondria. The first classifier was trained using this feature vector of size 164. The context features were computed using 5 by 5 patches at four scales (one at original resolution and three at coarser scales) that made the context feature vector of length 100. The remaining classifiers in the series had feature vector of size 264, which included both the input image features and the context features. The evolution of the results through the stages of multi-scale contextual model is shown in Fig. 10.16. It can be seen that the classifier is able to remove some undesired parts such as mitochondria from the interior of the cells.

Post-processing and Segmentation

For this dataset the number of iterations for the PDE post-processing was again optimized empirically using the 30 training images. The optimal number of iterations for this dataset was found to be 425. The remaining parameters were found to be the same because of the similarity in structure between the datasets. Following 425 iterations of the PDE, the result was thresholded with a threshold of 0 and all of the membrane areas were replaced with their values from a nonlocal means [101] denoised version of the original image. Following this replacement the watershed process was started using the resultant image. As for the watershed merge tree method, the initial water level was set as 1 % of the maximum value in each corresponding probability map. Regions smaller than $n_r = 50$ pixels were removed in the initial segmentation; 7×7 texture patches were used for generating texton features. A random forest with 500 trees was again used.

Table 10.2 illustrates the pixel accuracy and Rand error of the multi-scale contextual model alone and multi-scale contextual model followed by PDE

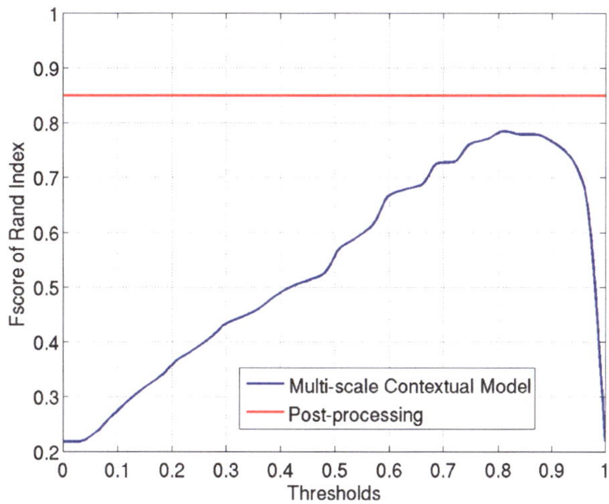

Fig. 10.15 F-value of Rand Index for the testing set in *C. elegans* VNC dataset

post-processing and watershed merge tree segmentation. Similar to section "*C. elegans* Ventral Nerve Cord ssTEM", post-processing worsens the pixel accuracy, it significantly improves the Rand error. Figure 10.17 illustrates the results of the various steps visually.

Figure 10.15 shows the improvement in Rand error provided by the post-processing step against the Rand error of the multi-scale contextual model at different thresholds.

Mouse Neuropil SBFSEM

Dataset

This dataset is a stack of 400 images from the mouse neuropil acquired using SBFSEM. It has a pixel resolution of 10 $\times$10 $\times$10 nm and each 2D section is 4, 096 by 4, 096 pixels. To train and test the segmentation framework, a subset of this data (700 $\times$700 $\times$70) was manually annotated by an expert electron microscopist. From those 70 images, 14 images were used for training and the 56 remaining images were used for testing. The training set contains 4. 5 million samples, which one third of them are positive samples and the remaining of them are negative samples.

Multi-scale Series-ANN Pixel Classifier

The same series classifier as the previous section was trained on this dataset. Figure 10.18 shows four examples of test images and their corresponding

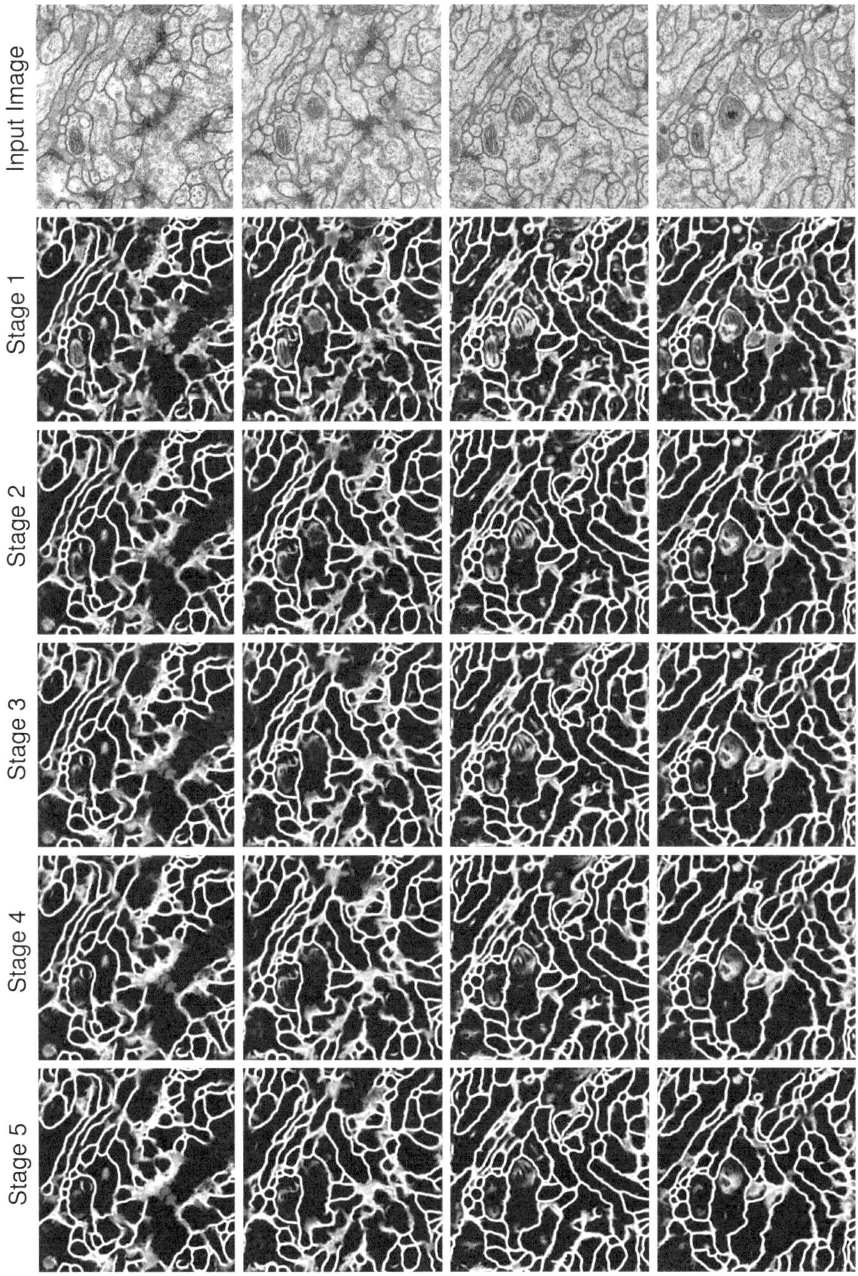

Fig. 10.16 Test results for membrane detection for four different input images from Drosophila VNC. The first row shows the input images, rows 2–5 show the series output at different stages of the multi-scale contextual model

Table 10.2 Testing performance of the multi-scale contextual model and post-processing methods (pde + watershed merge tree) for the Drosophila VNC ssTEM dataset

	Training		Testing	
Method	Rand error	Pixel error	Rand error	Pixel error
Multi-scale contextual model	0.2084	0.0527	0.1312	0.0752
Post-processing	0.0378	0.0599	0.0770	0.1026

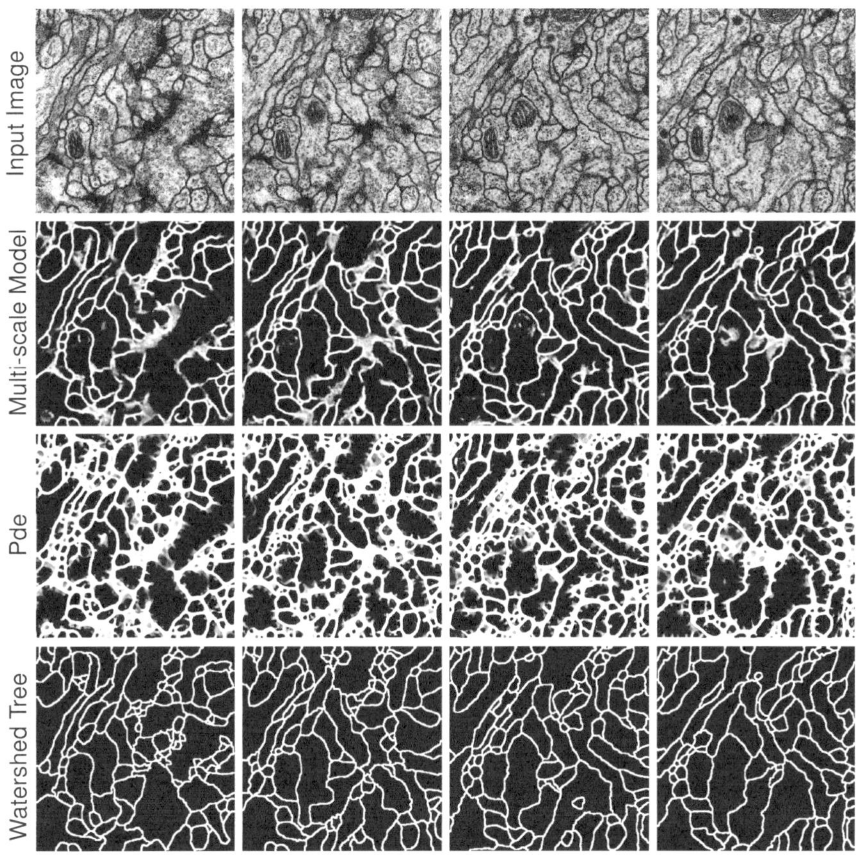

Fig. 10.17 Test results for membrane detection for four different input images from Drosophila VNC. The first row shows the input images, row 2 shows the multi-scale contextual model results, row 3 shows the PDE post-processing results (applied on the results in row 2), and row 4 shows the watershed merge tree results (applied on the results in row 3). The testing ground truth images for the ISBI challenge were not distributed to the contestants; therefore, we are unable to show them here

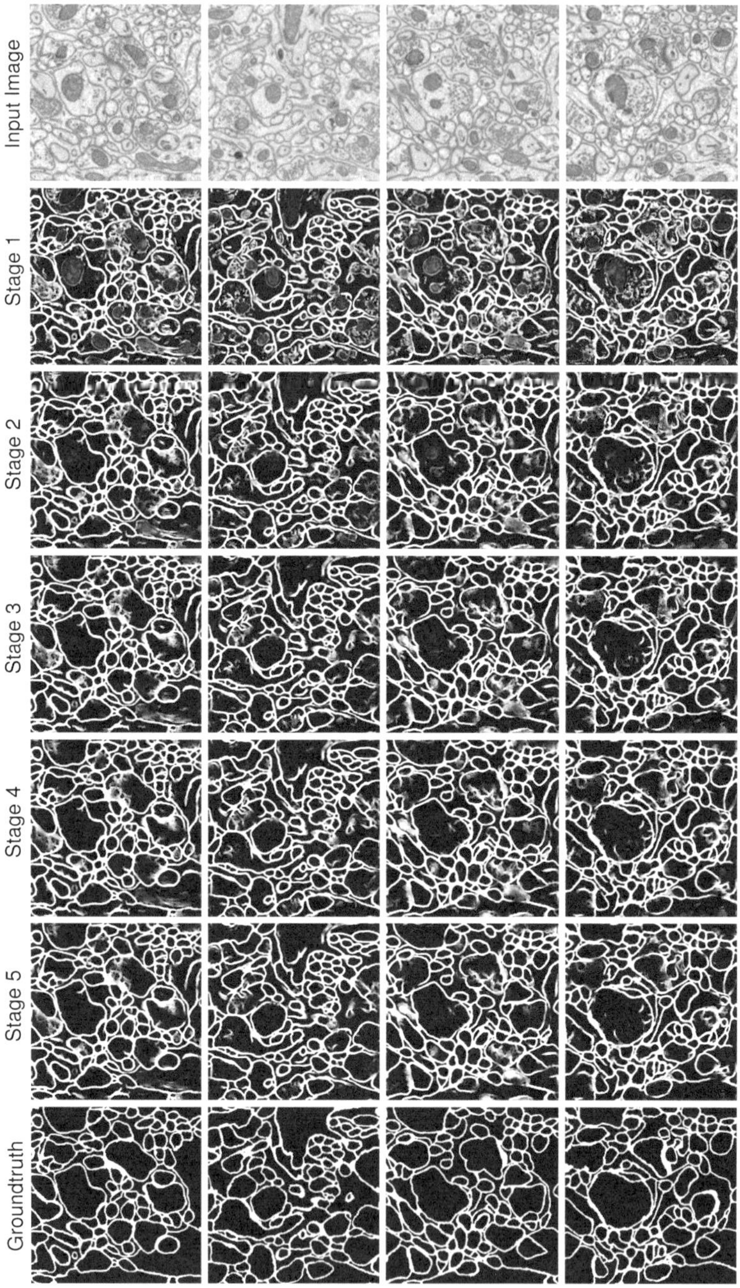

Fig. 10.18 Test results for membrane detection for four different input images from mouse neuropil. The first row shows the input images, rows 2–6 show the series output at different stages, and the last row shows the manually marked image

segmentation results at different stages of the multi-scale contextual model. The accuracy of the results is improved through the stages and cleaner images are obtained at later stages of the series (see Fig. 10.18). Four test images and corresponding membrane detection results for conventional ANN series and multi-scale contextual model are shown in Fig. 10.19. In comparison, multi-scale contextual model is more successful in removing undesired parts and generating cleaner results.

Post-processing and Segmentation

For this dataset the number of iterations was again optimized empirically using the 14 images from bin 1. The optimal number of iterations for this dataset was again found to be 288 while the remaining parameters remained the same. For this dataset, histogram equalization was performed prior to using the image for gradient calculation. The threshold used prior to replacement with the original image intensities in the membrane areas was again 0. Following this replacement the watershedding process was started using the resultant image. The parameters selection of the watershed merge tree classifier was identical to that of the drosophila VNC ssTEM dataset: the initial water level was 1 % of the maximum values correspondingly; regions smaller than $n_r = 50$ pixels were removed; 7 ×7 texton patches were used; and the random forest utilized 500 trees.

Figure 10.19 illustrates the results of the various steps visually. Table 10.3 shows the pixel accuracy and Rand error of the multi-scale contextual model alone and multi-scale contextual model followed by PDE post-processing and watershed merge tree segmentation. Again, notice that while the post-processing worsens the pixel accuracy slightly, it significantly improves the Rand error. Since Rand error is a measure of segmentation errors, this particular trade-off between the pixel accuracy and Rand error is desirable. Finally, Fig. 10.20 shows the Rand error of the multi-scale contextual model as a function of the final threshold applied to the classifier output. It also shows the Rand error of the post-processing step.

Discussion

In this chapter, we demonstrated a pipeline that utilizes several machine learning strategies to provide a reasonable solution to the problem of segmenting neurons in electron microscopy images. Both supervised and unsupervised techniques were used. The first step of the pipeline is a pixel-level classifier that attempts to mark each pixel in an image either as membrane or non-membrane. This supervised learning approach has clear advantages over traditional image processing methods that involve no learning: the learning approach can adapt to the data, requires no hand designed features, and outperforms the traditional methods. In our pixel-level classifier, we employed a series of ANNs. The ANNs directly use pixel intensities

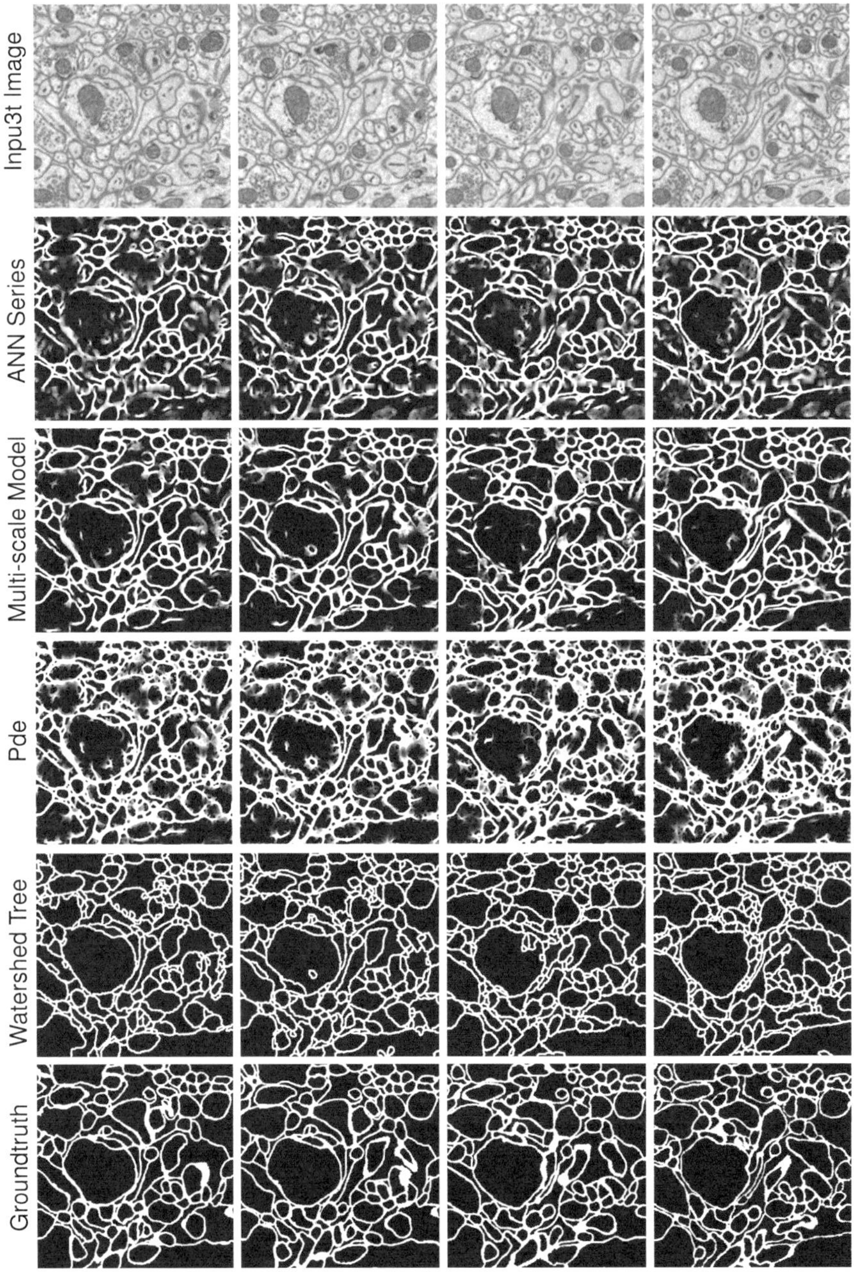

Fig. 10.19 Test results for membrane detection for four different input images from mouse neuropil. The first row shows the input images, the second row shows the conventional ANN series results, row 3 shows the multi-scale contextual model results, row 4 shows the PDE post-processing results (applied on the results in row 3), row 5 shows the watershed merge tree results (applied on the results in row 4), and the last row shows the corresponding grountruth images

Table 10.3 Performance of the multi-scale contextual model and post-processing methods (pde + watershed merge tree) for the mouse neuropil SBFSEM dataset

	Training		Testing	
Method	Rand error	Pixel error	Rand error	Pixel error
Multi-scale contextual model	0.2551	0.0512	0.2413	0.0510
Post-processing	0.1274	0.0716	0.1538	0.0745

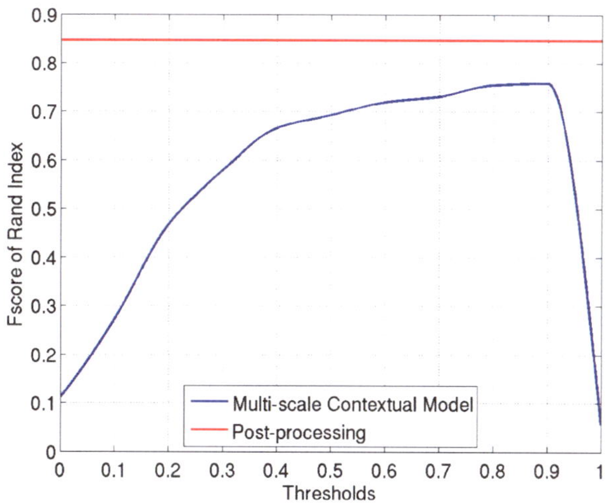

Fig. 10.20 F-value of Rand Index for different thresholds for the mouse neuropil SBFSEM dataset

in neighborhoods as features. Each ANN in the series learns to improve upon the previous ANNs's results by sampling neighborhoods from both the input image and the previous ANN's output (probability map). Intracellular structures such as mitochondria and synaptic vesicles are mostly removed from the membrane detection results and some small gaps in the membranes are filled. These improvements are observed both in training and in testing datasets. A multi-scale version of the series-ANN which can more effectively sample the images was shown to provide further improvement in accuracy. However, the main problem with the pixel-level classifiers is two-fold: (i) it optimizes pixel accuracy instead of segmentation accuracy and (ii) it cannot use region-based features. The first point is problematic because even a single pixel gap in the membrane map, which is negligible in view of pixel error, can create a large segmentation error. The next two steps of our pipeline aim to fix these problems. The second step is an unsupervised PDE which aims to fill small gaps in the membrane map hence favoring over-segmentation over under-segmentation. This is achieved mainly by using an inverse diffusion term directed along the eigenvector of the Hessian of the probability map associated with its larger eigenvalue, i.e. the direction perpendicular to the cell membrane. The over-segmentation created by the PDE step is finally fixed using the watershed merge tree. Similar to the pixel classifier step, this is also a supervised learning-based step. Incrementally raising the water level in the watershed algorithm creates a hierarchy of regions. Each time two regions merge in the tree due to rising water level, we have to ask the question: Is this merge salient or not? We train a classifier that we call the boundary classifier to answer this question. The advantage of the boundary classifier over the pixel-level classifier is that it can make use of potentially more powerful region-based features. Furthermore, the boundary classifier is trained to optimize segmentation accuracy as measure by the rand error. The saliency of each region is then defined as the probability that its children merge times 1 minus the probability that it doesn't merge with its sibling. Finally, we pick the salient regions from the watershed tree by using a greedy approach in search of the most salient regions. As expected the outcome of these post-processing steps significantly improves segmentation error over the pixel-level classifier. The pixel accuracy is slightly worsened over the pixel-level classifier; however, this is not considered important since the main goal is to improve better segmentations. One reason for the worsening of pixel accuracy is errors in the membrane width that might be introduced by the post-processing which optimizes segmentation error since such errors don't impact the segmentation error.

The pipeline introduced in this chapter can be used to automatically segment neurons in electron microscopy images. However, if perfect accuracy is required as is the case for most connectomics problems, manual proof-reading of the results by an expert will be necessary. To minimize the time that experts need to spend proof-reading results, future methods will focus on further improving the accuracy. Our pipeline also is a new example for how machine learning methods can benefit automatic image analysis.

Acknowledgments This work was supported by NIH R01 EB005832 and 1R01NS075314. The *C. elegans* dataset was provided by the Jorgensen Lab at the University of Utah. The mouse neuropil dataset was provided by the National Center for Microscopy Imaging Research. The retina dataset was provided by the Marc Lab at the University of Utah. The drosophila VNC dataset was provided by the Cardona Lab at HHMI Janelia Farm.

References

1. Suzuki K, Horiba I, Sugie N (2003) Neural edge enhancer for supervised edge enhancement from noisy images. IEEE Trans Pattern Anal Mach Intell 25:1582–1596
2. Suzuki K, Horiba I, Sugie N, Nanki M (2004) Extraction of left ventricular contours from left ventriculograms by means of a neural edge detector. IEEE Trans Med Imag 23:330–339
3. Sporns O, Tononi G, Ktter R (2005) The human connectome: A structural description of the human brain. PLoS Comput Biol 1:e42
4. Briggman KL, Denk W (2006) Towards neural circuit reconstruction with volume electron microscopy techniques. Curr Opin Neurobiol 16:562–570

5. Mishchenko Y (2008) Automation of 3D reconstruction of neural tissue from large volume of conventional serial section transmission electron micrographs. J Neurosci Methods 176 (2):276–289
6. Anderson J, Jones B, Yang J-H, Shaw M, Watt C, Koshevoy P, Spaltenstein J, Jurrus E, U V K, Whitaker R, Mastronarde D, Tasdizen T, Marc R (2009) A computational framework for ultrastructural mapping of neural circuitry. PLoS Biol 7(3):e74
7. Mishchenko Y, Hu T, Spacek J, Mendenhall J, Harris KM, Chklovskii DB (2010) Ultrastructural analysis of hippocampal neuropil from the connectomics perspective. Neuron 67:1009–1020
8. Cardona A, Saalfeld S, Preibisch S, Schmid B, Cheng A, Pulokas J, Tomančák P, Hartenstein V (2010) An integrated micro- and macroarchitectural analysis of the *Drosophila* brain by computer-assisted serial section electron microscopy. PLoS Biol 8(10):e1000502
9. Bock DD, Lee W-C, Kerlin AM, Andermann ML, Hood G, Wetzel AW, Yurgenson S, Soucy ER, Kim HS, Reid RC (2011) Network anatomy and in vivo physiology of visual cortial neurons. Nature 471:177–182
10. Briggman KL, Helmstaedter M, Denk W (2011) Wiring specificity in the direction-selectivity circuit of the retina. Nature 471:183–188
11. Marc RE, Jones BW, Watt CB, Vazquez-Chona F, Vaughan DK, Organisciak DT (2008) Extreme retinal remodeling triggered by light damage: implications for age related macular degeneration. Mol Vis 14:782–806
12. Marc RE, Jones BW, Watt CB, Strettoi E (2003) Neural remodeling in retinal degeneration. Progr Retin Eye Res 22:607–655
13. Sutula T (2002) Seizure-induced axonal sprouting: assessing connections between injury, local circuits, and epileptogenesis. Epilepsy Current 2:86–91
14. Koyama R, Yamada MK, Fujisawa S, Katoh-Semba R, Matsuki N, Ikegaya Y (2004) Brain-derived neurotrophic factor induces hyperexcitable reentrant circuits in the dentate gyrus. J Neurosci 24:7215–7224
15. Xiao YP, Wang Y, Felleman DJ (2003) A spatially organized representation of colour in macaque cortical area v2. Nature 421(6922):535–539
16. Minsky M (1961) Microscopy apparatus. U.S. Patent number 301,467, December 1961
17. Denk W, Strickler JH, Webb WW (1990) Two-photon laser scanning microscopy. Science 248:73–76
18. Egner A, Hell SW (2005) Fluorescence microscopy with super-resolved optical sections. Trends Cell Biol 15:207–215
19. Rust MJ, Bates M, Zhuang X (2006) Sub-diffraction-limit imaging by stochastic optical reconstruction microscopy (storm). Nat Meth 3:793–796
20. Betzig E, Patterson G, Sougrat R, Lindwasser O, Olenych S, Bonifacino J, Davidson M, Lippincott-Schwartz J, Hess H (2006) Imaging intracellular fluorescent proteins at nanometer resolution. Science 313(5793):1642–1645
21. White JG, Southgate E, Thomson JN, Brenner S (1986) The structure of the nervous system of the nematode caenorhabditis elegans. Philos Trans R Soc Lond B Biol Sci 314 (1165):1–340
22. Hall DH, Russell RL (1991) The posterior nervous system of the nematode caenorhaditis elegans: Serial reconstruction of identified neurons and complete pattern of synaptic interactions. J Neurosci 11(1):1–22
23. Chen BL, Hall DH, Chklovskii DB (2006) Wiring optimization can relate neuronal structure and function. Proc Natl Acad Sci USA 103(12):4723–4728
24. Chklovskii DB, Vitaladevuni S, Scheffer LK (2010) Semi-automated reconstruction of neural circuits using electron microscopy. Curr Opin Neurobiol 20(5):667–675
25. Anderson JR, Jones BW, Watt CB, Shaw MV, Yang JH, Demill D, Lauritzen JS, Lin Y, Rapp KD, Mastronarde D, Koshevoy P, Grimm B, Tasdizen T, Whitaker R, Marc RE (2011) Exploring the retinal connectome. Mol Vis 17:355–379

26. Varshney LR, Chen BL, Paniagua E, Hall DH, Chklovskii DB (2011) Structural properties of the *Caenorhabditis elegans* neuronal network. PLoS Comput Biol 7(2):e1001066
27. Deerinck TJ, Bushong EA, Thor A, Ellisman MH (2010) NCMIR methods for 3D EM: A new protocol for preparation of biological specimens for serial block face scanning electron microscopy. Microscopy and Microanalysis Meeting, Portland, OR, 1–5 August 2010
28. Hayworth K, Kasthuri N, Schalek R, Lichtman J (2006) Automating the collection of ultrathin serial sections for large volume TEM reconstructions. Microsc Microanal 12 (2):86–87
29. Tasdizen T, Koshevoy P, Grimm BC, Anderson JR, Jones BW, Watt CB, Whitaker RT, Marc RE (2010) Automatic mosaicking and volume assembly for high-throughput serial-section transmission electron microscopy. J Neurosci Meth 193(1):132–144
30. Saalfeld S, Cardona A, Hartenstein V, Tomančák P (2010) As-rigid-as-possible mosaicking and serial section registration of large ssTEM datasets. Bioinformatics 26(12):i57–i63
31. Tasdizen T, Koshevoy P, Grimm B, Anderson J, Jones B, Watt C, Whitaker R, Marc R (2010) Automatic mosaicking and volume assembly for high-throughput serial-section transmission electron microscopy. J Neurosci Meth 193:132–144
32. Anderson J, Mohammed S, Grimm B, Jones B, Koshevoy P, Tasdizen T, Whitaker R, Marc R (2011) The viking viewer for connectomics: scalable multi-user annotation and summarization of large volume data sets. J Microscopy 241:13–28
33. Knott G, Marchman H, Wall D, Lich B (2008) Serial section scanning electron microscopy of adult brain tissue using focused ion beam milling. J Neurosci 28(12):2959–2964
34. Soto GE, Young SJ, Martone ME, Deerinck TJ, Lamont S, Carragher BO, Hama K, Ellisman MH (1994) Serial section electron tomography: A method for three-dimensional reconstruction of large structures. NeuroImage 1(3):230–243
35. Chen X, Winters CA, Reese TS (2008) Life inside a thin section: Tomography. J Neurosci 28 (38):9321–9327
36. Hama K, Arii T, Katayama E, Marton M, Ellisman MH (2004) Tri-dimensional morphometric analysis of astrocytic processes with high voltage electron microscopy of thick golgi preparations. J Neurocytol 33:277–285. doi:10.1023/B:NEUR.0000044189.08240.a2
37. Kreshuk A, Straehle CN, Sommer C, Koethe U, Cantoni M, Knott G, Hamprecht FA (2011) Automated detection and segmentation of synaptic contacts in nearly isotropic serial electron microscopy images. PLoS One 6(10):e24899
38. Andres B, Köthe U, Helmstaedter M, Denk W, Hamprecht FA (2008) Segmentation of SBFSEM volume data of neural tissue by hierarchical classification. In: Rigoll G (ed) Pattern Recognition. LNCS, vol 5096. Springer, Berlin, Heidelberg, pp 142–152
39. Jain V, Murray J, Roth F, Turaga S, Zhigulin V, Briggman K, Helmstaedter M, Denk W, Seung H (2007) Supervised learning of image restoration with convolutional networks. IEEE 11th International Conference on Computer Vision, pp 1–8, Rio de Janeiro, Brazil, 14–21 October 2007
40. Jeong W-K, Beyer J, Hadwiger M, Blue R, Law C, Vazquez-Reina A, Reid RC, Lichtman J, Pfister H (2010) Secret and neurotrace: Interactive visualization and analysis tools for large-scale neuroscience data sets. IEEE Comput Graph 30(3):58–70
41. Jurrus E, Whitaker R, Jones B, Marc R, Tasdizen T (2008) An optimal-path approach for neural circuit reconstruction. In: Proceedings of the 5th IEEE International Symposium on Biomedical Imaging: From Nano to Macro, pp 1609–1612, Paris, France, 14–17 May 2008
42. Macke J, Maack N, Gupta R, Denk W, Schölkopf B, Borst A (2008) Contour-propagation algorithms for semi-automated reconstruction of neural processes. J Neurosci Meth 167:349–357
43. Allen BA, Levinthal C (1990) Cartos II semi-automated nerve tracing: Three-dimensional reconstruction from serial section micrographs. Comput Med Imag Graph 14(5):319–329
44. Jurrus E, Tasdizen T, Watanabe S, Davis MW, Jorgensen EM, Whitaker RT (2008) Semi-automated reconstruction of the neuromuscular junctions in the c. elegans. In: MICCAI

Workshop on Microscopic Image Analysis with Applications in Biology, New York, NY, 5–6 September 2008
45. Jurrus E, Watanabe S, Paiva A, Ellisman M, Jorgensen E, Tasdizen T (2012) Semi-automated neuron boundary detection and slice traversal algorithm for segmentation of neurons from electron microscopy images. Neuroinformatics 11(1):5-29
46. Funke J, Andres B, Hamprecht FA, Cardona A, Cook M (2011) Multi-hypothesis crf-segmentation of neural tissue in anisotropic em volumes. CoRR abs/1109.2449
47. Anderson JR, Mohamed S, Grimm B, Jones BW, Koshevoy P, Tasdizen T, Whitaker R, Marc RE (2010) The viking viewer for connectomics: scalable multi-user annotation and summarization of large volume data sets. J Microsc 241(1):1328
48. Vazquez L, Sapiro G, Randall G (1998) Segmenting neurons in electronic microscopy via geometric tracing. In: Proceedings of International Conference on Image Processing, pp 814–818, San Diego, CA, 12–15 October 1998
49. Bertalmío M, Sapiro G, Randall G (2000) Morphing active contours. IEEE Trans Pattern Anal Mach Intell 22:733–737
50. Jurrus E, Hardy M, Tasdizen T, Fletcher P, Koshevoy P, Chien CB, Denk W, Whitaker R (2009) Axon tracking in serial block-face scanning electron microscopy. Med Image Anal 13:180–188
51. Reina AV, Miller E, Pfister H (2009) Multiphase geometric couplings for the segmentation of neural processes. In: Proceedings of IEEE Conference on Computer Vision and Pattern Recognition, pp 2020–2027, Miami, FL, 20–25 June 2009.
52. Jeong W-K, Beyer J, Hadwiger M, Vazquez A, Pfister H, Whitaker RT (2009) Scalable and interactive segmentation and visualization of neural processes in em datasets. IEEE Trans Visual Comput Graph 15(6):1505–1514
53. Vazquez-Reina A, Miller E, Pfister H (2009) Multiphase geometric couplings for the segmentation of neural processes. In: Proceedings of IEEE Conference on Computer Vision and Pattern Recognition, pp 2020–2027, Miami, FL, 20–25 June 2009
54. Tasdizen T, Whitaker RT, Marc RE, Jones BW (2005) Enhancement of cell boundaries in transmission electron microscopy images. In: Proceedings of International Conference on Image Processing, vol 2, pp 129–132, Genoa, Italy, 11–14 September 2005
55. Kumar R, Va andzquez Reina A, Pfister H (2010) Radon-like features and their application to connectomics. In: IEEE Computer Society Conference on CVPRW, pp 186–193, San Francisco, CA, 13–18 June 2010
56. Akselrod-Ballin A, Bock D, Reid RC, Warfield SK (2009) Improved registration for large electron microscopy images. In: Proceedings of IEEE International Symposium on Biomedical Imaging, pp 434–437, Boston, MA, 28 June–1 July 2009
57. Preibisch S, Saafeld S, Tomancak P (2009) Globally optimal stitching of tiled 3d microscopic image acquisitions. Bioinformatics 25(11):1463–1465
58. Vu N, Manjunath B (2008) Graph cut segmentation of neuronal structures from transmission electron micrographs. In: Image Processing, 2008. ICIP 2008. 15th IEEE International Conference on, pp 725–728, San Diego, CA, 12–15 October 2008
59. Yang H-F, Choe Y (2009) Cell tracking and segmentation in electron microscopy images using graph cuts. In: Proceedings of IEEE International Symposium on Biomedical Imaging: From Nano to Macro, Boston, MA, 28 June–1 July 2009
60. Yang H-F, Choe Y (2009) 3D volume extraction of densely packed cells in em data stack by forward and backward graph cuts. Computational Intelligence for Multimedia Signal and Vision Processing, pp 47–52, Nashville, Tennessee, 30 March–2 April 2009
61. Kaynig V, Fuchs T, Buhmann JM (2010) Neuron geometry extraction by perceptual grouping in ssTEM images. In: IEEE Conference on Computer Vision and Pattern Recognition, San Francisco, CA, 13–18 June 2010
62. Venkataraju KU, Paiva A, Jurrus E, Tasdizen T (2009) Automatic markup of neural cell membranes using boosted decision stumps. In: EEE International Symposium on Biomedical Imaging (ISBI): From Nano to Macro, Boston, MA, 28 June–1 July 2009

63. Jurrus E, Paiva ARC, Watanabe S, Anderson J, Whitaker BWJRT, Jorgensen EM, Marc R, Tasdizen T (2010) Detection of neuron membranes in electron microscopy images using a serial neural network architecture. Med Image Anal 14(6):770–783
64. Geman S, Geman D (1984) Stochastic relaxation, gibbs distributions and the bayesian restoration of images. IEEE Trans Pattern Anal Mach Intell 6:721–741
65. Freeman WT, Pasztor EC, Owen T, Carmichael Y (2000) Merl a mitsubishi electric research laboratory. Int J Comput Vis 40:2000
66. Lafferty J, McCallum A, Pereira F (2001) Conditional random fields: Probabilistic models for segmenting and labeling sequence data. In: International Conference on Machine Learning, pp 282–289, Williams College, Williamstown, MA, 28 June–1 July 2001
67. Kumar S, Hebert M (2003) Discriminative random fields: A discriminative framework for contextual interaction in classification. In: ICCV, pp 1150–1157, Nice, France, 14–17 October 2003
68. Jain V (2010) Machine Larning of Image Analysis with Convolutional Networks and Topological Constraints. PhD Thesis, MIT
69. Turaga SC, Briggman KL, Helmstaedter M, Denk W, Seung HS (2009) Maximin learning of image segmentation. In: Advances in Neural Information Processing Systems, Vancouver, British Columbia, Canada, 7–10 December 2009
70. Turaga SC, Murray JF, Jain V, Roth F, Helmstaedter M, Briggman KL, Denk W, Seung HS (2010) Convolutional networks can learn to generate affinity graphs for image segmentation. Neural Comput 22(2):511–538
71. Jain V, Bollmann B, Richardson M, Berger DR, Helmstaedter MN, Brigmann KL, Bowden JB, Mendenhall JM, Abraham WC, Harris KM, Kasthuri N, Hayworth KJ, Schalek R, Tapia JC, Lichtmann JW, Seung HS (2010) Boundary learning by optimization with topological constraints. In: IEEE Conference on Computer Vision and Pattern Recognition, San Francisco, CA, 13–18 June 2010
72. Veeraraghavan A, Genkin AV, Vitaladevuni S, Scheffer L, Xu S, Hess H, Fetter R, Cantoni M, Knott G, Chklovskii D (2010) Increasing depth resolution of electron microscopy of neural circuits using sparse tomographic reconstruction. In: IEEE Conference on Computer Vision and Pattern Recognition, San Francisco, CA, 13–18 June 2010
73. Fukushima K (1982) Neocognitron: A new algorithm for pattern recognition tolerant of deformations and shifts in position. Pattern Recogn 15(6):455–469
74. Hubel D, Wiesel T (1962) Receptive fields, binocular interaction and functional architecture in the cat's visual cortex. J Physiol 160:106–154
75. LeCun Y, Bengio Y (1995) Convolutional networks for images, speech, and time series. The handbook of brain theory and neural networks. MIT Press, Cambridge, MA, pp 255–258
76. Garcia C, Delakis M (2004) Convolutional face finder: A neurl architecture for fast and robust face detection. IEEE Trans Pattern Anal Mach Intell 26(11):1408–1423
77. Osadchy R, Miller M, LeCun Y (2005) Synergistic face detection and pos estimation with energy-based model. In: Advances in Neural Information Processing Systems, Vancouver, British Columbia, Canada, 5–8 December 2005
78. Lawrence S, Giles CL, Tsoi AC, Back A (1997) Face recognition: A convolutional neural network approach. IEEE Trans Neural Network 8(1):98–113
79. LeCun Y, Huang FJ, Bottou L (2004) Learning methods for generic object recognition with invariance to pose and lighting. In: Proceedings of the 2004 I.E. Computer Society Conference on Computer Vision and Pattern Recognition, vol 2, pp II–97–104, Washington, DC, 27 June–2 July 2004
80. Huang FJ, LeCun Y (2006) Large-scale learning with svm and convolutional nets for generic object categorization. In: IEEE Conference on Computer Vision and Pattern Recognition, New York, NY, 17–22 June 2006
81. Ning F, Delhomme D, Lecun Y, Piano F, Bottou L, Barbano PE (2005) Toward automatic phenotyping of developing embryos from videos. IEEE Trans Image Process 14:1360–1371

82. Seyedhosseini M, Kumar R, Jurrus E, Guily R, Ellisman M, Pfister H, Tasdizen T (2011) Detection of neuron membranes in electron microscopy images using multi-scale context and radon-like features. In: Medical Image Computing and Computer-Assisted Intervention MICCAI 2011. Lecture Notes in Computer Science (LNCS), vol 6891. Springer, Berlin, Heidelberg, pp 670–677
83. Lee H, Grosse R, Ranganath R, Ng AY (2009) Convolutional deep belief networks for scalable unsupervised learning of hierarchical representations. In: International Conference on Machine Learning, vol. 382, pp 609–616, Montreal, Quebec, Canada, 2009
84. Norouzi M, Ranjbar M, Mori G (2009) Stacks of convolutional restricted boltzmann machines for shift-invariant feature learning. In: IEEE Conference on Computer Vision and Pattern Recognition, Miami, FL, 20–25 June 2009
85. Hinton GE, Osindero S (2006) A fast learning algorithm for deep belief nets. Neural Comput 18:2006
86. Ciresan D, Giusti A, Gambardella L, Schmidhuber J (2012) Neural networks for segmenting neuronal structures in EM stacks. In: ISBI Electron Microscopy Segmentation Challenge, Barcelona, Spain, 2–5 May 2012
87. Tu Z (2008) Auto-context and its application to high-level vision tasks. IEEE Conference on Computer Vision and Pattern Recognition, pp 1–8, Anchorage, Alaska, 24–26 June 2008
88. Tu Z, (2008) Auto-context and its application to high-level vision tasks. In: Proceedings of IEEE Computer Vision and Pattern Recognition, Anchorage, Alaska, 24–26 June 2008
89. Haykin S (1999) Neural networks: A comprehensive foundation, 2nd edn. Prentice-Hall, Upper Saddle River, NJ
90. Principe JC, Euliano NR, Lefebvre WC (2000) Neural and adaptive systems: Fundamentals through simulations. Wiley, New York
91. Pomerleau D (1993) Knowledge-based training of artificial neural networks for autonomous robot driving. In: Connell J, Mahadevan S (eds) Robot Learning. Kluwer Academic, Dordrecht, pp 19–43
92. Wells G, Venaille C, Torras C (1996) Promising research: Vision-based robot positioning using neural networks. Image Vis Comput 14:715–732
93. Cottrell G (1990) Extracting features from faces using compression networks: face, identity, emotion and gender recognition using holons. In: Connection models: Proceedings of the 1990 summer school. Morgan Kaufmann, San Mateo, CA, pp 328–337
94. Rabi G, Lu S (1998) Visual speech recognition by recurrent neural networks. J Electron Imag 7:61–69
95. Venkatataju KU, Paiva A, Jurrus E, Tasdizen T (2009) Automatic markup of neural cell membranes using boosted decision stumps. In: Proceedings of the 6th IEEE International Symposium on Biomedical Imaging, pp 1039–1042, Boston, MA, 28 June–1 July 2009.
96. Leung T, Malik J (2001) Representing and recognizing the visual appearance of materials using three-dimensional textons. Int J Comput Vision 43(1):29–44
97. Schmid C (2001) Constructing models for content-based image retrieval. In: Computer Vision and Pattern Recognition, 2001, CVPR 2001. Proceedings of the 2001 I.E. Computer Society Conference on, vol. 2, pp II–39–II–45, Kauai, HI, 8–14 December 2001
98. Varma M, Zisserman A (2003) Texture classification: are filter banks necessary? In: Computer Vision and Pattern Recognition, 2003. Proceedings of the 2003 I.E. Computer Society Conference on, vol. 2, pp II–691–8, Madison, WI, 16–22 June 2003
99. Awate SP, Tasdizen T, Whitaker RT (2006) Unsupervised Texture Segmentation with Nonparametric Neighborhood Statistics. In: Proceedings of the European Conference on Computer Vision. pp 494–507, Graz, Austria, 7–13 May 2006
100. Awate SP, Whitaker RT (2006) Unsupervised, information-theoretic, adaptive image filtering for image restoration. IEEE Trans Pattern Anal Mach Intell 28(3):364–376
101. Buades A, Coll B, Morel J-M (2005) A non-local algorithm for image denoising. In: Proceedings of IEEE Conference on Computer Vision and Pattern Recognition, pp 60–65, San Diego, CA, 20–26 June 2005

102. Tasdizen T (2008) Principal components for non-local means image denoising. In: Proceeding of International Conference on Image Processing, San Diego, California, 12–15 October 2008
103. Breiman L (2001) Random forests. Mach Learn 45(1):5–32
104. Jin Y, Hoskins R, Horvitz HR (1994) Control of type-D GABAergic neuron differentiation by *C. elegans* UNC-30 homeodomain protein. Nature 372:780–783
105. White JQ, Nicholas T, Gritton J, Truong L, Davidson ER, Jorgensen EM (2007) The sensory circuitry for sexual attraction in *C. elegans* males. Curr Biol 17:1847–1857
106. Cybenko G (1989) Approximation by superpositions of a sigmoidal function. Math Contr Signals Syst 2:303–314
107. Hornik K (1991) Approximation capabilities of multilayer feedforward networks. Neural Network 4(2):251–257
108. Cardona A, Saalfeld S, Schindelin J, Arganda-Carreras I, Preibisch S, Longair M, Tomancak P, Hartenstein V, Douglas RJ (2012) Trakem2 software for neural circuit reconstruction. PLoS One 7(6):e38011

Chapter 11
Image Analysis Techniques for the Quantification of Brain Tumors on MR Images

Nishant Verma, Matthew C. Cowperthwaite, Mark G. Burnett, and Mia K. Markey

Abstract Advances in neuro-imaging methods over the last few decades have enabled collection of detailed anatomical and functional information about the brain. Although functional imaging provides rich information for diagnosis and treatment planning, practical considerations such as cost and availability currently limit its clinical utility. As a result, structural imaging methods that provide detailed information about the anatomical structures of the brain are routinely used to manage brain tumors in the clinical setting. Typically, radiological images are visually inspected and interpreted by trained health professionals to detect gross anatomical abnormalities, which are associated with various types of brain tumors. This approach entails generally qualitative interpretations that do not fully realize the potential of modern imaging technologies. Furthermore, several types of brain tumors manifest with gross anatomical changes that are visually similar, which limits the use of MRI in differentiating between them. Computer-aided image analysis enables a quantitative description of brain anatomy and detection of subtle, but

N. Verma (✉)
Department of Biomedical Engineering, The University of Texas at Austin, 107 W Dean Keeton Street Stop, 1 University Station, C0800, Austin, TX 78712, USA

NeuroTexas Institute, St. David's HealthCare, 1015 East 32nd Street Suite 404, Austin, TX 78705, USA
e-mail: vnishant@utexas.edu

M.C. Cowperthwaite • M.G. Burnett
NeuroTexas Institute, St. David's HealthCare, 1015 East 32nd Street Suite 404, Austin, TX 78705, USA
e-mail: Matthew.Cowperthwaite@stdavids.com; mburnett@neurotexas.net

M.K. Markey
Department of Biomedical Engineering, The University of Texas at Austin, 107 W Dean Keeton Street Stop, 1 University Station, C0800, Austin, TX 78712, USA

Department of Imaging Physics, The University of Texas MD Anderson Cancer Center, Houston, TX 77030, USA
e-mail: Mia.Markey@austin.utexas.edu

K. Suzuki (ed.), *Computational Intelligence in Biomedical Imaging*,
DOI 10.1007/978-1-4614-7245-2_11,

important, anatomical changes that may be difficult to detect by visual inspection. Therefore, it's imperative to develop sophisticated image analysis tools that can handle the highly complex and varied organization of the brain across individuals. Such tools will form the foundation for decision support systems (DSSs) to aid health professionals in more precise and personalized management of brain tumors.

Introduction

Medical imaging plays a key role in the clinical management of brain tumors for diagnosis, treatment planning, and follow-up assessment. Magnetic resonance imaging (MRI) is the current standard of neuro-oncologic imaging and has become more widely used than computed tomography (CT) due to its advantages such as higher contrast resolution among soft tissues and absence of exposure to ionizing radiation. Typically, MR images are visually inspected and interpreted by trained radiologists. The information gathered through visual inspection generally consists of qualitative assessments of any gross anatomical abnormalities observed on the images and often does not include finer differences that may be difficult to detect by visual inspection. Visual inspection therefore limits the utility of MRI for diagnosing brain tumors that often manifest with similar gross anatomical characteristics. A final diagnosis is typically made by histological examination of tissue specimens by a pathologist following biopsy, which is time consuming, expensive and the risks involved may often outweigh the benefits.

A decision support system (DSS) is a sophisticated tool that helps a person consider multiple criteria in order to make a choice from among alternatives. In the medical context, a DSS provides clinicians, staff, patients, and other individuals with patient-specific information, intelligently filtered and presented at appropriate times, to enhance health and healthcare [1]. A radiological DSS can potentially help in the detection and quantification of the more subtle characteristics of radiologic images that are difficult to detect via visual inspection. DSS can assist radiologists with interpreting medical images in a variety of ways, such as through better presentation of important information or by providing a "second opinion" based on an objective and quantitative evaluation of tumor morphology. A radiological DSS could help reduce reading errors resulting from subtle but important anatomical changes, decrease radiologist variability, and increase the efficiency of reviewing and interpreting MR images.

Basic Overview of DSS for brain MRI

Noninvasive medical imaging is crucial for managing brain tumors. It is used not only for diagnosis of brain tumors but also for treatment planning and following patients to assess the effectiveness of their treatment and the status of their disease. Whereas most DSSs for cancer imaging have focused on earlier detection of cancer (such as detecting spiculated masses in mammograms [2] or solid lung nodules in lung CT images [3]), those developed for brain tumors have addressed all phases of care from diagnosis to post-treatment monitoring. There are generally three stages of care for brain tumor patients: diagnosis, treatment, and monitoring. These stages serve as a useful framework to broadly classify DSSs for brain tumors:

1. *Diagnostic DSS*: Accurate diagnosis is important both for treatment planning and for providing vital prognostic information to patients. Physicians often incorporate the morphological features observed on medical images to identify brain tumor type and grade. By extracting relevant features from radiologic images that may distinguish between brain tumor types, diagnostic DSSs can help physicians better diagnose patients with brain tumors. One possibility is a two-class categorization system may provide additional information to the radiologist about whether a candidate lesion is a brain tumor or not; for example, identifying whether a contrast-enhancing lesion observed on patient follow-up is due to tumor recurrence or side effect of radiation therapy. Another type of DSS could be a multi-class categorization system that could, for example, be used to classify lesions into brain tumor type and grade.
2. *Treatment DSS*: Accurately characterizing the extent of tumor invasion in the surrounding brain tissue is critical to successful planning of aggressive treatments such as surgery and radiation therapy. It enables more localized and efficient treatment not only to minimize radiation exposure but also reduce the risk of treatment side effects in brain tumor patients. DSSs may help physicians with treatment planning by more accurately delineating the extent of brain tumors and other surrounding structures (such as edema and necrosis) than is possible by visual inspection. Other DSSs that play important roles during the treatment stage are those that help with image-guided surgery and radiation therapy.
3. *Follow-up DSS*: An essential part of brain cancer management is the assessment of outcomes following treatment. Advances in neuro-imaging have enabled noninvasive methods for assessing patient outcomes based on serial imaging examinations. In the clinical setting, this is typically performed by comparing imaging data acquired at different time points while following the patient. However, this is a challenging task due to the amount of imaging data, variability in image-acquisition parameters (e.g., modality type, number of slices, and slice thickness), variability in patient orientation inside scanner, and the limitations of human vision to detect subtle changes in an image. The third category of DSSs, therefore, deals with computer-based detection of changes in images and better presenting this information to physicians by directing their attention to the potentially most informative regions of the imaging data. The characterization of the change can be performed using the classification DSS as discussed earlier.

   The earliest stages of recurrence are difficult to detect due to the small size of the growing tumor and may be missed on visual inspection of patient imaging data. Thus, another important role of DSS is follow-up monitoring of brain tumor patients. More accurate assessment of follow-up imaging would enable earlier detection of tumor recurrence at an asymptomatic stage, potentially improving patient prognosis and quality of life.

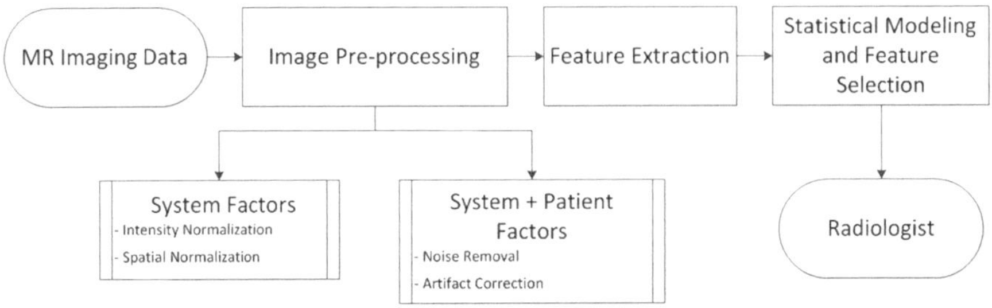

Fig. 11.1 Flowchart illustrating main image analyses steps involved in a typical DSS

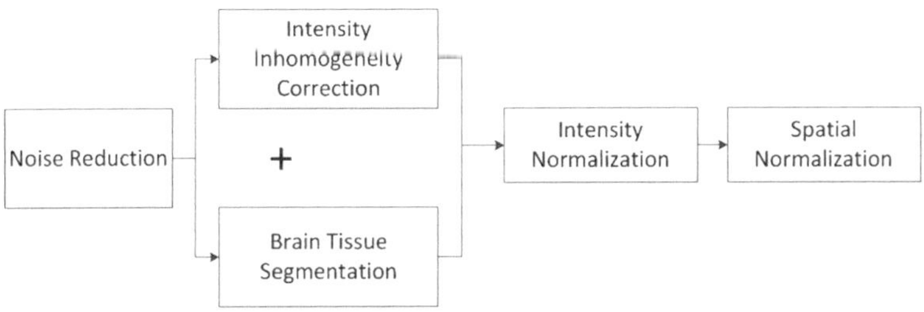

Fig. 11.2 Flowchart illustrating the sequence of important preprocessing steps required before any MR image analyses

Despite the different stages of brain tumor care during which a DSS can be utilized, they share several common aspects in their design (Fig. 11.1). Thus, the remainder of this chapter is organized by analysis techniques rather than application domain. Sections "MRI Preprocessing: Adjusting for System Factors" and "MRI Preprocessing: Adjusting for Patient Factors" describe preprocessing techniques such as methods for image normalization and artifact removal. For clarity, we separate preprocessing procedures necessitated by image corruptions that are solely due to issues concerning the imaging system itself (section "MRI Preprocessing: Adjusting for System Factors") from those that are also dependent on the patient anatomy (section "MRI Preprocessing: Adjusting for Patient Factors"). The flowchart in Fig. 11.2 indicates the ways in which these methods operate in sequence to facilitate subsequent analyses. Section "MRI Feature Extraction" reviews algorithms for feature extraction. Section "Statistical Modeling and Selection of Image Features" highlights the primary considerations in developing statistical models for feature selection and classification. We conclude the chapter (section "Conclusion") with a brief discussion of future directions.

MRI Preprocessing: Adjusting for System Factors

MRI preprocessing is an essential first step of any sophisticated image analysis. Acquiring MR images on different platforms results in different pixel intensity ranges, image resolutions, contrast-to-noise ratios, slice thicknesses, background details, and subject orientations that makes serial and inter-subject analysis problematic. These variations may confound comparisons of image features between brain tumor types and complicate a classification task. Therefore, preprocessing of MR images is essential to ensure that any information obtained from the images is standardized, comparable, and reproducible.

Intensity Normalization Methods

Intensity normalization is the most important preprocessing step when preparing to analyze a set of MR images because many of the morphological features used in classification or serial image comparisons are directly dependent on the image intensities. Several methods have been proposed for intensity normalization of MR images with varying success. In this section, we discuss some of the most popular and widely used normalization methods.

Kullback–Leibler Divergence-Based Intensity Normalization

Wiesenfeld et al. [4] proposed a Kullback–Leibler (KL) divergence-based technique to simultaneously estimate the intensity inhomogeneity and normalize the intensities in MR images. The method assumes a multiplicative model of intensity inhomogeneity,

$$O(x,y) = F(x,y) \times I(x,y) + n(x,y)$$

where $O(x, y)$ is the observed image, $F(x, y)$ is the multiplicative intensity inhomogeneity, $I(x, y)$ is the corrected image, and $n(x, y)$ is the acquisition noise. The method assumes that the noise has very little influence on the intensity normalization. The KL divergence between the intensity inhomogeneity corrected image $I \approx F^{-1}O$ and a target intensity histogram is iteratively minimized to estimate $F(x, y)$,

$$\underset{F^{-1}}{\operatorname{argmin}} \sum_k p_k log_2 \left(\frac{p_k}{q_k} \right)$$

Simultaneous perturbation stochastic approximation (SPSA) is used to generate gradient estimates of the KL-divergence. Although this method works well, pixel-wise estimation of the intensity inhomogeneity $F(x, y)$ reduces the performance of this normalization method such that it is much slower than the other methods presented in the following sections.

Consistent Intensity Correction

Consistent intensity correction operates by matching the observed intensity histogram to a target intensity histogram [5]. The two histograms are approximated using Gaussian mixture models (GMMs) and the expectation maximization (EM) method is used to estimate the model parameters. The intensities within specific anatomical regions are aligned and interpolated using a smooth polynomial function $f^p(x)$ of order p,

$$f^p(x) = \sum_{i=0}^{p} \theta^i x^i$$

The coefficients of the polynomial function θ^i are estimated by minimizing the following energy function,

$$E = \sum_{l=1}^{n} \left(f^p(\mu_l) - v_l\right)^2$$

where $l = 1, \ldots, n$ represents the anatomical regions, and μ_l and v_l are the mean intensity of the anatomical regions in the histogram of the image to be normalized and the target histogram, respectively. The advantage of this method is that it does not require a spatial alignment for the image(s) to be corrected. However, this method suffers from low generalizability and only average accuracy relative to other methods discussed in this section.

Intensity Normalization by Joint Histogram Registration

Jager et al. [6] proposed an intensity normalization method that minimizes a distance measure between the joint probability density functions (PDFs) of the tissue types from a set of MR images to be normalized and a set of reference images. The distance minimization is posed as a nonrigid registration problem with the images considered to be the joint PDFs. The minimization problem can be formulated as,

$$\tau(p_R, p_U; \boldsymbol{f}) = D(p_R, p_U; \boldsymbol{f}) + \alpha S(\boldsymbol{f})$$

where $\boldsymbol{f}$ is the deformation field mapping the PDF of the uncorrected images p_U to the PDF of the reference images p_R; $D(p_R, p_U; \boldsymbol{f})$ is a sum of squared differences (SSD) based distance measure; and $S(\boldsymbol{f})$ is a smoothness measure. The distance measure is defined as,

$$D^{SSD}(p_R, p_U; f) = \frac{1}{2}\int_{\Omega}\left(p_{U_\varphi}(i) - p_R(i)\right)^2 di$$

where $p_{U_\varphi}(i) = p_U \circ (i - f(i))$, and Ω represents the joint PDF image domain. A regularization measure based on curvature smoothness is defined as,

$$S^{curv}(f) = \frac{1}{2}\sum_{l=1}^{n}\int_{\Omega}(\Delta f_l)^2 dx$$

with $\Delta(.)$ being the Laplacian operator, and n as the dimensionality of joint PDF. The objective function $\tau(p_R, p_U; f)$ is minimized using a variational approach. The histogram registration method is applicable for multi-modality images, but requires at least two imaging sequences (e.g., T1 and T2 weighted images). The method has been reported to perform well and is fairly generalizable [7]. However, nonrigid registration makes this method considerably slower than approaches that normalize an image without using additional preprocessing steps.

Decile Normalization Method

Decile normalization (DN) [8, 9] is a widely used method for intensity normalization of brain MR images. This method works by setting percentile-based ten intensity landmarks (deciles) C_L,

$$C_L = \left\{p_{low}, m_{10}, m_{20}, m_{30}, m_{40}, m_{50}, m_{60}, m_{70}, m_{80}, m_{90}, p_{high}\right\}$$

where each m_i, $i = \{10, 20, \ldots, 90\}$ denotes pixel intensities of the ith percentile of the histogram corresponding to the foreground in the MR image. Since image artifacts and outliers typically have extreme image intensities, p_{low} and, p_{high} are used as the end percentiles instead of m_0, and m_{100} to reduce sensitivity to such image corruptions. The foreground extraction is performed through a thresholding approach that uses the mean intensity of the image (for intensities between p_{low} and p_{high}) as the intensity threshold. The landmarks of the template MR image C_L^{Temp} to be normalized are then transformed to landmarks calculated on a reference histogram C_L^{Ref} using a piecewise linear mapping. Piece-wise linear mapping (Fig. 11.3) helps reduce the sensitivity of normalization method to the presence of anatomical abnormalities such as lesions and treatment scars.

This method is very fast, easy to implement, and applicable to images from multiple modalities [8–10]. Gasser et al. [10] evaluated the effectiveness of DN on MR images containing pathology, obtained from multiple acquisition sites, scanners, and MR modalities. They quantitatively evaluated the effect of DN on tissue separation, and reported significantly improved accuracy when intensity normalization is performed.

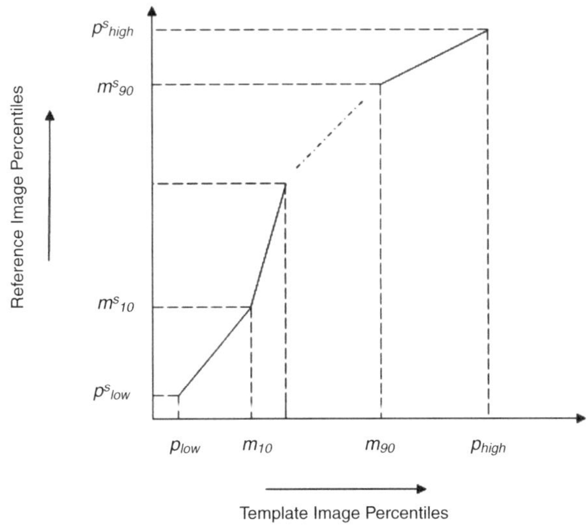

Fig. 11.3 Figure illustrating piecewise linear mapping between input image histogram and reference histogram

Spatial Normalization

The spatial location of brain tissue often does not correlate well across images and varies among different MR acquisitions. The variations in spatial location of brain tissue are due to differences in acquisition parameters, patient placement in the scanner, and patient motion. Therefore, spatial normalization is an important preprocessing step required before any comparison studies can be done. These can be both interpatient comparisons (between different patients) and intra-patient comparisons (change detection during follow-up to evaluate treatment outcomes). The spatial normalization involves alignment of MR imaging data to a standard reference dataset of images using image registration. The reference set of images used in existing normalization methods is often chosen as corresponding to tissue probability maps (Fig. 11.4). The alignment of imaging data to tissue probability maps has the additional benefit in brain tissue segmentation of introducing tissue-specific priors into probability-based models often used for voxel classification.

Spatial normalization using image registration is a difficult task since MR images may have been captured through multiple modalities and is further complicated by the presence of anatomical deviations in the brain such as pathology, resection scars, and treatment side effects. In this section, we discuss some of the most commonly used spatial normalization methods for brain MR images.

Unified Segmentation

Image registration is affected by changes in image intensities due to corruptions such as noise, intensity inhomogeneity, and partial volume effects. Unified segmentation combines the three interdependent tasks of segmentation, intensity

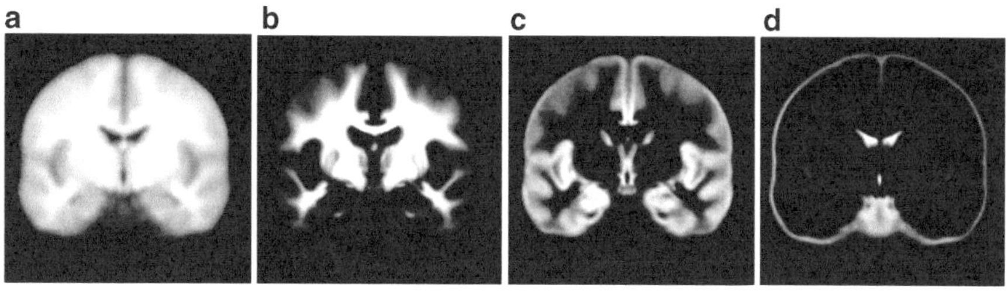

Fig. 11.4 Figure showing (**a**) template image, and probabilistic atlas maps of (**b**) white matter, (**c**) gray matter, and (**d**) cerebrospinal fluid obtained from International Consortium for Brain Mapping (ICBM)

inhomogeneity correction, and spatial normalization under the same iterative formulation [11]. As a rough fit, a tissue probability map is first aligned to the patient data using affine registration. The initial alignment is further refined using nonlinear deformations, which are modeled as linear combinations of discrete cosine transform basis functions. This spatial normalization is combined with the task of image segmentation using a principled Bayesian probabilistic formulation that utilizes tissue probability maps as priors. The intensity inhomogeneity correction is included within the segmentation model to account for smoothly varying intensities across the image domain. Once the method converges, the inverse of the transformation that aligns the tissue probability maps to the patient data can be used to normalize the patient MR images.

Diffeomorphic Anatomical Registration Through Exponentiated Lie Algebra

Diffeomorphic anatomical registration through exponentiated lie algebra (DARTEL) is another such normalization method that depends on image segmentation [12]. The reference imaging data is deformed to align them to the patient MR imaging data. However, unlike unified segmentation, DARTEL includes a much higher number of parameters in registration, which enables the modeling of more detailed and finer deformations. In DARTEL, the deformations are modeled using a flow field that is assumed to be constant in time. This enables a one-to-one inverse mapping of the deformation field from the reference imaging data that can be used for normalization of patient MR imaging data. DARTEL has been reported to be superior to unified segmentation for spatial normalization of MR images, including those with anatomical deviations such as tumors and resection scars [13, 14].

Automatic Registration Toolbox

Automatic registration toolbox (ART) [15] is based on a multi-scale neighborhood search to find the most similar image voxel between the patient MR images $\{I_P(v), v \in \Omega_\mathrm{p}\}$ and the reference images $\{I_R(v), v \in \Omega_\mathrm{R}\}$, where v corresponds to the image voxels belonging to image domains Ω_p and Ω_R, respectively. The patient MR images are resized and interpolated to match the dimensions of the reference MR data, followed by a neighborhood-based voxel search in the reference image. A similarity metric $S(w_1, w_1)$ between two vectors w_1 and w_1 is defined as,

$$S(w_1, w_2) = \frac{w_1^T H w_2}{\sqrt{w_2^T H w_2}}$$

where H is an idempotent symmetric centering matrix that removes the mean of the vector it pre-multiplies. For every voxel v_i in patient MR data, vector w_1 is defined as a vector of voxel intensities that are in a neighborhood N_{v_i} around v_i, $f_{v_i}^P = \{I_P(v), v \in N_{v_i}\}$. The corresponding voxel in the reference MR data I_R can be found by searching in a finite neighborhood ψ_i around and including voxel location v_i. Let voxel $v_j \in \psi_i$ be the voxel in this neighborhood when the similarity measure $S\left(f_{v_i}^P, f_{v_j}^R\right)$ is maximum,

$$S\left(f_{v_i}^P, f_{v_j}^R\right) = \max_{v \in \psi_i} S\left(f_{v_i}^P, f_v^R\right)$$

The initial estimate of the displacement field for voxel v_i is $w(i) = j - i$. The estimation is further refined by computing the displacement field at multiple resolution levels using the scale-space theory. In comparison studies performed on normal subjects, ART has been reported superior to other methods for reducing inter-subject anatomical variability [13, 15].

MRI Preprocessing: Adjusting for Patient Factors

The presence of noise and other image artifacts is often prominent in MRI and adversely affects any attempts at quantitative image analysis. The correction of such image corruptions is also an essential part of the image preprocessing required before any quantitative feature extraction can be performed. In this chapter, we divide preprocessing steps into two categories based on the source of the problem. While the methods discussed in section "MRI Preprocessing: Adjusting for System Factors" dealt specifically with problems that arise solely from system factors, this section deals with image corruptions that result from the combined effect of system and patient factors.

This raises the question of the sequence in which these two categories of preprocessing methods should be carried out. Both image normalization and removal of image corruptions utilize image intensity information and therefore are interdependent tasks. Madabhushi and Udupa [16] in an analysis of nearly 4,000 cases suggested that noise and artifact removal should precede image normalization. They also demonstrated that iterative adjustment of system and patient factors, as is often done, does not considerably improve the image quality (Fig. 11.2).

Image De-Noising

As with other medical imaging modalities, MR images contain significant amounts of noise that compromise the performance of the image analyses incorporated into any DSS. The main causes of noise in MRI are due to thermally driven Brownian motion of electrons within patient's conducting tissue (patient factor) and within reception coil (system factor). There is a trade-off between spatial resolution, signal-to-noise ratio (SNR), and acquisition time in MRI. While SNR can, in principle, be improved by increasing the acquisition time it is not a practical solution to implement in the clinic. Therefore, there is a need for de-noising algorithms that can improve image quality and reduce image noise after image acquisition.

Several de-noising algorithms have been proposed in the literature that are based on methods adapted from either general image processing or developed specifically for MRI specific noise. The distribution of noise in MR images is known to follow a Rician distribution, which, unlike Gaussian noise, is signal dependent and therefore much harder to remove. The noise in MR images is introduced during the calculation of the magnitude image from the complex Fourier domain data collected during an MRI scan. In this section, we discuss some of the most widely used de-noising methods in MRI.

Anisotropic Diffusion

Anisotropic diffusion is a widely used adaptive de-noising method that only locally smoothes the continuous regions of an image, while preserving the edges/boundaries between the image regions. The anisotropic diffusion model is defined by,

$$\begin{aligned}\partial_t u(x,y,t) &= div\left(g\left(\left|\nabla u(x,y,t)\right|^2\right)\nabla u(x,y,t)\right)\\ &= g\left(\left|\nabla u(x,y,t)\right|^2\right)\Delta u(x,y,t)\\ &\quad + \nabla\left(g\left(\left|\nabla u(x,y,t)\right|^2\right)\right).\nabla u(x,y,t)\end{aligned}$$

where $u(x,y,t)$ represents an image parameterized with the spatial coordinates (x, y) and an artificial time t that represents the number of smoothing iterations; $div(.)$, $\Delta(.)$ and $\nabla(.)$ are the divergence, the Laplacian, and the gradient operators, respectively; $g(|\nabla u(x,y,t)|^2)$ is a diffusivity term that controls the strength of smoothing. The following diffusivities $g(|\nabla u(x,y,t)|^2)$ were proposed by Perona and Malik [17],

$$g(s^2) = \frac{1}{1+\frac{s^2}{\lambda^2}}, \quad \text{and,} \quad g(s^2) = \exp(-(s^2/\lambda^2))$$

where $\lambda > 0$ is a scaling parameter that controls the edge enhancement threshold. Anisotropic diffusion works well for natural images with well-defined boundaries; however, their use in MR images is limited due to the presence of partial volume effects that result in smooth region boundaries.

Wavelet Analysis

In wavelet analysis, an image $u(x,y)$ is decomposed into discrete wavelets at different scales and translations defined as,

$$u(x,y) = \sum_{j=-\infty}^{\infty} \sum_{k=-\infty}^{\infty} d_{j,k} \Psi_{j,k}(x,y)$$

where $\Psi_{j,k}(x,y)$ are the wavelet basis functions, and j and k are the scale and translation parameters, respectively, and $d_{j,k}$ are the wavelet mixing coefficients estimated by,

$$d_{j,k} = \iint_{-\infty}^{\infty} u(x,y) \Psi_{j,k}(x,y) dxdy$$

De-noising an image with wavelet analysis involves thresholding wavelet coefficients $d_{j,k}$ to discard coefficients that do not have significant energy. Although successful in removing noise, wavelet-based methods do not preserve the finer details in MR images and thus further exacerbating any partial volume effects.

Rician-Adapted Non-Local Means Filter

The non-local (NL) means filter [18] removes noise by computing a weighted average of surrounding pixels. The weights are determined using a similarity measure between local neighborhoods around the pixels being compared. The NL-corrected version of an image $u(x)$ can be represented as,

$$NL(u(x_i)) = \sum_{x_j \in S_i} w(x_i, x_j) u(x_j)$$

where S_i represents the size of the neighborhood around any pixel x_i to be used to compute the weighted average. $w(x_i, x_j)$ are the assigned weights to pixels x_j belonging to space S_i defined as,

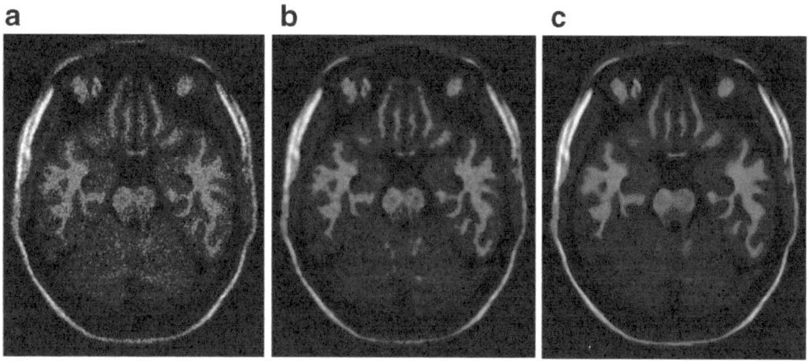

Fig. 11.5 Figure showing (**a**) sample MR image with Rician noise, (**b**) denoised image with anisotropic diffusion, and (**c**) denoised image obtained from Rician-adapted NLM filter

$$w(x_i, x_j) = \frac{1}{Z_i} exp\left(- \frac{||u(N_i) - u(N_j)||^2}{h^2} \right), \quad w(x_i, x_j) \in [0, 1]$$

where Z_i is a normalization constant such that $\sum_{x_j \in S_i} w(x_i, x_j) = 1$, h is a decay parameter determining the rate of decay in weighting, and N_i is the neighborhood image patch centered around pixel x_i of radius r.

Wiest-Daessle [19] proposed a Rician-adapted version of this NL-means filter using the properties of the second-order moment of a Rice law,

$$NL_R(u(x_i)) = \sqrt{\max\left(\left(\sum_{x_j \in S_i} w(x_i, x_j) u(x_j)^2\right) - 2\sigma^2, 0\right)}$$

where σ is the variance of the Gaussian noise in the complex Fourier domain of MR data and is estimated using pseudo-residual technique proposed by Gasser et al. [10].

Rician-adapted NL-means filter has been reported to outperform wavelet analysis, Gaussian smoothing, and anisotropic diffusion for de-noising MR images with Rician noise distribution [20–22] (Fig. 11.5).

Removal of MRI Artifacts

MR images suffer from several image artifacts such as partial volume effects, Gibbs's artifacts, chemical shifting, motion artifacts, and intensity inhomogeneities. These artifacts often produce an abnormal distribution of intensities in the image, thereby compromising the accuracy of automatic image analysis methods. Though some artifacts can be corrected during the image reconstruction phase, other artifacts must be corrected through post-acquisition image processing. In this section, we will discuss some of the post-processing methods to deal with partial

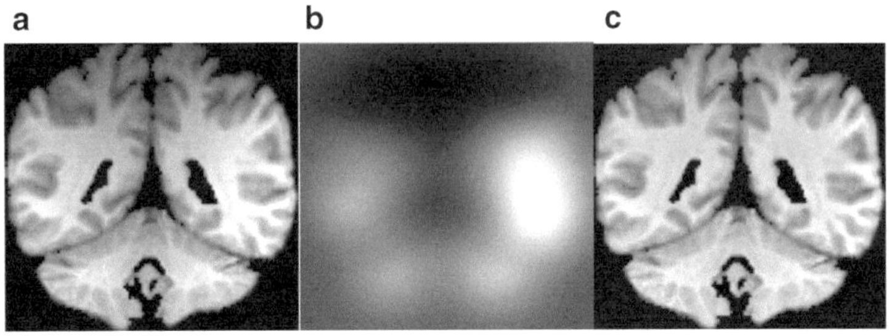

Fig. 11.6 Figure showing real MR image (**a**) corrupted from intensity inhomogeneity, (**b**) estimated intensity inhomogeneity, and (**c**) recovered image

volume effects and intensity inhomogeneities, two of the most prominent and widely studied artifacts that require post-processing.

Intensity inhomogeneity, also known as intensity nonuniformity (INU), the bias field, or shading, is one of the most prominently occurring artifacts in MR images. This adverse phenomenon appears as smooth intensity variations across the image domain (Fig. 11.6), which results in the intensity of voxels belonging to the same class varying with location within the image. INU artifacts in MR images are mostly due to acquisition imperfections such as nonuniform RF excitation, nonuniform coil receptor sensitivity, and standing wave effects [23]. Other minor factors that may also produce INU effects include eddy currents due to rapid switching of magnetic field gradients; patient-induced electromagnetic interactions, and geometric distortions. The INU artifacts become much more significant when scanners are operating at higher strength magnetic field strengths. Although INU artifacts have little effect on visual interpretation of an MR image by a radiologist, they significantly degrade the performance of automatic image analysis methods. For this reason, INU correction has been an active field of research and a number of methods have been proposed in the literature.

The correction of intensity inhomogeneities can be broadly classified into: *prospective* and *retrospective* methods. Prospective correction requires special imaging sequences with physical phantoms and multiple reception coils and involves recalibrating the scanner based on an assessment of the excitation field strength and the nonuniformity in reception coils. Although prospective methods can potentially correct for static INU artifacts resulting from scanner imperfections, they are unable to account for patient-induced intensity inhomogeneities. Furthermore, the longer scanning routines typically involved in prospective correction methods make them impractical in clinical settings. Retrospective correction, on the other hand, uses the intensity information contained within an acquired image to estimate INU artifacts and is therefore a more general solution than prospective correction. This makes them much more useful for clinical use; however, they are unable to distinguish between scanner and patient-induced intensity inhomogeneities.

Spectrum Filtering Methods

Due to their slowly varying nature across image domain, correction methods generally assume that INU artifacts are low-frequency signals that can be removed from the higher frequency spectrum of anatomical structures. The two main filtering approaches are *homomorphic filtering* and *homomorphic unsharp masking*.

Homomorphic filtering takes the difference between the log transformed image log($I(x,y)$) and a low-pass filtered (*LPF*) version of the logarithmic image, with a mean-preserving normalization constant (C) [24]. The corrected image $\widetilde{I}(x,y)$ can be obtained by taking the exponential of the difference image,

$$\widetilde{I}(x,y) = \exp(\log(\mathrm{I}(x,y)) - LPF(\log(I(x,y))) + C)$$

Homomorphic unsharp masking corrects an image by dividing the acquired image $I(x, y)$ with the *LPF* version of the image, scaled by a mean-preserving normalization constant [25].

$$\widetilde{I}(x,y) = \frac{I(x,y)}{LPF(I(x,y))/c}$$

Although widely used, low-pass filtering methods are thought to have rather limited ability to correct for INU artifacts in brain MR images. The limited effectiveness of these methods is due to the significant overlap of the frequency spectrums of INU artifacts and brain structures, which does not fit the assumption underlying these techniques.

Intensity Histogram-Based Methods

Histogram-based methods operate on the principle that the information content in an image is changed by artifacts such as intensity inhomogeneities. Sled et al. [26] proposed a non-parametric nonuniformity normalization (N3) method that iteratively corrects for INU artifacts by maximizing the frequency content of the intensity distributions in the corrected image. N3 is a fully automated method, does not include any assumptions about the anatomical structures present, and has been reported to be one of the most successful methods for INU correction.

Histogram-based methods have also been developed that propose the information content of an image increases when corrupted by INU artifacts. These methods assume that INU artifacts can be corrected by minimizing the entropy (information content) of the image, subject to some constraints. Several researchers have explored this concept by minimizing energy functions that combine image entropy, INU smoothness constraints and mean-preserving regularization terms to correct for INU artifacts [27–30]. An advantage is that these information minimization methods are highly generalizable and thus can be used on any MR image.

Spline Fitting Methods

The smooth varying nature of INU artifacts has motivated the use of polynomial and spline surfaces on a set of extracted image features to estimate INU artifacts. In these methods, a spline function is least squares fitted to a set of image pixels belonging to a major tissue type and distributed throughout the image. Both manual and automatic candidate image feature selection methods have been investigated, and manual selection was reported to be more accurate than automatic selection [31]. A major limitation of this approach is the extrapolation of INU computed from a single tissue class to estimate the INU artifacts across the entire image. This framework may be sufficient to correct INU artifacts due to scanner imperfections, but patient-induced INU artifacts that may vary between tissue types are not handled appropriately. The time consuming manual selection of points in every image slice is another limitation, and also potentially introduces user subjectivity.

INU Correction Combined with Brain Tissue Segmentation

Combining INU correction with image segmentation is commonly used for retrospective correction of intensity inhomogeneities in MR images. INU correction and image segmentation depend on one another, and, therefore, better segmentation and INU correction can be achieved by simultaneously utilizing information from these tasks. Furthermore, one result of these approaches is brain tissue segmentation, which is often essential for subsequent quantitative MR image analysis. A common theme of these methods is the minimization/maximization of an objective function that contains a data fitting term that is regularized with an INU artifact smoothness term.

Several probabilistic approaches using maximum likelihood (ML) and maximum a posteriori (MAP) have been proposed to define data fitting terms for image voxel classification. The intensity distributions inside each image region are modeled using assumed parametric models that incorporate effects from intensity corruptions due to INU. A common choice of parametric models has been the finite Gaussian mixture (FMM) models over the image domain with the model parameters estimated using popular expectation maximization (EM) algorithm. FMM are often defined with every tissue class described using a single Gaussian component [32, 33], or as a combination of multiple components [34–36]. The class priors are often included to improve the segmentation and INU artifact estimation using either probabilistic atlases or hidden Markov random field (HMRF) defined priors. Other approaches have also been proposed including non-parametric segmentation based on *max-shift* and *mean-shift* clustering for INU estimation [37, 38], and fuzzy C-means (FCM)-based methods that assume each voxel can belong to multiple tissue classes. Since there is significant overlap in the algorithms used for segmentation and INU estimation, we refer readers to see "Brain Tissue Segmentation" section of this chapter.

The data fitting term is regularized with a smoothness term that ensures that the estimate INU artifact is smoothly varying across the image domain. The smoothness term is often defined in terms of the first and second order derivatives of the intensity inhomogeneity field. The minimization of the smoothness term accounts for the smoothly varying nature of INU artifacts in MR images. For numerical convenience, polynomial and spline surfaces have been widely used for modeling intensity inhomogeneity. When combined with the tissue segmentation process, selection of candidate points can be performed automatically. This addresses the major limitation suffered by spline fitting methods as discussed in earlier sections.

Brain Tissue Segmentation

Segmentation of brain MR images into tissue types is often an important and essential task in the study of many brain tumors. It enables quantification of neuroanatomical changes in different brain tissues, which may be informative for diagnosis and treatment follow-up of brain tumor patients. Besides brain tumors, brain tissue segmentation is useful in management of neurodegenerative and psychiatric disorders such as schizophrenia, and epilepsy. Multiple sclerosis (MS), for instance, requires accurate quantification of lesions in the white matter part of the brain for assessment of drug treatment. Even though MRI produces high quality volumetric images, the presence of image corruptions (noise, intensity inhomogeneities, and partial-volume effects) makes the segmentation of brain MR images complicated and challenging. Due to these reasons, brain MR segmentation has been an active field of research with a variety of methods proposed in literature. Traditional methods such as image thresholding and region growing usually fail due to the complex distribution of intensities in medical images. Furthermore, the presence of intensity inhomogeneity and noise significantly impact these intensity-based methods. In this section, we discuss some of the most widely explored methods for medical image segmentation.

Fuzzy C-Means-Based Segmentation Methods

FCM is based on calculating fuzzy membership of image voxels to each of multiple classes. The following objective function is iteratively minimized,

$$E = \sum_{i=1}^{N} \sum_{j=1}^{C} w_{i,j}^{k} d(x_i, \mu_j), \quad 0 < w_{i,j}^{k} < 1$$

where $w_{i,j}^{k}$ is the fuzzy membership of observation x_i in cluster c_j satisfying $\sum_{j=1}^{C} w_{i,j} = 1$, k represents the fuzziness degree in clustering, $d(x_i, \mu_j)$ is the distance between observation x_i and center μ_j of cluster c_j, N and C represent the number of observations and clusters, respectively. Conceptually, FCM seems suitable for modeling partial volume effects in MR images. However, FCM is extremely sensitive to noise and intensity inhomogeneities. Several studies have proposed variants of FCM that are less sensitive to noise and artifacts, but they still do not perform well in comparison with parametric methods [39–43].

Mixture Modeling and MAP/ML Estimation

Mixture models have been widely used for modeling intensity distributions in MR images. In GMMs, the likelihood of a D-dimensional observation x belonging to class C is defined as,

$$p(x|C) = \sum_{i=1}^{N} w_i g(x|\mu_i, \Sigma_i)$$

where N is the number of mixture components to model class C, w_i are the prior probabilities of mixture components, $g(x|\mu_i, \Sigma_i)$ is the likelihood of observation x belonging to i^{th} mixture component,

$$g(x|\mu_i, \Sigma_j) = \frac{1}{(2\pi)^{D/2}|\Sigma|^{1/2}} \exp\left(-\frac{1}{2}(x-\mu_i)'\Sigma_i^{-1}(x-\mu_i)\right)$$

The parameters of the mixture model are: (μ_i,Σ_i), $i = 1,..., n$, where μ_i and Σ_i represent the mean and covariance matrices of mixture components, respectively. The parameters are estimated using the expectation-maximization (EM) algorithm that maximizes the joint likelihood of the observed data with the mixture model. EM requires prior information on the number of mixture components to estimate the model parameters. Several studies have used a single Gaussian component for each of four classes: white matter (WM), gray matter (GM), cerebrospinal fluid (CSF), and background (BG) [32, 33]. In the presence of intensity inhomogeneities and partial volume effects, some studies have proposed using multiple Gaussian components for modeling each tissue type [34–36]. Several variants of ML and EM algorithm have also been proposed that additionally account for image corruptions [44–46]. Some researchers have also proposed estimation of parameters based on MAP instead of ML by introducing class priors in the probabilistic model [36]. Prior probabilities can be introduced by using probabilistic atlas maps; however, this requires complex medical image registration that is time consuming and an active area of research in itself. Another type of class priors often used for image segmentation is based on HMRF that introduces spatial contextual information in the classification model [47, 48]. HMRF priors help reduce the sensitivity of segmentation model to noise by incorporating neighborhood information in the segmentation process (neighboring pixels tend to belong to the same tissue class).

Edge-Based Active Contour Models

In active contour models (also commonly known as "snakes"), a parametric curve $C(s) = [x(s), y(s)]$ evolves on the image domain Ω under the influence of an energy function of the form,

$$E = \int \frac{1}{2}\left(\alpha\left|X'(s)\right|^2 + \beta\left|X''(s)\right|^2\right) + E_{ext}(X(s))ds$$

where $s \in [0,1]$ is the arc length, the first two terms $\alpha|X'(s)|^2$ and $\beta|X''(s)|^2$ represent regularizations on the evolving curve, and $E_{ext}(X(s))$ represents an external force driving the evolution of the curve $C(s)$.

A Gaussian-smoothed gradient force is often used for the external force term and thus this method is relatively insensitive to the contour initialization parameters and boundary concavities,

$$E_{ext}(X(s)) = -|G_\sigma * \nabla I|^2$$

Region-Based Active Contour Models and Level Set Formulation

Region-based active contours define an energy functional based on the region statistics rather than local image gradient,

$$E(C) = \mu.Length(C) + v.Area(C_{in}) + \lambda.F_{ext}$$

where μ, v, $\lambda \geq 0$ are fixed parameters, the first two regularization terms in the energy functional enforce local constraints on the curve C, while F_{ext} denotes the external force that drives the evolution of the curve. The image domain Ω is partitioned by the curve C into two image regions: C_{in} and C_{out} corresponding to the image regions within and outside of curve C. Chan and Vese [49] proposed a piecewise-constant model for image segmentation, defining the external force term as,

$$F_{ext} = \int_{C_{in}} \left|I(x,y) - c_1\right|^2 dxdy + \int_{C_{out}} \left|I(x,y) - c_2\right|^2 dxdy$$

where c_1 and c_2 are the average intensities of pixels inside image regions C_{in} and C_{out}, respectively. Minimizing the energy functional is difficult in terms of image regions C_{in} and C_{out}. Level set formulations [50] enable representing image regions C_{in}, C_{out} and the evolving curve C in terms of a higher dimensional Lipchitz function $\Phi : \Omega \rightarrow R$ such that,

$$\Phi(x,y) = \begin{cases} = 0 & at \quad C \\ > 0 & inside \quad C(C_{in}), \\ < 0 & outside \quad C(C_{out}) \end{cases} \quad (x,y) \in \Omega$$

Using the Heaviside function H and Dirac measure δ defined as,

$$H(z) = \begin{cases} 1 & \text{if } z \geq 0 \\ 0 & \text{if } z < 0 \end{cases}, \quad \delta(z) = \frac{\partial}{\partial z} H(z)$$

The region-based formulation proposed by Chan and Vese [49] can therefore be rewritten as,

$$\begin{aligned} E(\Phi, c_1, c_2) = {} & \mu \int_\Omega \delta(\Phi) |\nabla \Phi| dxdy \\ & + v \int_\Omega H(\Phi) dxdy + \lambda \int_\Omega |I(x,y) - c_1|^2 H(\Phi) dxdy \\ & + \lambda \int_\Omega |I(x,y) - c_2|^2 (1 - H(\Phi)) dxdy \\ E(\Phi, c_1, c_2) = {} & \int_\Omega F(\Phi, \Phi_x, \Phi_y) dxdy \end{aligned}$$

Minimizing the energy functional $E(\Phi, c_1, c_2)$ with respect to $\Phi(x,y)$ gives the associated Euler–Lagrange equation,

$$\frac{\partial E(\Phi, c_1, c_2)}{\partial \Phi} = F_\Phi - \frac{\partial}{\partial x} F_{\Phi_x} - \frac{\partial}{\partial y} F_{\Phi_y}$$

Parameterization by an artificial time $t \geq 0$ gives the update equation of $\Phi(x,y,t)$ in the steepest gradient descent direction,

$$\frac{\partial \Phi(x,y,t)}{\partial t} = -\frac{\partial E(\Phi, c_1, c_2)}{\partial \Phi}$$

The regularization terms that impose local constraints on the curve C make this segmentation method relatively insensitive to noise and the curve initialization parameters. The active contour framework in a level set formulation is a powerful tool that can be used to solve complex objective functions using an iterative scheme. Herein we give an example of such an approach.

In [51], we proposed a probabilistic region-based active contour model for automatic segmentation of brain MR images. A decision theory-based approach that assigns a particular penalty/loss value to every decision/classification on an image voxel is used to drive the voxel classification. A loss matrix L can therefore be defined in which each element L_{ij} corresponds to the loss incurred if a voxel belong to the ith class is misclassified into j^{th} class. For a two-class classification problem, the loss matrix can therefore be defined as $L = \begin{bmatrix} L_{11} & L_{12} \\ L_{21} & L_{22} \end{bmatrix}$. The external force F_{ext} that drives the evolution of the curve is defined via a Bayesian approach of minimizing the expected loss incurred due to voxel misclassification over the entire image,

$$F_{ext} = E[L] = \sum_k \sum_j \iint_{(x,y)\in R_j} L_{kj} \times P((x,y), C_k)dxdy$$

where R_j denotes image region j and, $P((x, y), C_k)$ represents the joint likelihood of voxel (x, y) belonging to class C_k. Therefore, for a two-class classification problem,

$$F_{ext} = \iint_{C_{in}} L_{21}P((x,y), C_{out})dxdy + \iint_{C_{out}} L_{12}P((x,y), C_{in})dxdy$$

Most existing segmentation methods assume a Gaussian distribution of intensities and utilize piecewise-constant approximation inside each image region. Although such an assumption is valid for natural images, its not appropriate for MR images due to significant amount of noise and image artifacts such as intensity inhomogeneity and partial volume effects. The presence of such image corruptions produces arbitrary intensity distributions within image regions that are difficult to model with a single Gaussian distribution. Instead of making implicit assumptions regarding the underlying intensity distribution, the arbitrary intensity distributions are modeled using mixture models. The joint likelihoods $P((x, y), C_k)$ can therefore be represented as,

$$P((x,y), C_j) = P((x,y|C_j) \times P(C_j) = \sum_{i=1}^{M} w_i g((x,y)|\mu_i, \Sigma_i) \times P(C_j)$$

where $g((x,y)|\mu_i, \Sigma_i)$ is a multi-variate Gaussian mixture component with μ_i and Σ_i as the mean and the covariance matrices, respectively, and w_i are the mixture priors or weights of each Gaussian component. The prior probabilities for the different brain tissue types $P(C_j)$ are obtained using probability atlas maps (Fig. 11.4). The energy functional driving evolution of the active contour can therefore be represented as,

$$\begin{aligned} F(C, \lambda_1, \lambda_2) = {} & \mu.Length(C) + v.Area(C_{in}) \\ & + \iint_{(x,y)\in C_{in}} L_{21} \sum_{j=1}^{M_2} w_j g((x,y)|\mu_j, \Sigma_j) P(C_{out})dxdy \\ & + \iint_{(x,y)\in C_{out}} L_{12} \sum_{i=1}^{M_1} w_i g((x,y)|\mu_i, \Sigma_i) P(C_{in})dxdy \end{aligned}$$

This energy functional is converted into a level set formulation by using the Heaviside H and Dirac measure δ functions,

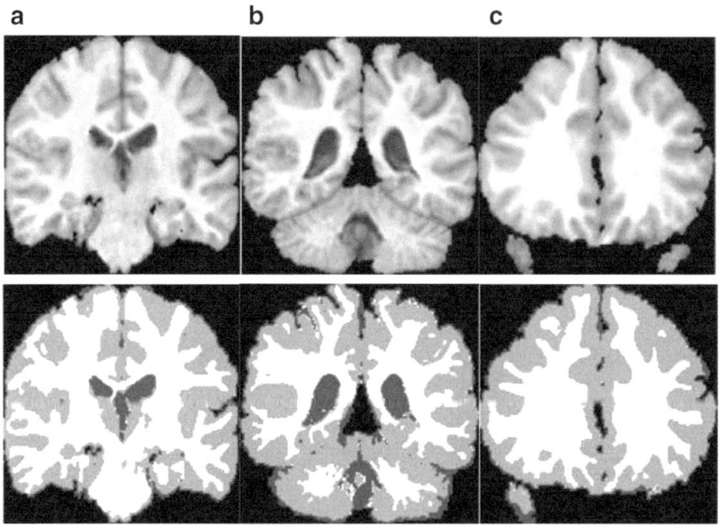

Fig. 11.7 Figure showing real MR images (*first row*) and corresponding soft tissue segmentations (*second row*) into white matter, gray matter, and cerebrospinal fluid using method proposed in [51]

$$
\begin{aligned}
F(\phi,\lambda_1,\lambda_2) = {} & \mu\int_\Omega \delta(\phi)|\nabla\Phi|dxdy \\
& + v\int_\Omega H(\Phi)dxdy \\
& + \iint\limits_\Omega L_{21}\sum_{j=1}^{M_2} w_j g\big((x,y)\big|\mu_j,\Sigma_j\big)P(C_{out})(H(\phi))dxdy \\
& + \iint\limits_\Omega L_{12}\sum_{i=1}^{M_1} w_i g\big((x,y)\big|\mu_i,\Sigma_i\big)P(C_{in})(1-H(\phi))dxdy
\end{aligned}
$$

Minimizing the energy functional with respect to $\phi(x, y)$ and parametrization by $t > 0$ gives the following update equations for $\phi(x, y, t)$ (Fig. 11.7),

$$
\begin{aligned}
\frac{\partial\phi(x,y,t)}{\partial t} = {} & \delta(\phi)[\mu.div\left(\frac{\nabla\phi}{|\nabla\phi|}\right) - v \\
& +L_{12}\sum_{i=1}^{M_1} w_i g\big((x,y)\big|\mu_i,\Sigma_i\big)P(C_{in}) \\
& -L_{21}\sum_{j=1}^{M_2} w_j g\big((x,y)\big|\mu_j,\Sigma_j\big)P(C_{out})]
\end{aligned}
$$

MRI Feature Extraction

Radiological DSSs typically use image-derived features along with relevant clinical variables to generate predictions and classifications. Shape, texture, and intensity are the most informative visual cues in medical images and are often used by physicians in a qualitative manner for image interpretation. The visual cues observed on medical images can be quantified using automated techniques, which address some of the limitations associated with conventional methods for medical image interpretation. However, quantifying image features using automatic techniques requires careful selection of objective definitions to represent image features. While some image features (such as tumor volume) require absolute quantification to be physically meaningful, relative definitions may be required for other features (such as extent of contrast enhancement). One desirable property for many image-derived features is invariance to transformations such as translation, rotation, and scaling (TRS). In this section, we discuss some of the well-established techniques for the quantification of shape, texture, and intensity features in medical images.

Shape Features

The shapes of the anatomical changes observed on brain MR images (such as lesion, necrosis inside lesion, and associated edema) provide important information about the growth patterns of tumors in different brain tissues and are often used qualitatively by physicians to identify the type and grade of a brain tumor. For example, while meningiomas are often characterized by more regular shapes with sharp boundaries delimiting them from the surrounding normal brain tissue, glioblastoma multiforme (GBM) tumors frequently exhibit more convoluted shapes with diffuse boundaries.

The shape of brain tumors and the surrounding structures can be quantified using established shape descriptors. Although these shape descriptors may not be able to entirely reconstruct the shape, they are sufficiently specific to discriminate between different shape types. Shape description techniques are typically classified into two major categories—*region-based* and *contour-based* methods, depending on whether the shape features are extracted from the entire region or only from the shape boundary. We discuss shape descriptors that have been used in many studies to describe lesion shapes in medical images.

Simple Shape Features

Several simple shape features have been put forth in the literature to describe the shape of an object in a global sense. However, these simplistic features have

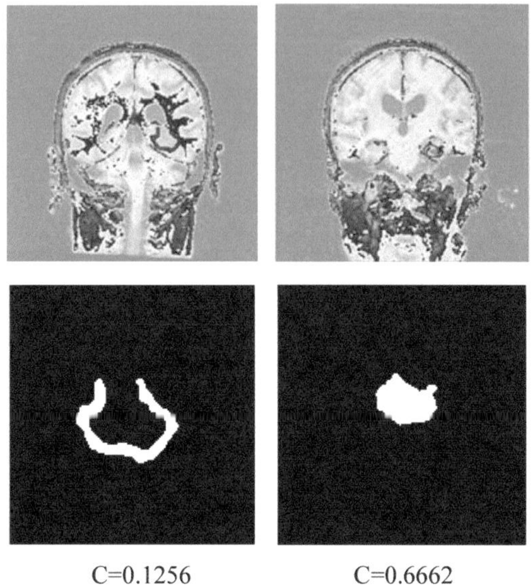

Fig. 11.8 Examples illustrating compactness measures for real 2D MR image slices

relatively limited power and can only discriminate between shapes that are substantially different. Therefore, simple shape features are typically used in combination with other more sophisticated descriptors to classify shapes. Some commonly used simple shape features are *circularity*, *eccentricity*, *rectangularity*, *principal axis orientation*, *bending energy*, and *convexity*.

1. *Circularity*: Circularity or compactness is a common measure used to define the shape of objects and quantify the similarity of the object to the most compact shape, i.e., a circle in 2D and a sphere in 3D. In two-dimensional case,

$$Circularity(C) = \frac{4\pi \times Area}{(Perimeter)^2}, C \in [0, 1]$$

where a value of $C = 1$ corresponds to the circle. C decreases with decreasing similarity to a circle in symmetry (Fig. 11.8). In three dimensions, compactness can be represented as,

$$Circularity(C) = \frac{36\pi \times (Volume)^2}{(Surface\ Area)^3}, C \in [0, 1]$$

Although circularity is straightforward to calculate for the two-dimensional case, calculating the surface area of an object in three dimensions is complicated and requires defining a neighborhood connectedness system. A numerically efficient method for calculating the surface area in 3D is to use the spatial moments $\mu_{p,q,r}$ as defined in the next section "Geometric Moment Invariants."

$$C = \frac{3^{5/3}}{5(4\pi)^{2/3}} \times \frac{{\mu_{0,0,0}}^{5/3}}{\mu_{2,0,0} + \mu_{0,2,0} + \mu_{0,0,2}}$$

Although C represents similarity to the most symmetric shape, it does not accurately represent the irregularity of shape boundaries.

Other simple shape descriptors commonly used to define global shapes are:

2. *Eccentricity*: The ratio of the distance between the two foci to the length of the semi-major axis.
3. *Rectangularity*: The degree of similarity to a rectangle, calculated as the ratio of the object area to the area of the smallest rectangular bounding box.
4. *Principal Axis Orientation*: The orientation along which the object is most elongated.
5. *Bending Energy*: The integration of the squared curvature along the entire contour of the object shape.
6. *Convexity*: The ratio of the area enclosed inside the shape contour to the area of convex hull.

Other types of simple shape descriptors often used to characterize brain tumors are relative volumes of tissue necrosis, edema, and enhancing region [52, 53]. These are calculated as the ratio of the absolute structure volume to the total tumor volume.

Geometric Moment Invariants

Geometric moment invariants are region-based shape descriptors that are defined using nonlinear combinations of image moments and can be used to characterize the roughness or irregularity of a shape's boundary. The image moment $m_{p,q}$ of order $(p + q)$ for an image $I(x,y)$ of size $M \times N$ is defined as,

$$m_{p,q} = \sum_{x=1}^{M} \sum_{y=1}^{N} x^p y^q I(x, y) dx dy$$

The image moments can be defined both for binary and gray-scale images. For binary images, the moments strictly quantify the shape of the object, whereas in gray-scale images moments include additional information describing the intensity distributions. The following TRS invariant descriptors can be defined using these image moments [54],

$$\phi_1 = \eta_{2,0} + \eta_{0,2}$$

$$\phi_2 = \left(\eta_{2,0} - \eta_{0,2}\right)^2 + 4\eta_{1,1}^2$$
$$\phi_3 = \left(\eta_{3,0} - 3\eta_{1,2}\right)^2 + \left(3\eta_{2,1} - \eta_{0,3}\right)^2$$
$$\phi_4 = \left(\eta_{3,0} + \eta_{1,2}\right)^2 + \left(\eta_{2,1} + \eta_{0,3}\right)^2$$
$$\phi_5 = \left(\eta_{3,0} - 3\eta_{1,2}\right)\left(\eta_{1,2} + \eta_{3,0}\right)\left[\left(\eta_{1,2} + \eta_{3,0}\right)^2 - 3\left(\eta_{2,1} + \eta_{0,3}\right)^2\right]$$
$$+ 3\left(\eta_{2,1} - \eta_{0,3}\right)\left(\eta_{2,1} + \eta_{0,3}\right)\left[3\left(\eta_{1,2} + \eta_{3,0}\right)^2 - \left(\eta_{2,1} + \eta_{0,3}\right)^2\right]$$
$$\phi_6 = \left(\eta_{2,0} - \eta_{0,2}\right)\left[\left(\eta_{1,2} + \eta_{3,0}\right)^2 - \left(\eta_{2,1} + \eta_{0,3}\right)^2\right]$$
$$+4\eta_{1,1}\left(\eta_{1,2} + \eta_{3,0}\right)\left(\eta_{2,1} + \eta_{0,3}\right)$$
$$\phi_7 = \left(3\eta_{2,1} - \eta_{0,3}\right)\left(\eta_{1,2} + \eta_{3,0}\right)\left[\left(\eta_{1,2} + \eta_{3,0}\right)^2 - 3\left(\eta_{2,1} + \eta_{0,3}\right)^2\right]$$
$$+\left(3\eta_{1,2} - \eta_{3,0}\right)\left(\eta_{2,1} + \eta_{0,3}\right)\left[3\left(\eta_{1,2} + \eta_{3,0}\right)^2 - \left(\eta_{2,1} + \eta_{0,3}\right)^2\right)$$

where $\eta_{p,q} = \frac{\mu_{p,q}}{\left(\mu_{0,0}\right)^{(p+q+2)/2}}$ are the normalized central moments, and

$$\mu_{p,q} = \sum_{x=1}^{M}\sum_{y=1}^{N}(x - x_c)^p(y - y_c)^q I(x,y)dxdy$$
$$x_c = \frac{m_{1,0}}{m_{0,0}}, \quad and \quad y_c = \frac{m_{0,1}}{m_{0,0}}$$

The shape features of an object can then be defined as a vector of geometric moment invariants $\{\phi_1, \ldots, \phi_7\}$. Image moments contain important information about the spatial distribution of intensities in an image and can be used to calculate other simple shape descriptors such as eccentricity and principal axis orientations.

$$Eccentricity\ (\varepsilon) = \frac{\left(\mu_{2,0} - \mu_{0,2}\right)^2 + 4\mu_{1,1}^2}{\left(\mu_{2,0} + \mu_{0,2}\right)^2}$$

$$Principal\ axis\ orientation\ (\theta) = \frac{1}{2}tan^{-1}\frac{2\mu_{1,1}}{\mu_{2,0} - \mu_{0,2}}$$

Higher irregularity or roughness of a lesion shape corresponds to higher values of invariant descriptors. Geometric moments provide important information about the irregularity or roughness of a lesion's boundary in 2D images. However, some applications require quantifying a lesion's shape in 3D using volumetric neuro-imaging data, which is difficult using shape descriptors from multiple 2D image slices. Therefore, 3D geometric moments are defined for volumetric images as well [55–57].

$$m_{p,q,r} = \sum_{x=1}^{M}\sum_{y=1}^{N}\sum_{z=1}^{L} x^p y^q z^r \times \rho(x,y,z)$$

where $\rho(x,y,z)$ is volumetric image of size $M \times N \times L$. TRS shape descriptors using geometric moments $m_{p,q,r}$ can be defined as

$$J_1 = \eta_{2,0,0} + \eta_{0,2,0} + \eta_{0,0,2}$$

$$J_2 = \eta_{2,0,0}\eta_{0,2,0} + \eta_{2,0,0}\eta_{0,0,2} + \eta_{0,2,0}\eta_{0,0,2} - \eta_{1,1,0}^2 - \eta_{1,0,1}^2 - \eta_{0,1,1}^2$$

$$J_3 = \eta_{2,0,0}\eta_{0,2,0}\eta_{0,0,2} + 2\eta_{1,1,0}\eta_{1,0,1}\eta_{0,1,1} - \eta_{0,0,2}\eta_{1,1,0}^2 - \eta_{0,2,0}\eta_{1,0,1}^2 - \eta_{2,0,0}\eta_{0,1,1}^2$$

$$J_4 = \eta_{3,0,0} + \eta_{0,3,0} + \eta_{0,0,3} + 3\eta_{2,1,0} + 3\eta_{2,0,1} + 3\eta_{1,2,0} + 6\eta_{1,1,1} + 3\eta_{1,0,2} + 3\eta_{0,2,1} + 3\eta_{0,1,2}$$

where $\eta_{p,q,r} = \frac{\mu_{p,q,r}}{\mu_{0,0,0}^{(p+q+r+3)/3}}$ are the normalized central moments with,

$$\mu_{p,q,r} = \sum_{x=1}^{M}\sum_{y=1}^{N}\sum_{z=1}^{L} (x - x_c)^p (y - y_c)^q (z - z_c)^r \times \rho(x,y,z)$$

$$x_c = \frac{m_{1,0,0}}{m_{0,0,0}}, y_c = \frac{m_{0,1,0}}{m_{0,0,0}}, \quad and, \quad z_c = \frac{m_{0,0,1}}{m_{0,0,0}}$$

Similar to the 2D case, shape features for a lesion's shape in 3D can be defined as vector of moment invariants, $\{J_1, J_2, J_3, J_4\}$.

Shape Signatures and Boundary Moments

Shape signatures represent the shape of an object by a one-dimensional function derived from the boundary points. A common signature is based on the measurement of Euclidean radial distance $d(n)$ of each pixel $(x(n), y(n))$ on the boundary from the centroid of the shape (x_c, y_c) (Fig. 11.9). Other shape signatures that are common in practice include complex coordinates, tangent angle, curvature, chain codes, and chord-length.

The shape signatures are typically normalized with respect to their magnitude to make them scale and translation invariant. The boundary statistical moments can then be used to reduce the dimensions of the boundary representation.

$$m_r = \frac{1}{N}\sum_{n=1}^{N} [z(n)]^r, \quad and, \quad \mu_r = \frac{1}{N}\sum_{n=1}^{N} [z(n) - m_1]^r$$

where μ_r is the central moment of order r, N is the number of boundary points, and $z(n)$ represents the normalized shape signature. Contour-based TRS invariant descriptors can be obtained for shape representations,

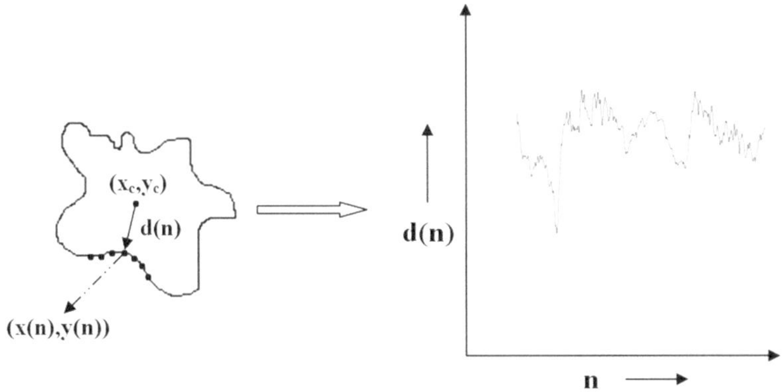

Fig. 11.9 Schematic diagram illustrating the object contour by a one-dimensional function

$$\overline{m_r} = \frac{m_r}{(\mu_2)^{r/2}}, \quad and, \quad \overline{\mu_r} = \frac{\mu_r}{(\mu_2)^{r/2}}$$

Moments of order higher than 4 are highly sensitive to noise and therefore the use of $\overline{m_1}, \overline{\mu_3}$ and $\overline{\mu_4}$ has been recommended for low noise-sensitive shape descriptors. Another shape descriptor that has been reported to have good invariance properties and accurately capture shape complexity is [58],

$$F_1 = \frac{\mu_4^{1/4}}{m_1} - \frac{\mu_2^{1/2}}{m_1}$$

Boundary moments increase with increasing roughness or irregularity of the shape boundary.

Fourier Descriptors

Fourier descriptors are another type of contour-based method for describing the shapes of objects. Every pixel on the object boundary is represented as a complex number $P(n)$, with the real part as the x-coordinate and the imaginary part as the y-coordinate.

$$P(n) = x(n) + iy(n), n = 1, .., N$$

where N is the number of pixels on the object boundary. The object boundary can therefore be represented as a one-dimensional sequence of complex numbers by selecting some pixel as the starting point. The essential shape information of the object boundary is contained in the lower order coefficients of DFT of this sequence,

$$F(t) = \frac{1}{N}\sum_{n=1}^{N} P(n)\exp(-i2\pi nt/N)$$

However, the coefficients of $F(t)$ depend on the pixel selection for the starting point on the object boundary to create the complex number sequence. The starting point, translation, scale, and rotation invariant descriptors are obtained as,

$$F_{inv}(t) = \frac{F(1+t)F(1-t)}{F^2(1)}$$

The lower order coefficients can be used as shape descriptors for the object. Another descriptor that has been reported to have low noise sensitivity and invariance to translation, rotation, scale, and starting point is [59],

$$FF = 1 - \frac{\sum_{t=-\frac{N}{2}+1}^{N/2} \|F(t)\|/\|t\|}{\sum_{t=-\frac{N}{2}+1}^{N/2} \|F(t)\|}$$

The value of FF is limited to (0, 1) and increases with the complexity of the object's shape and the roughness or irregularity of the boundary.

Angular Radial Transform

Angular radial transform (ART) decomposes an image into a set of orthogonal complex basis functions. The ART coefficients of order p and q, $F_{p,q}$ of an image $I(\rho,\theta)$ are defined as,

$$F_{p,q} = \int_0^{2\pi}\int_0^1 B^*_{p,q}(\rho,\theta) \times I(\rho,\theta)\rho d\rho d\theta$$

where $B_{p,q}(\rho,\theta)$ represents the ART basis functions, which are separable along the angular and radial directions as,

$$B_{p,q}(\rho,\theta) = R_p(\rho) \times A_q(\theta)$$

For rotationally invariant features, a complex exponential function can be used as an angular basis function, and a cosine function as the radial basis function.

$$\mathrm{R}_p(\rho) = \begin{cases} 1 & p = 0 \\ 2\cos(\pi p\rho) & p \neq 0 \end{cases}, \qquad \textit{and}, \qquad A_q(\theta) = \frac{1}{2\pi}\exp(iq\theta)$$

A vector of ART coefficients $F_{p,q}$ normalized with $F_{0,0}$ can then be used as shape feature for the object.

$$I_{6\times 6} = \begin{bmatrix} 2 & 2 & 3 & 2 & 2 & 1 \\ 3 & 0 & 1 & 0 & 0 & 0 \\ 1 & 3 & 2 & 1 & 1 & 2 \\ 1 & 2 & 0 & 3 & 0 & 0 \\ 0 & 1 & 0 & 0 & 3 & 2 \\ 3 & 3 & 3 & 2 & 0 & 3 \end{bmatrix} \longrightarrow H_{\sqrt{2},45^\circ} = \begin{array}{c|cccc} - & 0 & 1 & 2 & 3 \\ \hline 0 & 1 & 2 & 4 & 2 \\ 1 & 4 & 0 & 1 & 1 \\ 2 & 1 & 0 & 1 & 1 \\ 3 & 3 & 3 & 1 & 0 \end{array}$$

Fig. 11.10 Example showing calculation of $H_{\sqrt{2},45^\circ}$ from a 6 × 6 image

Textural Features

Examining the appearance of brain tissues, lesions, and surrounding structures is often an important part of medical image interpretation. The appearance is visually understood through local intensity variations and can therefore be quantified using texture metrics.

Spatial Co-occurrence Matrix Features

Co-occurrence matrices enable calculation of textural features based on the relative spatial co-occurrence information of image pixels. A co-occurrence matrix $H_{d,\theta}$ (i, j), $i, j = \{1,\ldots,K\}$ is generated by tabulating the pairwise spatial co-occurrence of image pixels separated by a particular orientation θ and separation distance d over the K gray levels in the image $I(x, y)$under consideration.

Therefore, a co-occurrence matrix is a $K \times K$ matrix in which each element $H_{d,\theta}$ (i,j) represents the number of times that pixels with intensity i and j are located in the image at a relative position defined by d,θ (Fig. 11.10). A common choice for relative position is $d = 1$, and θ =0, 45, 90, and 135°, respectively. The co-occurrence matrix $H_{d,\theta}$ is often normalized with $\Sigma_{i,j} H_{d,\theta}(i,j)$ to obtain measures of the probability of having pixel pairs at that relative position,

$$C_{d,\theta}(i,j) = \frac{H_{d,\theta}(i,j)}{\sum_{i,j} H_{d,\theta}(i,j)}$$

The probability co-occurrence matrix $C_{d,\theta}(i,j)$ can then be used to derive several textural measures:

- *Energy*: The energy, or angular second moment, quantifies the extent of heterogeneity inside the region and decreases with higher heterogeneity of the region.

$$Energy = \sum_{i=1}^{K} \sum_{j=1}^{K} [C_{d,\theta}(i,j)]^2$$

- *Inertia*: The inertia is a texture measure that weights each element $C_{d,\theta}(i,j)$ with gray level difference $(i - j)$and quantifies texture contrast. Inertia increases with higher heterogeneity of the region and accounts for the contrast between pixel pairs.

$$Inertia = \sum_{i=1}^{K} \sum_{j=1}^{K} (i - j)^2 C_{d,\theta}(i,j)$$

- *Inverse Different Moment* (*IDM*): IDM is a texture measure that can distinguish between near-constant intensity patches from regions with high contrasts in intensity.

$$IDM = \sum_{i=1}^{K} \sum_{j=1}^{K} \frac{C_{d,\theta}(i,j)}{1 + (i - j)^2}$$

- *Entropy*: The entropy quantifies the level of randomness in a region and can be used to distinguish a structurally textured region from region with less organization.

$$Entropy = -\sum_{i=1}^{K} \sum_{j=1}^{K} C_{d,\theta}(i,j) \times log(C_{d,\theta}(i,j))$$

- *Correlation*: The correlation of intensities in an image region can be computed using marginal distributions derived from the co-occurrence matrices.

$$Correlation = \frac{\sum_{i=1}^{K} \sum_{j=1}^{K} (ij) C_{d,\theta}(i,j) - \mu_{i'} \mu_{j'}}{\sigma_{i'} \sigma_{j'}}$$

$$\mu_{i'} = \sum_{i=1}^{K} \sum_{j=1}^{K} i C_{d,\theta}(i,j), \quad and, \quad \mu_{j'} = \sum_{i=1}^{K} \sum_{j=1}^{K} j C_{d,\theta}(i,j)$$

$$\sigma_{i'}^2 = \sum_{i=1}^{K} \sum_{j=1}^{K} (i - \mu_{i'})^2 C_{d,\theta}(i,j), \quad and, \quad \sigma_{j'}^2 = \sum_{i=1}^{K} \sum_{j=1}^{K} \left(j - \mu_{j'}\right)^2 C_{d,\theta}(i,j)$$

A vector of texture features obtained at different relative positions can be used as a descriptor of texture for the entire image.

Fractal Dimension

Objects in Euclidean geometry are defined in integer dimensions that may not adequately describe the morphology of complex objects. Fractal dimensions can be used to characterize more complex characteristics of objects. In this approach, objects are described in non-integer dimensions,

$$N = ar^{-D}$$

where N is the number of self-similar pieces, r represents the dimension of piece (diameter for spheres and side for cubes), a is a scaling factor, and D is the fractal dimension of the object. The fractal dimensions characterize complex objects with a fractional dimensionality higher than its Euclidean dimensionality.

If an image is considered as a surface with intensity value representing the height of the surface, the area of the surface can be represented as,

$$Area(r) = N \times r^2 = ar^{2-D},$$
$$or, \quad \log\big(Area(r)\big) = \big(2 - D\big)log\big(r\big) + log\big(a\big)$$

Box counting [60] can be used to estimate values of Area(r) at different values of r, followed by estimation of fractal dimensions D using linear regression. Another method of estimating Area(r) is triangular–prism–surface area (TPSA) proposed by Clarke [61]. TPSA averages gray-scale values at four corners of a box to find the center elevation value, dividing the box into four triangles that can be used to find surface area. This procedure is repeated for different box sizes followed by linear regression to estimate fractal dimension.

Fractional-Brownian motion model is another such method proposed by Mandelbrot and Ness [62] that regards rough image surface as the result of random walks such that,

$$E[\Delta I_d] = bd^{3-D}$$

where $E(.)$ is the expectation operator, b is a proportionality constant, d is the Euclidean distance between two pixels (x_1,y_1) and (x_2,y_2), and ΔI is the absolute difference between the intensity values $I(x_1,y_1)$ and $I(x_2,y_2)$. The value of fractal dimension D can be estimated using linear regression,

$$\log(E[\Delta I_d]) = \log(b) + (3 - D)\log(d)$$

Higher values for fractal dimension D are obtained for rougher textures in an image. Fractal dimensions have been used to characterize the vital parts of tumors by considering difference between fractal dimensions of inner and outer contours [63].

Intensity Histogram Features

Intensity features derived from brain tumors and surrounding structures are often correlated with physiological processes in the brain. Analysis of intensity features becomes even more important in contrast-enhanced imaging studies as the dynamics of intensity changes provide important information regarding physiology at the site of brain tumor. Intensity features have been widely used for classification of brain tumors [52, 53].

A common preprocessing step that prepares intensity data from the image to calculate intensity features is construction of the intensity histogram. Several intensity features can be calculated using statistical moments of the image histogram. The statistical moment of order n for an image $I(x,y)$ is defined as,

$$m_n = \frac{1}{K}\sum_{t=1}^{K} t^n h(t)$$

where $h(t)$, $t = 1, \ldots, K$ is the histogram of image $I(x,y)$ with K gray levels. First order statistical moment m_1 is the mean μ of image intensities. We can also define central statistical moments that provide important information about intensity variations inside image regions,

$$M_n = \frac{1}{K}\sum_{t=1}^{K} (t-\mu)^n h(t)$$

The second moment M_2 describes the variance of intensities inside the image region. The third and fourth central moments M_2 and M_3, skewness and kurtosis, represent asymmetry and uniformity of the histogram.

Statistical Modeling and Selection of Image Features

Morphological features extracted from MR images along with relevant clinical covariates are combined as independent variables $X = \{x_1,x_2, \ldots,x_n\}$ in a statistical model to obtain a prediction Y,

$$Y = f(X) + \varepsilon, \qquad \varepsilon \tilde{} N\left(0, \sigma^2 V\right)$$

where $f(.)$ is a function combining the independent variables $X = \{x_1, \ldots,x_n\}$, ε is noise in the observed data Y with zero offset, and $\sigma^2 V$ as the covariance. The objective of model training is to determine the appropriate form of $f(.)$ by fitting available data such that it generalizes well to future data. Once we obtain the model $f(.)$, further analysis such as the significance of each independent variable in the prediction variable Y can be evaluated. While the relationship between Y and some of the independent variables may be known *a priori*, it is often unknown for most of the independent variables under consideration. Previous studies have employed a variety of models ranging from simple linear models to complicated models such as artificial neural networks (ANNs) and support vector machines (SVMs) to combine morphological features and other relevant covariates for prediction and classification tasks. Although complex models may show a good fit on the training data, they may not be generalizable to the unseen test data. Such cases of data over-fitting are often observed in the literature and, therefore bring into attention the significance of appropriate model selection. Typically, model selection is performed using cross-validation experiments by dividing the available data into training and validation sets. However, the sample size available for imaging studies is often small and therefore limits the use of such cross-validation methods for model selection. The use of analytical model selection methods such as Akaike information criterion (AIC), Schwarz Bayesian information criterion (BIC), and minimum description length (MDL) that regularize data fitting with penalty terms is beneficial in such scenarios. While the type of model being fit is dependent on the task at hand, the significance of model complexity selection is highly important for performing any further analysis on correlation and significance of independent variables under consideration.

The selection of an appropriate statistical model also plays an important role in the performance of a medical imaging task. A wide variety of statistical models have been considered in literature, with varying complexities. Each model has its strengths and weaknesses and therefore there is no single statistical model that works best for all supervised learning problems ("no free lunch theorem" [64]). The choice of appropriate statistical model is mainly dependent on the specific task at hand (classification or prediction) and nature of data (such as type of independent variables, data heterogeneity, redundancy, outliers, and co-linearity). The characteristics of independent variables play an important role in the selection of the statistical model. The independent variables are typically either categorical (nominal or ordinal) or continuous in nature. While some statistical models perform well for continuous data (such as SVM, linear regression, logistic regression, and ANN), other models (such as decision trees) handle categorical data better. Typically, DSS for medical imaging tasks include a mixture of continuous (morphological image features) and categorical (such as clinical variables and survey) independent variables. This makes heterogeneity in the type of independent variables an important consideration for selection of the statistical model. Statistical models that employ distance cost functions (such as SVM, ANN, linear regression, and logistic regression) are particularly sensitive to heterogeneity in data and may require the independent variables to be numerically scaled. Prior information regarding redundancy in data, presence of outliers, and co-linearity between independent variables are also important factors that affect the selection of statistical model. In fields where extensive amounts of data are available, the selection of appropriate model type can be performed using cross-validation experiments. However, the evaluation of DSS often suffers from limited sample sizes that makes careful selection of appropriate model even more important for medical imaging tasks.

Feature selection is an important part of any DSS that helps reduce the effects of curse of dimensionality and co-linearity between the independent variables. Although essential for DSS, important considerations should be given to the associated physical significance of transformed model features obtained after feature selection. Dimensionality reduction techniques such as principal component analysis (PCA) or equivalently singular value decomposition (SVD) result in transformed model features that are linear combinations of original independent variables. Although the reduced feature space captures the most variation in data, the transformed variables may not be of any physical significance. This makes physicians hesitant towards using such tools and therefore user-understandability of the statistical model should be kept in mind while designing of DSS.

Conclusion

Current methods for interpretation of brain MR images are qualitative in nature and therefore suffer from several limitations. The use of DSSs enables quantification of anatomical changes observed on radiologic images and therefore can help physicians better manage brain tumor patients. In this chapter, we have discussed state-of-the-art image analysis methods and statistical modeling methods necessary to develop individual components that are generally part of any DSS. The use of image analysis methods has also been investigated in the management of other neurodegenerative and psychiatric disorders such as schizophrenia and epilepsy. Although in this chapter we deal specifically with brain tumors, the translation of methods used for other brain diseases may benefit the advancement of quantitative image analysis of brain tumors.

References

1. Berner ES (2009) Clinical decision support systems: state of the art. Agency for Healthcare Research and Quality (AHRQ), Rockville (publication no. 09-0069-EF)
2. Noble M, Bruening W, Uhl S, Schoelles K (2009) Computer-aided detection mammography for breast cancer screening: systematic review and meta-analysis. Arch Gynecol Obstet 279 (6):881–890
3. Chan H-P, Hadjiiski L, Zhou C, Sahiner B (2008) Computer-aided diagnosis of lung cancer and pulmonary embolism in computed tomography—a review. Acad Radiol 15(5):535–555
4. Weisenfeld NL, Warfteld SK (2004) Normalization of joint image-intensity statistics in MRI using the Kullback–Leibler divergence. Paper presented at IEEE international symposium on biomedical imaging: nano to macro, 15–18 April 2004, pp 101–104
5. Hellier P (2003) Consistent intensity correction of MR images. In: Proceedings of the international conference on image processing (ICIP), vol 1, Rennes, 14–17 September 2003, pp 1–1109
6. Jager F, Deuerling-Zheng Y, Frericks B, Wacker F, Hornegger J (2006) A new method for MRI intensity standardization with application to lesion detection in the brain. In: Kobbelt L et al (eds) Vision modeling and visualization 2006 proceedings. IOS Press, pp 269–276
7. Bergeest J-P, Jäger F, Tolxdorff T et al (2008) A comparison of five methods for signal intensity standardization in MRI, bildverarbeitung für die medizin 2008. Springer, Berlin, pp 36–40
8. Nyul LG, Udupa JK, Xuan Z (2000) New variants of a method of MRI scale standardization. IEEE Trans Med Imaging 19(2):143–150

9. Nyúl LG, Udupa JK (1999) On standardizing the MR image intensity scale. Magn Reson Med 42(6):1072–1081
10. Gasser T, Sroka L, Jennen-Steinmetz C (1986) Residual variance and residual pattern in nonlinear regression. Biometrika 73(3):625–633
11. Ashburner J, Friston KJ (2005) Unified segmentation. Neuroimage 26:839–885
12. Ashburner J (2007) A fast diffeomorphic image registration algorithm. Neuroimage 38:95–113
13. Klein A, Andersson J, Ardekani BA et al (2009) Evaluation of 14 nonlinear deformation algorithms applied to human brain MRI registration. Neuroimage 46(3):786–802
14. Ripollés P, Marco-Pallarés J, de Diego-Balaguer R et al (2012) Analysis of automated methods for spatial normalization of lesioned brains. Neuroimage 60(2):1296–1306
15. Ardekani BA, Guckemus S, Bachman A, Hoptman MJ, Wojtaszek M, Nierenberg J (2005) Quantitative comparison of algorithms for inter-subject registration of 3D volumetric brain MRI scans. J Neurosci Methods 142(1):67–76
16. Madabhushi A, Udupa JK (2005) Interplay between intensity standardization and inhomogeneity correction in MR image processing. IEEE Trans Med Imaging 24(5):561–576
17. Perona P, Malik J (1990) Scale-space and edge detection using anisotropic diffusion. IEEE Trans Pattern Anal Mach Intell 12(7):629–639
18. Buades A, Coll B, Morel JM (2005) A non-local algorithm for image denoising. In: IEEE Computer Society conference on computer vision and pattern recognition (CVPR), vol 2, 20–25 June 2005, pp 60–65
19. Wiest-Daessle N, Prima S, Coup P, Morrissey SP, Barillot C (2008) Rician noise removal by non-local means filtering for low signal-to-noise ratio MRI: applications to DT-MRI. In: Proceedings of the 11th international conference on medical image computing and computer-assisted intervention, part II, Springer, New York, pp 171–179
20. Manjón JV, Carbonell-Caballero J, Lull JJ, García-Martí G, Martí-Bonmatí L, Robles M (2008) MRI denoising using non-local means. Med Image Anal 12(4):514–523
21. Gal Y, Mehnert AJH, Bradley AP, McMahon K, Kennedy D, Crozier S (2010) Denoising of dynamic contrast-enhanced MR images using dynamic nonlocal means. IEEE Trans Med Imaging 29(2):302–310
22. Anand CS, Sahambi J (2010) Wavelet domain non-linear filtering for MRI denoising. Magn Reson Imaging 28:842–861
23. Simmons A TP, Barker GJ, Arridge SR (1994) Sources of intensity nonuniformity in spin echo images at 1.5 T. Magn Reson Med 32(1):121–128 (Wiley Subscription Services, Inc.)
24. Johnston B, Atkins MS, Mackiewich B, Anderson M (1996) Segmentation of multiple sclerosis lesions in intensity corrected multispectral MRI. IEEE Trans Med Imaging 15(2):154–169
25. Axel L, Costantini J, Listerud J (1987) Intensity correction in surface coil MR imaging. Amer J Roentgenol 148:418–420
26. Sled JG, Zijdenbos AP, Evans AC (1998) A nonparametric method for automatic correction of intensity nonuniformity in MRI data. IEEE Trans Med Imaging 17(1):87–97
27. Likar B, Viergever MA, Pernuˇs F (2001) Retrospective correction of MR intensity inhomogeneity by information minimization. IEEE Trans Med Imaging 20(12):1398–1410
28. Mangin J-F (2000) Entropy minimization for automatic correction of intensity nonuniformity. Presented at the IEEE workshop on mathematical methods in biomedical image analysis, Hilton Head Island, pp 162–169
29. Bansal R, Staib LH, Peterson BS (2004) Correcting nonuniformities in MRI intensities using entropy minimization based on an elastic model. In: Medical image computing and computer-assisted intervention (MICCAI 2004). Springer, Berlin, pp 78–86
30. Likar B, Viergever M A, Pernus F (2000) Retrospective correction of MR intensity inhomogeneity by information minimization. In: Medical image computing and computer-assisted intervention (MICCAI 2000). Springer, Berlin, pp 375–384
31. Dawant BM, Zijdenbos AP, Margolin RA (1993) Correction of intensity variations in MR images for computer-aided tissues classification. IEEE Trans Med Imaging 12(4):770–781

32. Van Leemput K, Maes F, Vandermeulen D, Suetens P (1999) Automated model-based tissue classification of MR images of the brain. IEEE Trans Med Imaging 18(10):897–908
33. Marroquin J, Vemuri B, Botello S, Calderon E, Fernandez-Bouzas A (2002) An accurate and efficient Bayesian method for automatic segmentation of brain MRI. IEEE Trans Med Imaging 21(8):934–945
34. Bach Cuadra M, Cammoun L, Butz T, Cuisenaire O, Thiran J (2005) Comparison and validation of tissue modelization and statistical classification methods in T1-weighted MR brain images. IEEE Trans Med Imaging 24(12):1548–1565
35. Ferreira da Silva AR (2007) A dirichlet process mixture model for brain MRI tissue classification. Med Image Anal 11(2):169–182
36. Greenspan H, Ruf A, Goldberger J (2006) Constrained Gaussian mixture model framework for automatic segmentation of MR brain images. IEEE Trans Med Imaging 25(9):1233–1245
37. Likar B, Derganc J, Pernuˇs F (2002) Segmentation-based retrospective correction of intensity non-uniformity in multi-spectral MR images. In: Proceedings of SPIE medical imaging, image process, San Diego, vol 4684, pp 1531–1540
38. Derganc J, Likar B, Pernuˇs F (2002) Nonparametric segmentation of multispectral MR images incorporating spatial and intensity information. In: Proceedings of SPIE medical imaging, image process, San Diego, vol 4684, pp 391–400
39. Hall LO, Bensaid AM, Clarke LP, Velthuizen RP, Silbiger MS, Bezdek J (1992) A comparison of neural network and fuzzy clustering techniques in segmenting magnetic resonance images of the brain. IEEE Trans Neural Netw 3:672–682
40. Zhang DQ, Chen SC (2004) A novel kernelized fuzzy C-means algorithm with application in medical image segmentation. Artif Intell Med 32(1):37–50
41. Acton ST, Mukherjee DP (2000) Scale space classification using area morphology. IEEE Trans Image Process 9(4):623–635
42. Siyal M, Yu L (2005) An intelligent modified fuzzy C-means based algorithm for bias estimation and segmentation of brain MRI. Pattern Recogn Lett 26(13):2052–2062
43. Horváth J (2006) Image segmentation using fuzzy c-means. In: Proceedings of SAMI, pp 144–151
44. Diplaros A, Vlassis N, Gevers T (2007) A spatially constrained generative model and an EM algorithm for image segmentation. IEEE Trans Neural Netw 18(3):798–808
45. Wang J (2007) Discriminative Gaussian mixtures for interactive image segmentation. In: IEEE international conference on acoustics, speech and signal processing, vol 1, pp 1–601
46. Sethian JA (1996) A fast marching level set method for monotonically advancing fronts. Proc Natl Acad Sci 93(4):1591–1595
47. Li SZ (1994) Markov random field models in computer vision. Lect Notes Comput Sci 801:361–370
48. Zhang Y, Brady M, Smith S (2001) Segmentation of brain MR images through a hidden Markov random field model and the expectation maximization algorithm. IEEE Trans Med Imaging 20(1):45–57
49. Chan TF, Vese LA (2001) Active contours without edges. IEEE Trans Image Process 10 (2):266–277
50. Osher S, Sethian JA (1988) Fronts propagating with curvature dependent speed: algorithms based on Hamilton–Jacobi formulations. J Comput Phys 79(1):12–49
51. Verma N, Muralidhar GS, Bovik AC, Cowperthwaite MC, Markey MK (2011), Model-driven, probabilistic level set based segmentation of magnetic resonance images of the brain. In: Annual international conference of the IEEE Engineering in Medicine and Biology Society (EMBC), pp 2821–2824
52. Zacharaki E, Kanas V, Davatzikos C (2011) Investigating machine learning techniques for MRI-based classification of brain neoplasms. Int J Comput Assist Radiol Surg 6(6):821–828
53. Zacharaki EI, Wang S, Chawla S et al (2009) Classification of brain tumor type and grade using MRI texture and shape in a machine learning scheme. Magn Reson Med 62 (6):1609–1618

54. Ming-Kuei H (1962) Visual pattern recognition by moment invariants. IEEE Trans Inf Theory 8(2):179–187
55. Sadjadi FA, Hall EL (1980) Three-dimensional moment invariants. IEEE Trans on Pattern Anal Mach Intell 2(2):127–136
56. Ng B, Abugharbieh R, Huang X, McKeown MJ (2006) Characterizing fMRI activations within regions of interest (ROIs) using 3D moment invariants. In: Conference on computer vision and pattern recognition workshop (CVPRW'06), June 2006, pp 63–63
57. Reiss TH (1992) Features invariant to linear transformations in 2D and 3D. In: Proceedings of 11th international conference on pattern recognition (ICPR'92), IEEE Computer Society Press, Hague, vol III, pp 493–496
58. Shen L, Rangayyan RM, Desautels JEL (1994) Application of shape analysis to mammographic calcifications. IEEE Trans Med Imaging 13(2):263–274
59. Rangayyan RM, El-Faramawy NM, Desautels JEL, Alim OA (1997) Measures of acutance and shape for classification of breast tumors. IEEE Trans Med Imaging 16(6):799–810
60. Barnsley M (1988) Fractals everywhere: the first course in deterministic fractal geometry. Academic
61. Clarke KC (1986) Computation of the fractal dimension of topographic surfaces using the triangular prism surface area method. Computers &Amp; Geosciences 12(5):713–722
62. Mandelbrot BB, Ness JWV (1968) Fractional brownian motions, fractional noises and applications. SIAM Rev 10(4):422–437
63. Rossmanith C, Handels H, Pöppl SJ, Rinast E, Weiss HD (1996) Characterisation and classification of brain tumours in three-dimensional MR image sequences. In: Visualization in biomedical computing. Springer, Berlin, pp 429–438
64. Duda RO, Hart PE, Stork DG (2001) Pattern classification. Wiley, New York (Section, 10, 1)

Chapter 12
Respiratory and Cardiac Function Analysis on the Basis of Dynamic Chest Radiography

Rie Tanaka and Shigeru Sanada

Abstract Dynamic chest radiography with computer analysis is expected to be a new type of functional imaging system. This chapter presents computerized methods for quantifying and visualizing cardiopulmonary function on dynamic chest radiographs. The measurement parameters are diaphragm motion, heart wall motion, pulmonary ventilation, and blood circulation. We will first introduce evaluation items, physiology, and diagnostic findings and then describe image analysis methods for each evaluation item. We pay particular attention to interframe subtraction and mapping technique, which play a critical role in the evaluation of pulmonary ventilation and blood circulation. We also discuss features, future perspectives, and issues related to dynamic chest radiography on the basis of preliminary clinical study.

Background

Functional information is of assistance in the diagnosis of diseases and determination of treatment strategy, along with anatomical information. In the diagnosis of pulmonary diseases, the pulmonary functional test (PFT) with a spirometer evaluates total function in both lungs, such as vital capacity, functional residual capacity, and diffusion capacity. To evaluate local cardiopulmonary function, we have a choice of functional imaging methods, e.g., nuclear scanning [1, 2], dynamic computed tomography (CT) [3, 4], and dynamic magnetic resonance imaging (MRI) [5–8]. Recent advancements in technology facilitated pulmonary functional imaging without the use of contrast agents. Dynamic CT allows cross-sectional

R. Tanaka (✉) • S. Sanada
Department of Radiological Technology, School of Health Sciences, College of Medical, Pharmaceutical and Health Sciences, Kanazawa University, 5-11-80 Kodatsuno, Kanazawa 920-0942, Japan
e-mail: rie44@mhs.mp.kanazawa-u.ac.jp

K. Suzuki (ed.), *Computational Intelligence in Biomedical Imaging*, 317
DOI 10.1007/978-1-4614-7245-2_12,

analysis of pulmonary ventilation based on respiratory-induced changes in CT values. On the other hand, dynamic MRI provides observations of diaphragmatic and lung motion in all sections. Although these examinations provide a definitive diagnosis based on anatomical and functional findings, they have certain disadvantages; in the CT approach, the patients are exposed to a large dose of radiation, while the MRI and nuclear scanning approaches are costly and time-consuming. If cardiopulmonary functional information becomes more readily available, it will be very helpful for determining an appropriate examination procedure and for patient follow-up.

Therefore, we focused on cardiopulmonary functional evaluation with dynamic chest radiography. There have been many reports demonstrating the feasibility of pulmonary densitometry [9–13]. These methods have not been adopted in clinical use because of technical limitations, such as poor image quality and small field of view (FOV) [14]. Dynamic flat-panel detectors (FPDs) allow acquisition of sequential chest radiographs with a large FOV and high image quality. Whereas image-intensifier (I.I.) systems are now being replaced with FPD systems, they are also expected to be useful as a new type of functional imaging system. Dynamic chest radiography using a dynamic FPD combined with computer analysis may overcome the difficulties encountered in the above-mentioned studies and provide quantitative functional information. In the following, we will introduce dynamic chest radiography using an FPD system and describe computerized methods for the evaluation of cardiopulmonary function along with the results of the preliminary clinical study.

Evaluation Items, Physiology, and Diagnostic Finding

Diaphragm Shape, Position, and Motion

Pulmonary function is estimated on the basis of the shape and position of the diaphragm on conventional chest radiographs [15, 16]. For example, in a patient with chronic obstructive pulmonary disease (COPD), the diaphragm position is lower and flatter than that in normal subjects because of pulmonary hyperinflation. Impaired function is also observed as limited diaphragm motion. In general, additional imaging at the expiration level is performed to assess diaphragm motion, in addition to conventional imaging at the inspiratory level. Dynamic chest radiography provides information regarding the motion process so that radiologists and surgeons can develop a more appropriate treatment strategy. Furthermore, large FOV of FPD permits simultaneous right-and-left evaluation of the diaphragm. Information regarding diaphragm motion is useful for the diagnosis of pulmonary impairments such as phrenic nerve stroke, foreign bodies in the bronchus, and COPD as well as patient selection for lung reduction surgery [17].

Cardiac Function

The cardiothoracic ratio (CTR) is the ratio of the transverse diameter of the heart to the internal diameter of the chest at its widest point just above the dome of the diaphragm as measured on a posteroanterior (PA) chest radiograph. The heart size is considered too large when the CTR is >50 % on a PA chest radiograph and an increased cardiac silhouette is almost always the result of cardiomegaly [18]. Heart wall motion is observed on dynamic chest radiographs. Amplitude and cycle length are directly measured so that cardiac function can be evaluated more precisely.

Pulmonary Ventilation

The pulmonary condition is evaluated on the basis of X-ray translucency in the lung area. An increase in X-ray translucency indicates localized air space that may represent anomalies like lung cyst, emphysema, and pneumothorax. In contrast, a decrease in X-ray translucency indicates decreased pulmonary air or enhanced tissues, suggestive of conditions like pulmonary inflammation, fibrosis, edema, or sclerosis [16]. Temporal changes in X-ray translucency during respiration depend on relative increases and decreases in air and lung vessel volume per unit volume, as shown in Fig. 12.1a [19, 20]. Figure 12.2 depicts measured pixel value and electrocardiogram (ECG) findings in a normal control. The pixel value decreases (X-ray translucency↑) according to increase in air volume in the lung during inspiratory phase; in contrast, the pixel value increases (X-ray translucency↓) according to decrease in air volume in the lung during expiratory phase. The slight change in synchrony with ECG findings is the results of changes caused by cardiac pumping and pulmonary blood circulation. The impact of cardiac motion is identified to be less than 10 % against the respiratory changes in pixel value [21]. It is possible to evaluate relative ventilation quantitatively from respiratory changes in X-ray translucency on dynamic chest radiographs. For example, COPD patients take time to expire, and also ventilate insufficiently due to trapped air. Therefore, it is possible to detect abnormalities such as delayed and decreased changes in pixel values. However, the present method does not directly measure the gas exchanges in lung alveoli; rather, it provides relative functional information related to pulmonary ventilation.

It is also well known that there are regional differences in ventilation in respiratory physiology [19]. Ventilation per unit volume is greatest near the bottom of the lung and becomes progressively smaller toward the top with symmetrical right-and-left distribution. Therefore, ventilatory impairment can be detected based on deviation from the normal pattern of ventilation distribution. In the case of dynamic chest radiography, ventilatory impairment could be detected by comparing respiratory-induced changes in pixel value in symmetrical positions in both lungs [22].

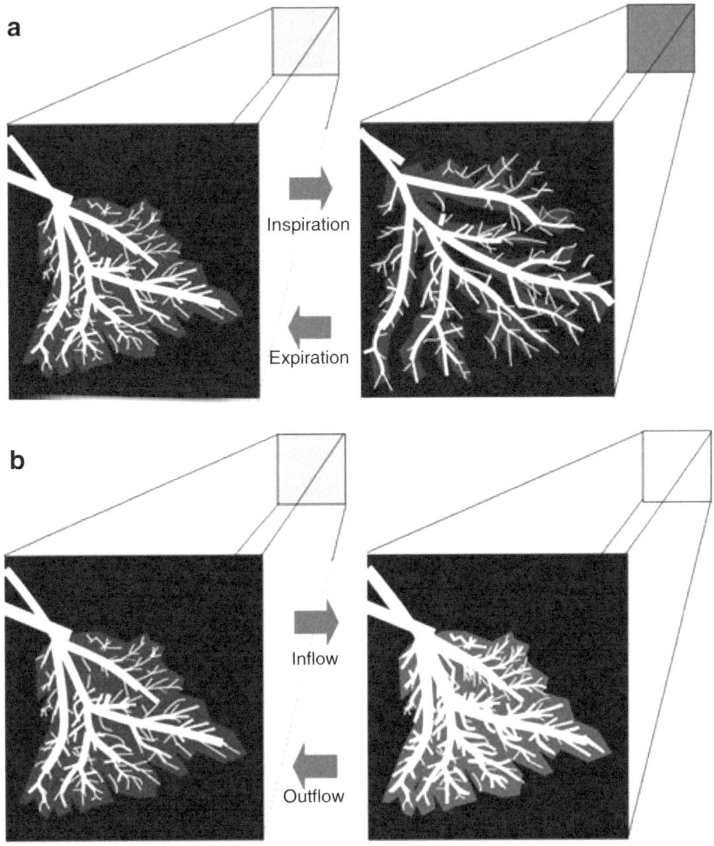

Fig. 12.1 Relationship between X-ray translucency and (**a**) air and lung vessel volume and (**b**) pulmonary blood volume per unit volume

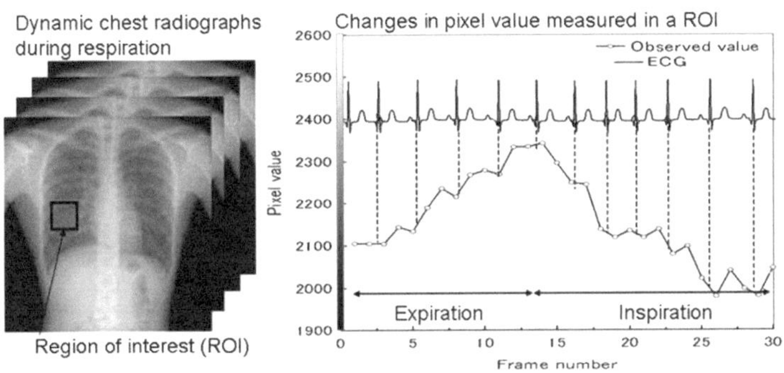

Fig. 12.2 Measured pixel value and electrocardiogram in a normal control

Other measurements showed that, at the end of expiration, the lower airway closes earlier than the upper airway due to the differences in air pressure of the thoracic cavity, i.e., airway closure, and the ventilation in the upper area becomes greater than that in the lower area. The lung volume when airway closure occurs is defined as the "closing volume," which is a very effective index for diagnosing pulmonary diseases. For example, in subjects with COPD and restrictive pulmonary disease, airway closure appears in early expiratory phase, and as a result closing volume becomes large. Therefore, abnormalities can be detected by evaluating the timing of "airway closure" [23].

Pulmonary Blood Circulation

Circulation dynamics is reflected on chest radiographs and abnormalities appear as shape changes or shifts in the distribution of pulmonary vessels [20, 24, 25]. These are effective indices for diagnosing specific cardiac diseases and determining an appropriate examination procedure: redistribution or cephalization of pulmonary blood flow indicating the presence of pulmonary venous hypertension [26]; a centralized pulmonary blood flow pattern, indicating pulmonary arterial hypertension [27]; or widening of the vascular pedicle indicating an increase in circulating blood volume [28]. Circulation dynamics is also reflected on fluoroscopic images as changes in X-ray translucency [10, 11, 29] (Fig. 12.1b), which provide functional information. This is because the lungs contain a constant volume of about 500 mL of blood, with 75 mL distributed variably across the vasculature due to cardiac pumping [18].

Figure 12.3 shows changes in pixel value measured in a normal subject, in ROIs as shown in Fig. 12.4. There is a strong correlation between the cardiac cycle and changes in pixel value, which are measured in the ventricles, atria, aortic arch, and pulmonary arteries. The changes in pixel values measured in each ROI can be explained by normal circulation dynamics as indicated below: (1) at the end of the diastole phase, the ventricles are at the maximum volume, as shown by large pixel values in the ventricles. (2) In the early ventricular systole phase, from closure of the atrioventricular (AV) valves to opening of the aortic valve, the ventricular volume remained constant, shown as the absence of a significant change in pixel values during this period. (3) After opening of the aortic arch, blood is pumped from the ventricles into the aortic arch and pulmonary arteries. This was shown as a decrease in pixel values in the ventricles and an increase in pixel values in the aortic arch and pulmonary arteries. (4) In the late ventricular systole phase, ventricular volume and aortic blood flow decrease, shown as a continuous decrease in pixel values. (5) In the early ventricular diastole phase, from closure of the aortic valve to opening of the AV valves, the ventricular volume remains constant. Thus, there is no significant change in the pixel value. (6) Blood rapidly moves from the atria to the ventricles in response to opening of the AV valves; this is why the pixel values in the ventricles increase while, in contrast, those in the atria and pulmonary veins decrease.

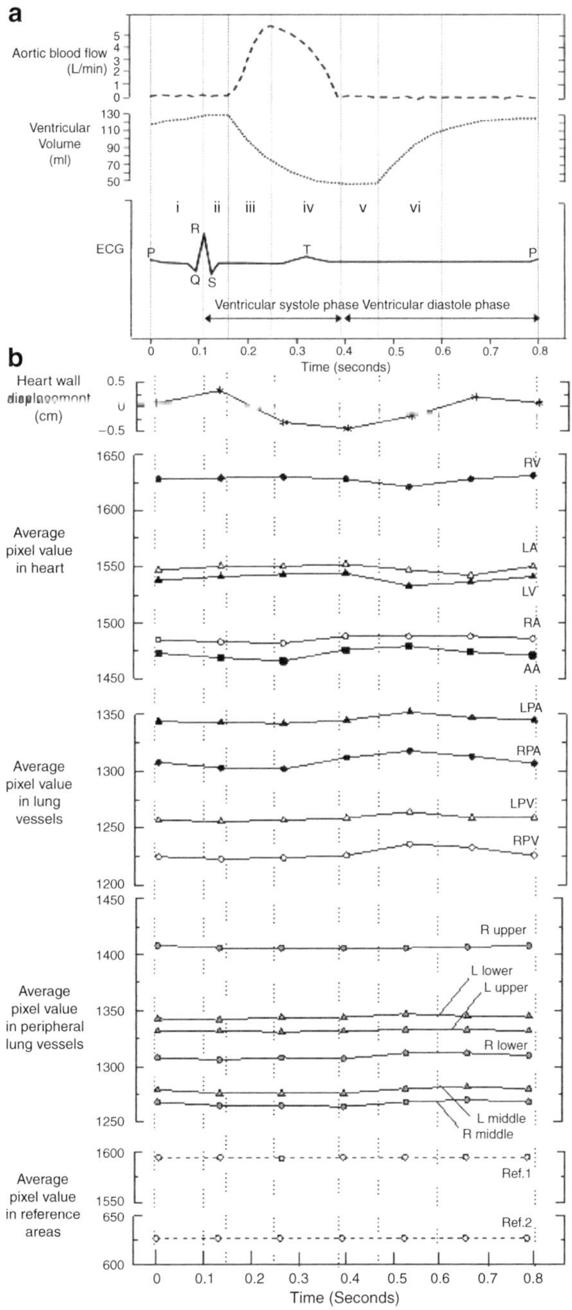

Fig. 12.3 Relationship between cardiac cycle and changes in pixel values. (**a**) Normal circulation determined by cardiac physiology, (**b**) measured pixel values in each ROI in the present study (normal, 22-year-old man)

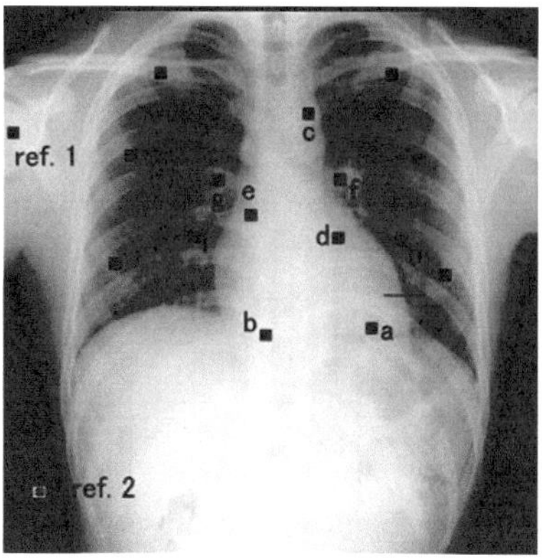

Fig. 12.4 Measurement location. *Small squares* show ROIs for measuring average pixel value, and the *horizontal line* shows a profile for measuring left-ventricle motion [*a*, left ventricle (LV); *b*, right ventricle (RV); *c*, aortic arch (AA); *d*, left atrium (LA); *e*, right atrium (RA); *f*, left pulmonary artery (LPA); *g*, right pulmonary artery (RPA); *h*, left pulmonary veins (LPV); *i*, right pulmonary veins (RPV); *other ROIs*, peripheral vessel; *ref. 1*, shoulder; *ref. 2*, air]

Fig. 12.5 Average changes in pixel values measured in each ROI. *Error bars* show ±SD (n = 7) (SD: standard deviation, N.S.: not significant)

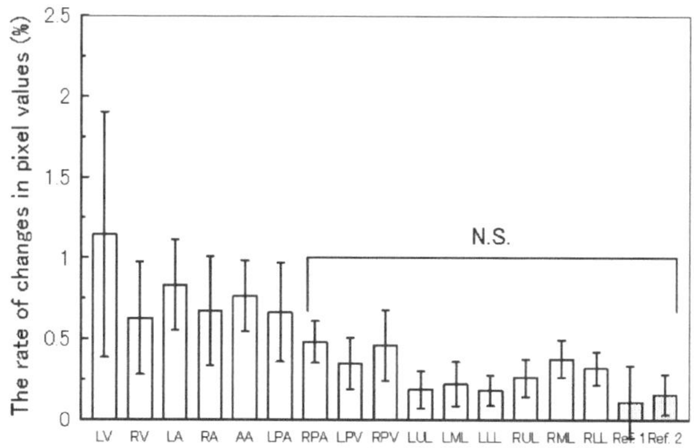

Figure 12.5 shows the average rate of change in pixel value for all subjects. The results measured in each ROI decrease in the following order: left ventricle > left atrium > aortic arch > right atrium > right ventricle > left pulmonary artery. These findings indicate that pulmonary blood circulation is reflected on dynamic chest radiographs and that the present method has the potential to evaluate local blood circulation.

Dynamic Chest Radiography

Sequential chest radiographs during respiration are obtained using a dynamic FPD system. Imaging is performed in the standing position and PA direction. For accurate evaluation of cardiopulmonary function, it is crucial to include the entire series of motions within a limited amount of time with good reproducibility. Therefore, it is recommended to use an automatic voice system and conduct pre-training for patients. The total patient dose can be less than the dose limit for lateral chest radiography recommended by the International Atomic Energy Agency (IAEA) (1.5 mGy) [30], and it can be set by adjusting the imaging time, imaging rate, and source to image distance (SID) [21, 29, 31–37]. Cardiopulmonary function is evaluated separately in each respiratory phase, inspiratory, expiratory, and breath-holding phase. The imaging rate should be greater than 7.5 frames per seconds (FPS) to permit accurate evaluation of cardiac function. If the focus is on the evaluation of respiratory function, a lower imaging rate is acceptable by taking into account the patient dose. However, an imaging time of greater than 10 s is required to induce maximum voluntary respiration.

Quantification of Cardiopulmonary Function

Analysis of dynamic chest radiographs comprises quantification, visualization, and detection of abnormal findings. Such processing permits the quantitative evaluation of diaphragm motion, cardiac function, pulmonary ventilation, and blood circulation. Figure 12.6 depicts the overall image analysis. The process in detail is outlined in the following sections. Low pixel values were related to dark areas in the images, and these in turn were related to high X-ray translucency in this chapter.

Measurement of Diaphragm Motion

Lung area was determined by edge detection using the first derivative technique and iterative contour-smoothing algorithm [38, 39]. Figure 12.7 depicts the measurement points for assessing diaphragm motion. The lung apex and diaphragm are determined in the first frame and traced by the template-matching technique after the second frame. The distance between the lung apex to the diaphragm is measured, and excursion of the diaphragm is then calculated by subtracting the distance at the maximum inspiratory level from that at the expiratory level [36, 37]. Abnormalities are detected by comparison with normal excursion or side-by-side comparison in each individual.

Measurement of Cardiac Wall Motion

Temporal–spatial cross-section images interpolated linearly are created from dynamic chest radiographs (Fig. 12.8) [34, 37]. These images could be obtained

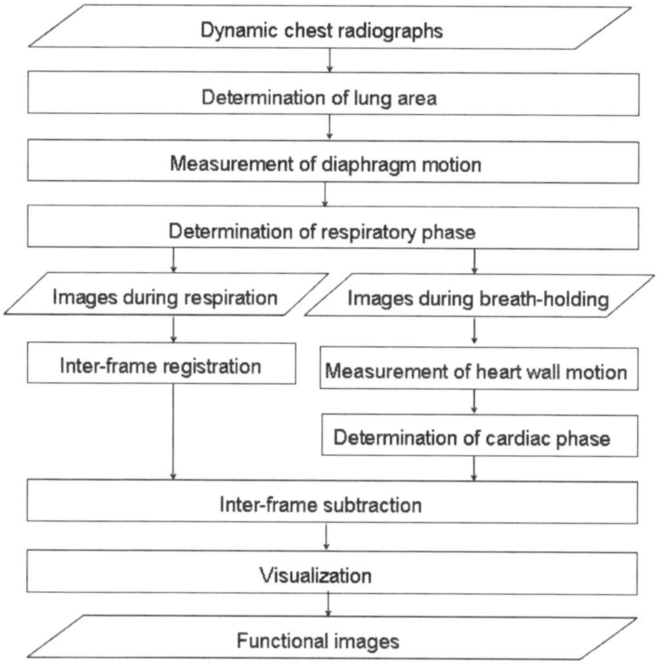

Fig. 12.6 Overall scheme of image analysis

Fig. 12.7 Measurement points for evaluating diaphragm motion

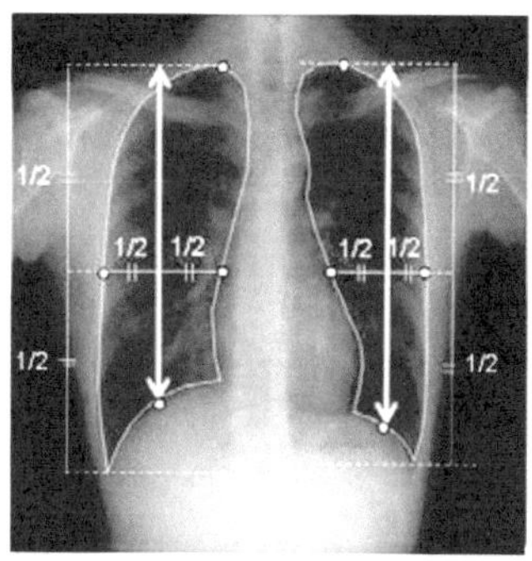

at any position of chest image and provide a visual observation of heart wall and diaphragm motion. Cardiac wall motion is also assessed by the profile curve analysis as shown in Figs. 12.3 and 12.4.

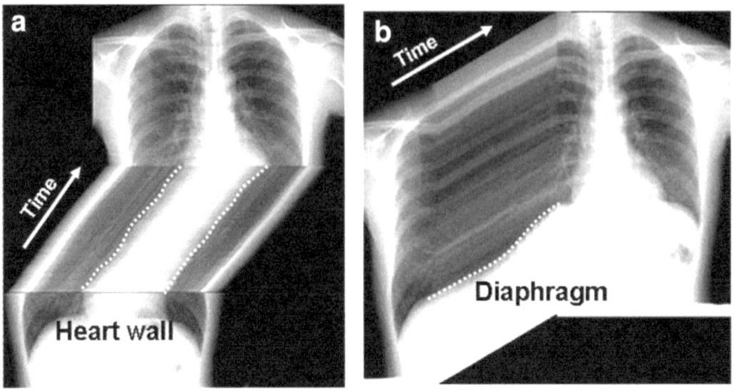

Fig. 12.8 Temporal cross-section images created from dynamic chest radiographs. (**a**) sagittal and (**b**) axial section images, respectively

Determination of the Respiratory Phase

Respiratory phase is determined based on the distance from the lung apex to diaphragm (Fig. 12.7). The frames in the maximum and minimum distance are determined as the maximum inspiratory and expiratory frames, respectively [35].

Determination of Cardiac Phase

The cardiac phase can be estimated on the basis of the change in pixel values measured near the left heart wall. Average pixel value is measured in an ROI located just outside of the left ventricular wall throughout all frames [31]. Increase in pixel values is determined as the diastole phase and decrease in pixel values as the systole phase. The frames composing a whole cardiac phase are determined and the first complete cycle is selected for evaluation of cardiac function. The cardiac phase is also determined using the results of profile curve analysis as shown in Fig. 12.3.

Measurement of Change in Pixel Value

Pulmonary function is assessed in images during respiration, whereas cardiac function is assessed in images during breath-holding. Pulmonary ventilation and blood circulation are indicated as changes in pixel values on the dynamic chest radiographs. However, it is difficult to evaluate the slight changes by observing images. Furthermore, accurate interpretation requires a great deal of knowledge regarding respiratory and cardiac physiology. Interframe subtraction is useful to

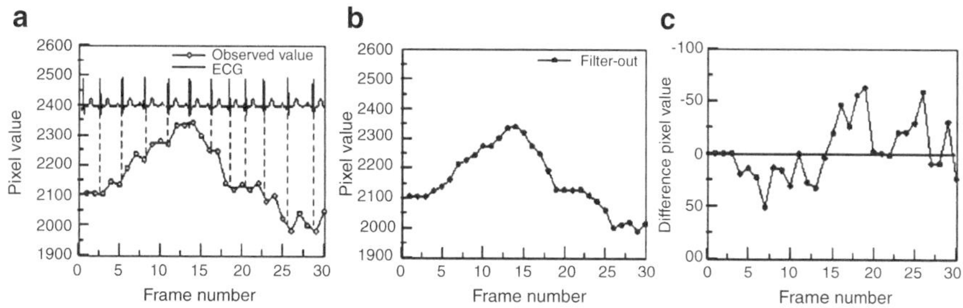

Fig. 12.9 Noise rejection and color table. (**a**) Measured pixel value and electrocardiogram (ECG). (**b**) Smoothed pixel value in the time axis direction. (**c**) Interframe difference of smoothed pixel value and color bar used to create functional images

identify slight changes in pixel value. There are two main approaches for the evaluation and visualization of pulmonary ventilation and blood circulation: a velocity-based approach by interframe subtraction and a distribution-based approach that accumulate differences in pixel values. The analysis algorithm is presented as follows.

Analysis of Pulmonary Air Flow

The velocity-based approach consists of an interframe subtraction and mapping technique [21, 32, 33]. First, smoothing of pixel values is performed in the time axis direction to reduce the change due to the heartbeat and artifacts due to rib movement (Fig. 12.9a, b). To evaluate respiratory changes in pixel values in each lung unit, average pixel value is calculated in each lung, the interframe differences of the average pixel value are calculated, then superimposed on dynamic chest radiographs in the form of color display as shown in Fig. 12.9c. The color display uses a color table in which negative changes (X-ray translucency ↑) are shown in warm colors and positive changes (X-ray translucency ↓) are shown in cold colors.

Analysis of Ventilation Distribution

Chest radiographs are divided into blocks to measure average pixel value in each local area (Fig. 12.10). The measurement in block units is to reduce the influence of slight movement, dilation, and contraction of lung structures, and also to facilitate comparison of local changes and statistical analysis. In Fig. 12.10, the block size is set to be slightly smaller than the intercostal space, so that each block is deformed in response to the changes in texture resulting from dilation and contraction of

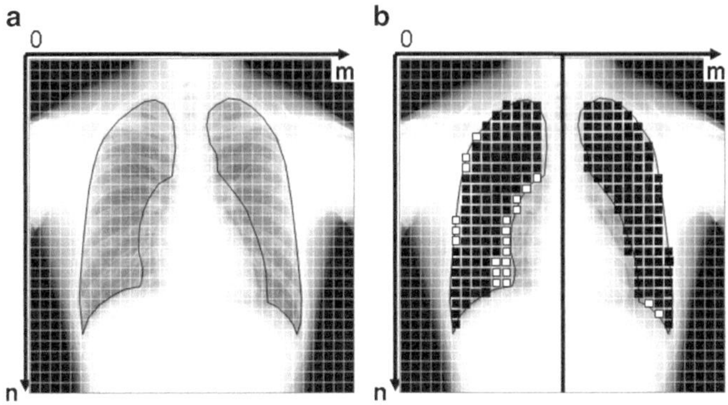

Fig. 12.10 One frame of sequential chest radiographs divided into 32 × 32 blocks that were slightly smaller than the intercostal space in size. (**a**) The *black lines* show the lung area determined for measurement of pixel values. The hilar regions are excluded from the lung area manually. (**b**) The *bold vertical line* shows the center of symmetry. "Symmetric positions" are pairs of blocks the same distance from the center of symmetry. The small *black* and *white squares* show the blocks with and without a pair for comparison, respectively

the pulmonary blood vessels and bronchi. The displacement of lung structures at the imaging rate of 7.5 fps is quite small, 0–3 pixels per frame, mainly in the craniocaudal direction. Thus, each block can be deformed geometrically using the affine transformation algorithm based on magnification percentages calculated from differences in displacement between adjacent blocks, as described elsewhere in detail [32, 40].

Average pixel values are measured in each block, tracking and deforming the region of interest (ROI). Interframe differences are then calculated, and the absolute values are summed in each block through all the frames. Interframe subtraction and summation of the absolute values are performed instead of subtraction between the maximum inspiration and expiration frames to reduce the influence of errors in image tracking and deformation.

The percentage of interframe differences of the pixel values to the summation of the results in all blocks is then calculated as below:

$$P_{\%}(m,n) = \frac{P_{total}(m,n)}{\sum_{n=0}^{N-1}\sum_{m=0}^{M-1} P_{total}(m,n)} \times 100 \qquad (12.1)$$

where M and N are the number of blocks in the horizontal and vertical directions, respectively. In addition, m and n represent the coordinates of the blocks in the horizontal and vertical directions, respectively. P_{total} (m, n) is the summation of the absolute interframe differences in each block. To facilitate visual evaluation, $P_{\%}$ (m, n) is mapped on the original image using a grayscale (hereafter called "Distribution map").

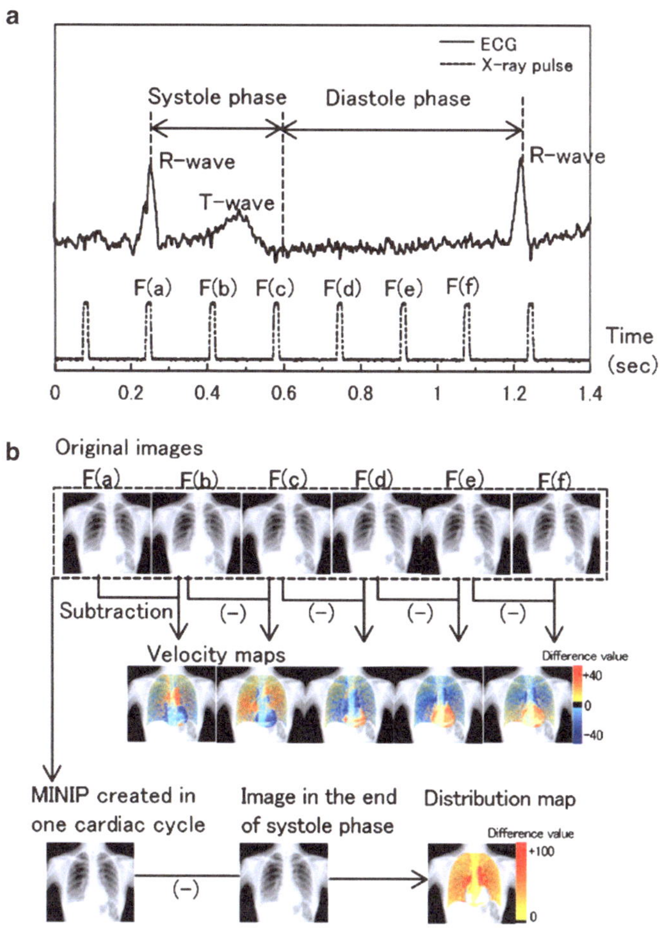

Fig. 12.11 Computer scheme for creating velocity and distribution maps of blood circulation. (**a**) ECG and pulse-wave, (**b**) processing process

Analysis of Pulmonary Blood Flow

Velocity maps of blood circulation are created by interframe differences in pixel values due to cardiac pumping. Thus, these images can provide information on blood flow velocities during each cardiac phase. Figure 12.11 shows the overall scheme of the computer algorithm for quantifying changes in pixel value due to pulmonary blood circulation. After determination of the lung area, the interframe difference is determined throughout all frames. Velocity maps of blood circulation are then created by superimposing of difference values on dynamic chest radiographs in the form of a color display, by use of a color table in which positive changes (lower X-ray translucency) are shown in warm colors and negative changes (higher X-ray translucency) are shown in cool colors.

Analysis of Circulation Distribution

Distribution maps of blood circulation are created by differences in pixel values between a frame in the minimum blood volume during one cardiac cycle and a frame at the end of the systole phase. Thus, the image can provide information on relative blood volumes during one cardiac cycle. Dilation and contraction of vessels would not be considered to affect the measurement of pixel values in projected images with a relatively large size because the rate of change is reported to be approximately ± 10 % [18]. In addition, a minimum-intensity projection (MINIP) image is created in one cardiac cycle, which is composed of pixel values showing the least blood during one cardiac cycle. Temporal subtraction is performed between a MINIP image and a frame at the end of the systole phase. The blood distribution in one cardiac cycle is also created by superimposing of the difference values on dynamic chest radiographs in the form of a color display.

To reduce the influence of movement, dilation, contraction of vessels as well as the influence of image noise, analysis in block units is recommended. A velocity-based approach in block units was reported by Tanaka et al. [32]. First, the images are divided into block units, and the average pixel value in each block $P_k(m, n)$ is calculated, as shown in Fig. 12.12. Here, m and n are the coordinates of blocks in the horizontal and vertical directions, respectively, and k is the frame number. The block size is the smallest determined experimentally in which defects in the blood flow could be detected by the present method under ideal conditions without the influence of the ribs [29]. When fluctuation is noted in adjacent frames in $P_k(m, n)$ due to X-ray output and image noise, it can be eliminated by smoothing pixel values, averaging adjacent values, in the time axis direction, as shown in Fig. 12.12. $P_{ave}(m, n)$, the average pixel value of $P_k(m, n)$ in one cardiac cycle, is then calculated, and the differences between $P_k(m, n)$ and $P_{ave}(m, n)$ are determined throughout one cardiac cycle in each block, representing the difference from the average state in blood volume. The sum of the absolute differences is finally output as $P_{total}(m, n)$, representing the total changes in pixel values in each block in one cardiac cycle. $P_{ave}(m, n)$ and $P_{total}(m, n)$ are defined as follows:

$$P_{ave}(m,n) = [P_0(m,n) + P_1(m,n) + \ldots. + P_k(m,n)]/K \ (0 < k < K) \tag{12.2}$$

$$P_{total}(m,n) = \sum |P_k(m,n) - P_{ave}(m,n)| \ (0 < k < K), \tag{12.3}$$

where K is the number of frames in one cardiac cycle. The percentage of the results in each block to the summation of the results in all the blocks in lung areas is then calculated as,

$$P_{\%}(m,n) = \frac{P_{total}(m,n)}{\sum_{n=0}^{N-1}\sum_{m=0}^{M-1} P_{total}(m,n)} \times 100, \tag{12.4}$$

where M and N are the number of blocks in the horizontal and vertical directions, respectively, and the computation is limited to lung areas.

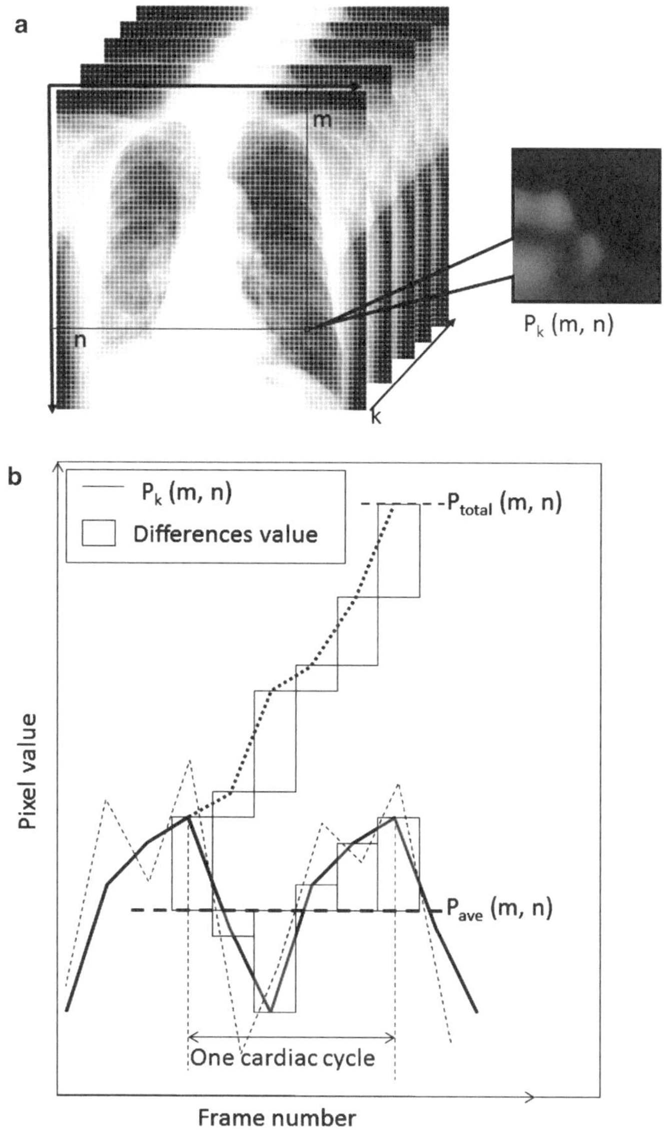

Fig. 12.12 Process for quantifying changes in pixel value. (**a**) One frame divided into 64 × 64 blocks and enlarged view of a block. (**b**) Average pixel value measured during one cardiac cycle in a block. The *broken* and *solid lines* are unprocessed and smoothed P_n (m, n), respectively. The *horizontal broken line* and *bar graphs* are P_{ave} (m, n) and the differences between P_{ave} (m, n) and P_n (m, n), respectively. The *dotted line* is the final output, P_{total} (m, n)

To facilitate visual evaluation, $P_{\%}(m, n)$ is mapped on the original image by use of a grayscale in which small changes are shown in white and large changes are shown in black (hereafter called the "Distribution map").

V/Q Study

Ventilation-perfusion (V/Q) ratio is very important diagnostic information to develop a treatment strategy in a patient with pulmonary diseases. V/Q ratio is usually calculated from radioactive count in lung scintigraphy. Functional imaging with a dynamic FPD has a potential for evaluating V/Q ratio [41]. A V/Q map based on changes in pixel value is provided using the resulting images of (b) analysis of ventilation distribution and (d) analysis of circulation distribution, as shown in Fig. 12.13. V/Q is calculated as a ratio of ventilation to perfusion as below;

$$V/Q_{PV}(m,n) = \frac{P_{\%ventilation}(m,n)}{P_{\%perfusion}(m,n)} \tag{12.5}$$

$V/Q_{pv}(m, n)$ is calculated using the results of $P_{\%ventilation}(m, n)$ measured in images during respiration and $P_{\%\ perfusion}(m, n)$ measured in breath-holding frames.

Results of the Preliminary Clinical Study

All patient data in this chapter were obtained at Kanazawa University Hospital in Japan. Approval for the study was obtained from our institutional review board, and the subjects gave their written informed consent to participation.

Analysis of Pulmonary Air Flow [21]

Figure 12.14 shows the results in a normal control (22-year-old man). The right and left diaphragms showed synchronous movement as shown in Fig. 12.14b. Average right and left diaphragm excursions in the normal controls ($n = 58$) were 4.2 ± 1.3 and 4.6 ± 1.2 cm, respectively. There were no significant differences between the left and right diaphragm. Figure 12.14c shows respiratory changes of the average pixel value in each lung. In the expiratory phase, interframe differences in pixel values were positive resulting from the decrease in X-ray translucency and were seen as cold colors on velocity maps, whereas in the inspiratory phase, interframe differences in pixel values were negative resulting from the increase in X-ray translucency and were shown as warm colors on velocity maps. On the velocity maps, the interframe differences were seen to be distributed symmetrically in both lungs throughout all respiratory phases and larger interframe differences were distributed in the lower area in some parts of the respiratory phase (Fig. 12.14d, e). The distribution of interframe differences in pixel value was consistent with well-known properties in respiratory physiology, such as regional differences in ventilation [19, 20].

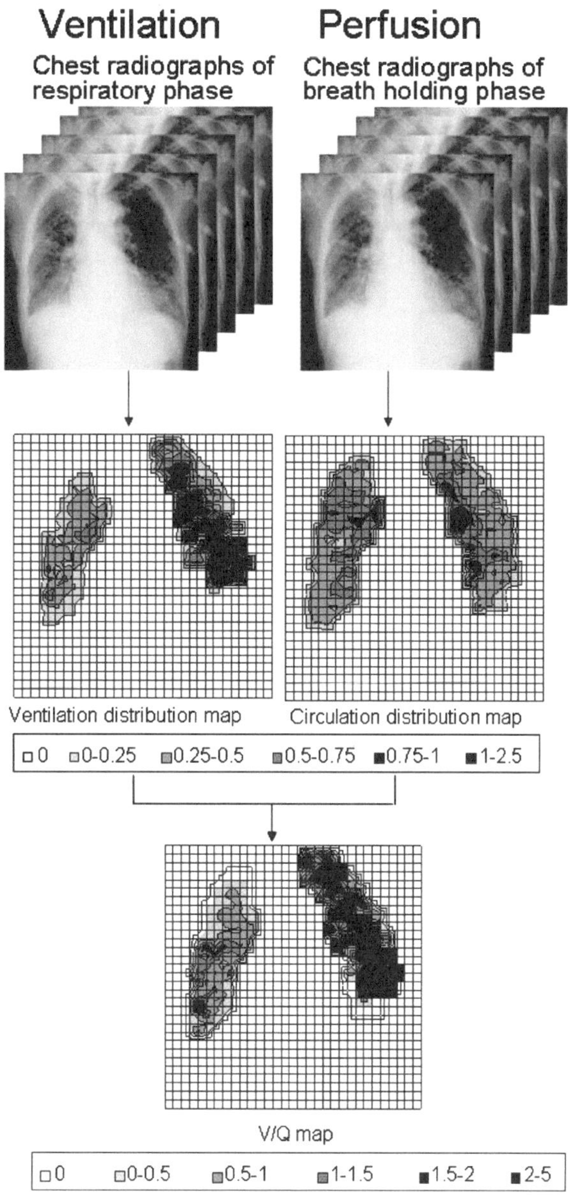

Fig. 12.13 The process of creating the V/Q map on the basis of changes in pixel value

Figure 12.15 shows the results in a patient with bilateral air trapping (31-year-old man, emphysema). PFT indicated low FEV1.0 % and %VC, which indicates mixed ventilatory impairment. It was expected that pulmonary airflow would be decreased in the areas with air trapping. Our method showed that the flat diaphragm pressured by air trapping moved dynamically and synchronously (Fig. 12.15d).

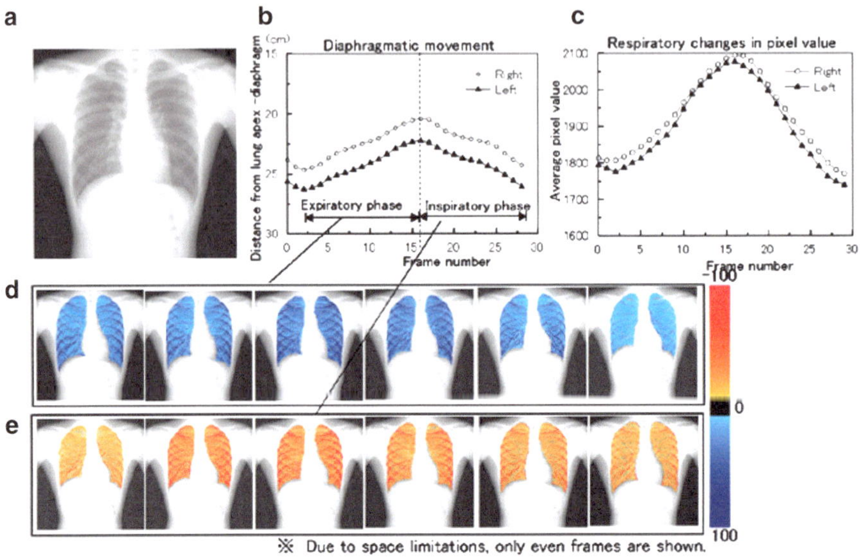

Fig. 12.14 Results in a normal control (22-year-old man). (**a**) Dynamic chest radiograph in the maximum inspiratory frame. (**b**) Distance from the lung apex to the diaphragm. (**c**) Average pixel values measured in each lung. (**d**) Velocity maps in the expiratory phase. (**e**) Velocity maps in the inspiratory phase

Excursion of the right diaphragm was 4.3 cm and that of the left diaphragm was 4.9 cm, which were the same or better than the average values of the normal controls. However, there were some areas with interframe differences near zero, i.e., showing little or no respiratory changes in pixel value, indicated as colorless areas on the velocity maps corresponding to the areas with air trapping on CT images (Fig. 12.15b, c, f, g).

Figure 12.16 shows the results in a patient with asthma (56-year-old man). Although there were no abnormal findings in CT images, as shown in Fig. 12.16b, c, PFT indicated obstructive abnormality. Thus, it was expected that the reduced regional pulmonary airflow would be seen as a colorless area on velocity maps resulting from interframe differences near zero. Our results showed that the excursions of the diaphragm were relatively small (2.4 cm on the right and 2.7 cm on the left) (Fig. 12.16d). However, some areas continuously showed interframe differences near zero in the upper lung, which appear as areas defective in color on the velocity maps as expected (Fig. 12.16f, g).

These results indicated that our method was useful for evaluating local pulmonary airflow in COPD and asthma, diseases associated with abnormalities in regional ventilation. However, some issues remain to be resolved. The velocity maps sometimes contained artifacts that could have been caused by misalignment of lung structures. Thus, it is necessary to develop a computer algorithm to reduce artifacts.

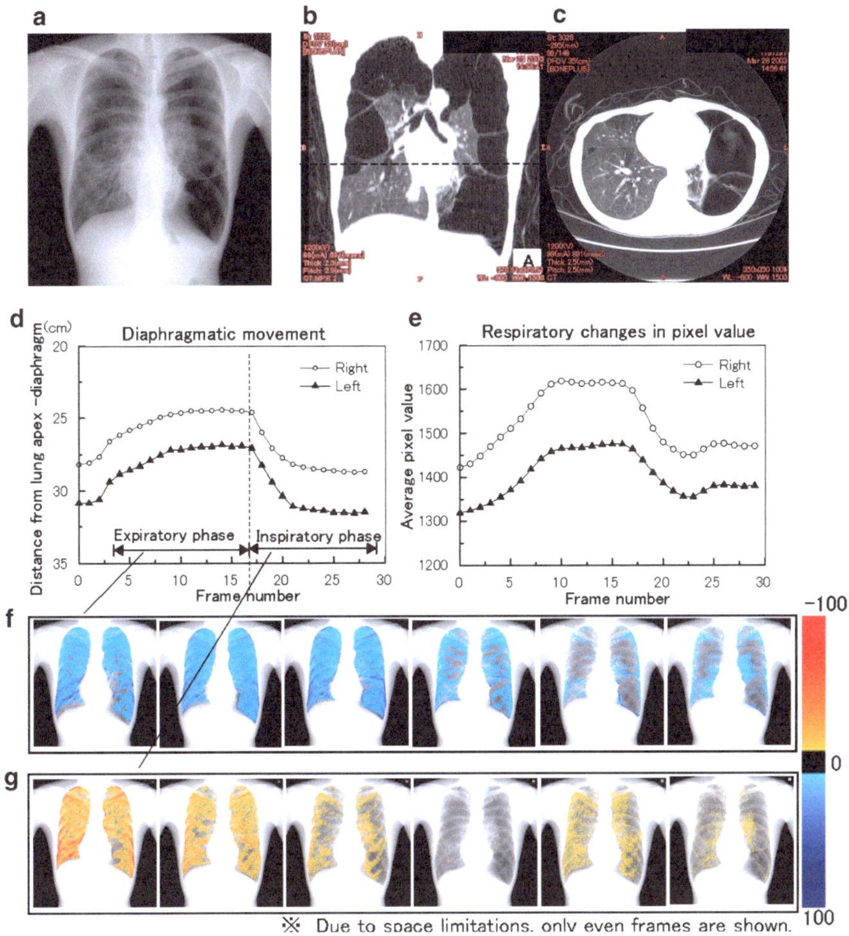

Fig. 12.15 Results in a patient with emphysema (31-year-old man). (**a**) Dynamic chest radiograph in the maximum inspiratory frame. (**b**) CT (coronal section). (**c**) CT (axial section). (**d**) Distance from the lung apex to the diaphragm. (**e**) Average pixel values measured in each lung. (**f**) Velocity maps in the expiratory phase. (**g**) Velocity maps in the inspiratory phase

Analysis of Ventilation Distribution [32]

Figure 12.17 shows the distribution map in a normal control (22-year-old man). The results showed the symmetrical distribution of $P_{\%}$ throughout the whole lung (Fig. 12.17b) and consistent with normal ventilation distribution, which decreases gradually and symmetrically from the upper region to the basal regions [19, 40]. In addition, a strong correlation was observed between right and left $P_{\%}$ (r = 0.70) (Fig. 12.17c). In normal controls (n = 6), $P_{\%}$ decreased from the lung apex to the

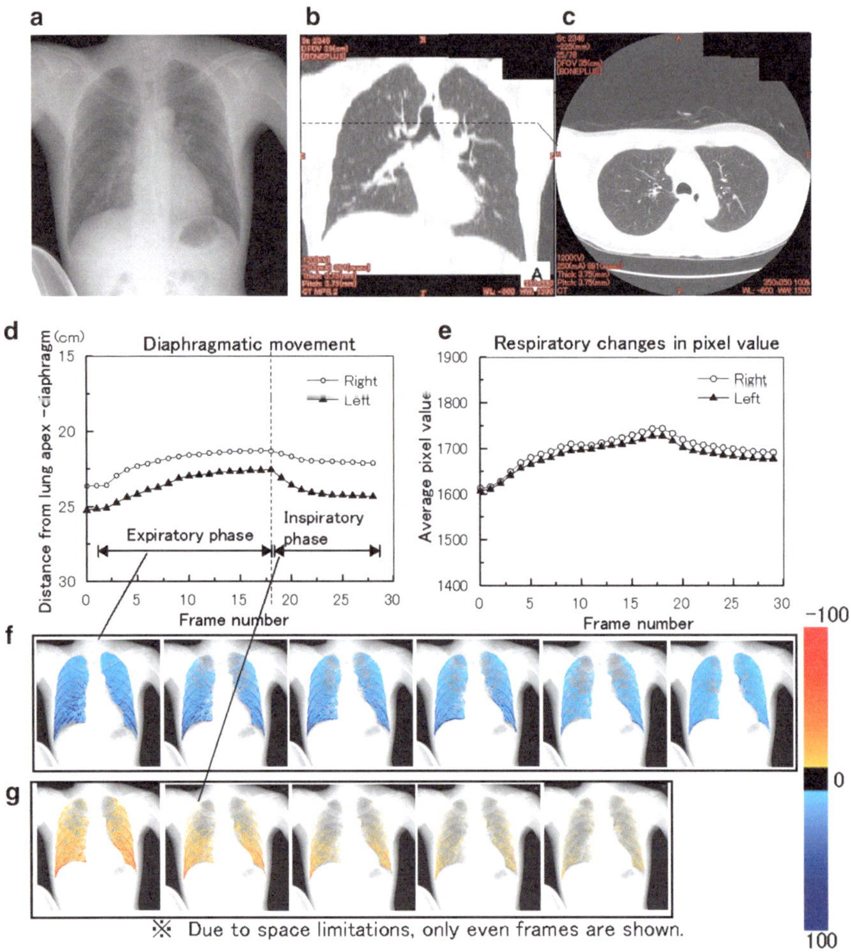

Fig. 12.16 Results in a patient with asthma (56-year-old man). (**a**) Dynamic chest radiograph in the maximum inspiratory frame. (**b**) CT (coronal section). (**c**) CT (axial section). (**d**) Distance from the lung apex to the diaphragm. (**e**) Average pixel values measured in each lung. (**f**) Velocity maps in the expiratory phase. (**g**) Velocity maps in the inspiratory phase

basal area with a symmetrical distribution. In contrast, many abnormal cases showed nonuniform distributions of $P_{\%}$, which were different from the normal pattern. Figure 12.18 shows the results in a patient with pleural adhesions in the left lung, resulting in middle restricted ventilatory abnormality (72-year-old woman). There were several findings of pleural adhesions in CT images (Fig. 12.18b, c). Lung scintigraphy showed marked reduction of ventilation in the left lung in comparison with the right lung (Fig. 12.18d). The distribution map of $P_{\%}$ also showed reduced changes in pixel value over the left lung (Fig. 12.18e), and there was no relationship between right and left $P_{\%}$ (r = 0.01) (Fig. 12.18f).

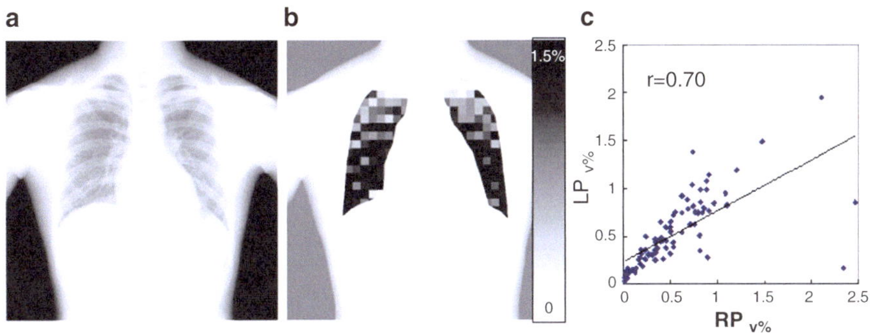

Fig. 12.17 Results in a normal control (22-year-old man). (**a**) One frame of dynamic chest radiograph. (**b**) Distribution map (**c**) Scatter chart of right and left $P_{\%}$ (r = 0.7). This symmetrical distribution of $P_{\%}$ was commonly observed in all normal controls

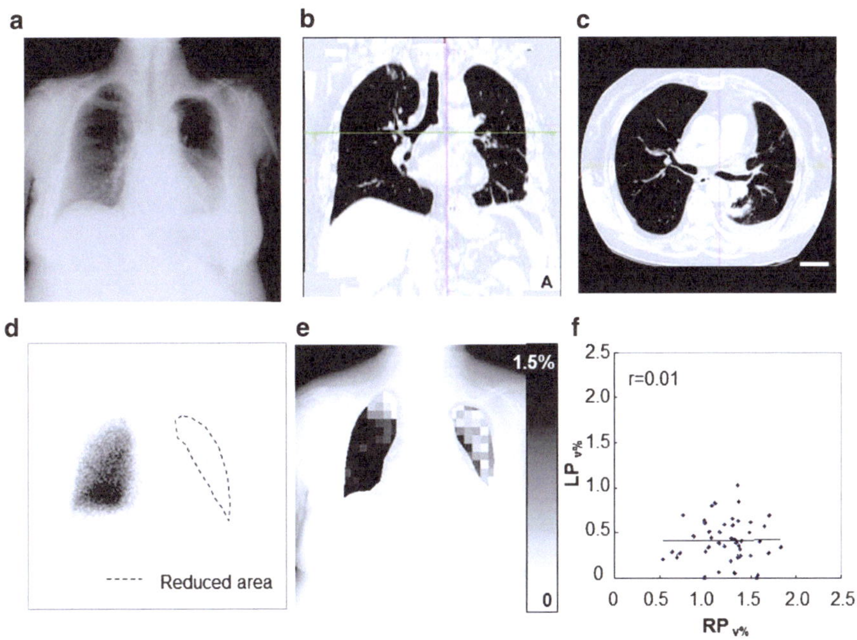

Fig. 12.18 Results in a subject with no correlation between right and left $P_{\%}$ (pleural adhesions, 72-year-old woman). (**a**) One frame of dynamic chest radiograph. Computed tomography in (**b**) coronal and (**c**) axial sections. There were no morphological anomalies associated with ventilation impairment in the lung scintigram. (**d**) Lung scintigram. Ventilation in the left whole lung showed marked reduction. (**e**) Distribution map. The left whole lung and right upper lung area had small $P_{\%}$. (**f**) Scatter chart of right and left $P_{\%}$ (r = 0.01). There was no relationship between right and left $P_{\%}$ at symmetrical positions

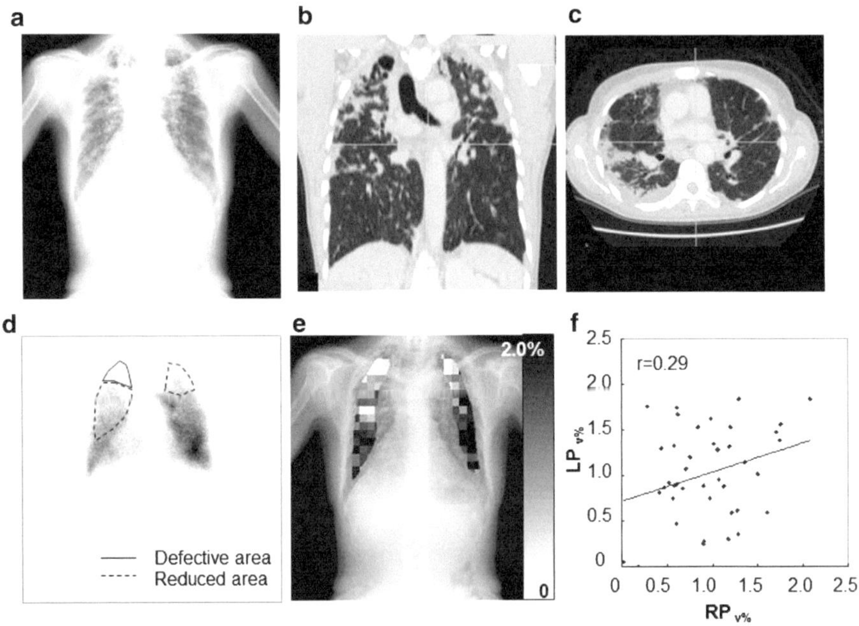

Fig. 12.19 Results in a subject with poor correlation between right and left $P_{\%}$ (pulmonary fibrosis, 56-year-old woman). (**a**) One frame of dynamic chest radiograph. There were areas of no or reduced ventilation in the right upper and middle lung, and the left upper lung. Computed tomography in (**b**) coronal and (**c**) axial sections. (**d**) Lung scintigram. There were several areas with advanced pulmonary fibrosis for ventilation impairment. (**e**) Distribution map. The right upper and middle, and left upper regions are indicated as small $P_{\%}$. (**f**) Scatter chart of right and left $P_{\%}$ (r = 0.29). There is a weak relationship between right and left $P_{\%}$ at symmetrical positions

Figure 12.19 shows the results in a patient with upper-predominant pulmonary fibrosis, resulting in middle restricted ventilatory abnormality (56-year-old woman). In CT images, there were several areas with advanced pulmonary fibrosis for ventilatory impairment (Fig. 12.19b, c). Lung scintigraphy also showed that there were areas of no ventilation in the upper right lung and of reduced ventilation in the left upper and right middle lung (Fig. 12.19d). These areas showed reduced changes in pixel value in the distribution map of $P_{\%}$ (Fig. 12.19e), and there was a low correlation coefficient between right and left $P_{\%}$ (r = 0.29) (Fig. 12.19f).

These results indicated that pulmonary ventilatory impairment could be detected as a deviation from the symmetry of respiratory-induced changes in pixel value. However, there were several limitations of the present method. They were classified into two groups, i.e., bilateral ventilation abnormalities or differences in lung size. If a lung is recognized in a smaller size for some reason, e.g., heart enlargement and atelectasis, some blocks in another lung had no pair for comparison, even though there are abnormalities. To detect bilateral abnormalities, multistratified analysis of the $P_{\%}$ distribution pattern should be performed by combining several methods, such as comparison with the normal distribution pattern of $P_{\%}$, time series

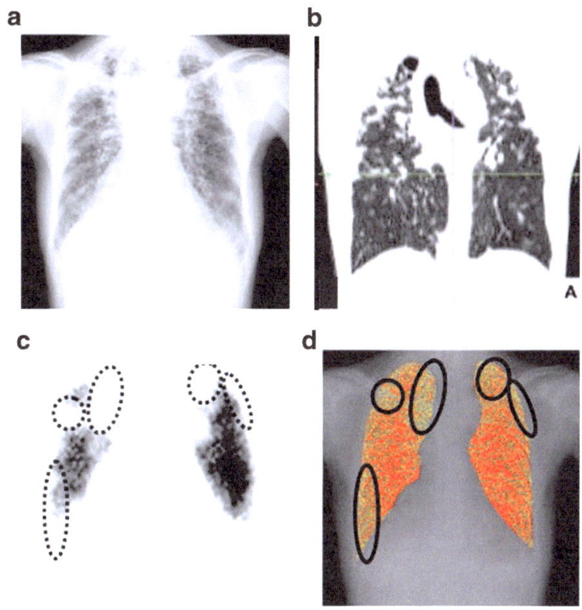

Fig. 12.20 Results of our method and the other clinical examinations in a subject with pulmonary fibrosis (56 years old, female). (**a**) Chest radiograph, (**b**) computed tomography (coronal section), (**c**) lung perfusion scintigraphy, and (**d**) distribution map. In the blood distribution map, there were some reductions of changes in pixel value (*solid-line circles*), which were consistent with defect in blood flow as indicated by scintigraphic test [*broken-line circles* in (**c**)]

analysis, examination of craniocaudal variation, and pattern analysis considering lung structures. Furthermore, it is also necessary to evaluate the detection method in larger numbers of patients along with investigation of analysis parameters, such as block size and shape.

Analysis of Pulmonary Blood Flow [29]

Figure 12.11 shows the results in a normal control. Slight changes in pixel value were visualized as velocity and distribution maps without contrast media (Fig. 12.11). The resulting images showed a normal pattern determined by the physiology of pulmonary blood circulation, which diffuses from around the pulmonary arteries to the peripheral area, with no perfusion defects throughout the entire lung region. In contrast, the results in an abnormal case showed that abnormalities, such as a decrease or defect in blood circulation, would be shown as defects in color. Figure 12.20 shows results in a patient with lung fibrosis (56 years old, female). The chest radiograph and CT (coronal section) showed advanced fibrosis of the lung in the upper area (Fig. 12.20a, b). The results of perfusion scintigraphy of the lung showed some areas of decreased blood flow, as seen in Fig. 12.21c. The distribution map showed some areas with decreased changes in pixel value (Fig. 12.20d), which were coincident with the abnormal area in perfusion scintigraphy of the lung.

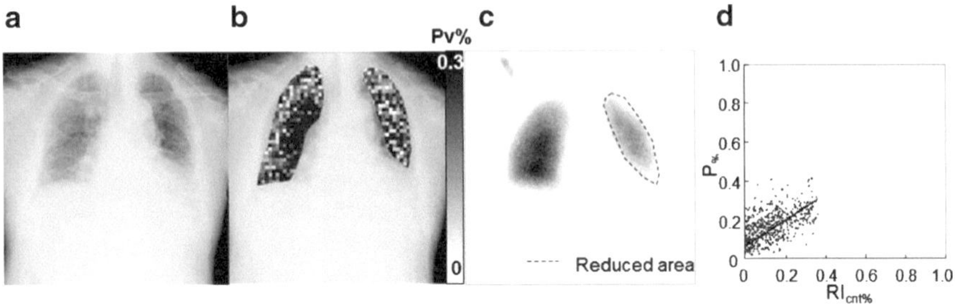

Fig. 12.21 Results in restrictive lung disease (pulmonary fibrosis, 82-year-old man). (**a**) One frame of dynamic chest radiograph. (**b**) Distribution map. (**c**) Lung perfusion scan (^{99m}Tc-MAA). The area surrounded by *broken lines* shows reduced blood flow. (**d**) Scatter diagram of $P_{\%}$ – $RIcnt_{\%}$ (r = 0.70). The *regression line* is shown. $RIcnt_{\%}$ was calculated on the basis of RI count using Eq. (12.4)

These findings indicated that dynamic chest radiography with a dynamic FPD has potential for functional imaging. The present method is expected to be a rapid and simple method for evaluation of blood circulation in general chest radiography, because dynamic FPDs are now widely available. However, there is not enough clinical evidence supporting the usefulness of the present method. Further studies in larger numbers of subjects with abnormalities in blood flow, such as pulmonary embolism, pulmonary hypertension, pulmonary edema, and general heart diseases, are required along with investigations into the ability of this method to detect abnormalities. The errors due to vessel misalignment and the reproducibility of the present method should also be addressed.

Analysis of Circulation Distribution

Figure 12.21 shows the results for a patient with pulmonary fibrosis (82-year-old man) [32]. The area surrounded by broken lines in the perfusion scan shows the area with reduced blood flow determined by a radiologist specializing in nuclear medicine. The perfusion scan showed a marked reduction of blood flow in the left lung in comparison with the right lung (Fig. 12.21c). The distribution map also showed reduced total changes in pixel value over the left lung (Fig. 12.21b). There was a strong correlation between distribution map and lung perfusion (r = 0.70) (Fig. 12.21d).

Figure 12.22 shows the results for a patient with obstructive pulmonary disease (62-year-old man) [32]. The perfusion scan showed that there were areas of no blood flow in the upper right lung and of reduced blood flow in the left upper and middle lung (Fig. 12.22c). These areas showed reduced changes in pixel value in the distribution map (Fig. 12.22b). There was an intermediate correlation between distribution map and lung perfusion (r = 0.63) (Fig. 12.22d).

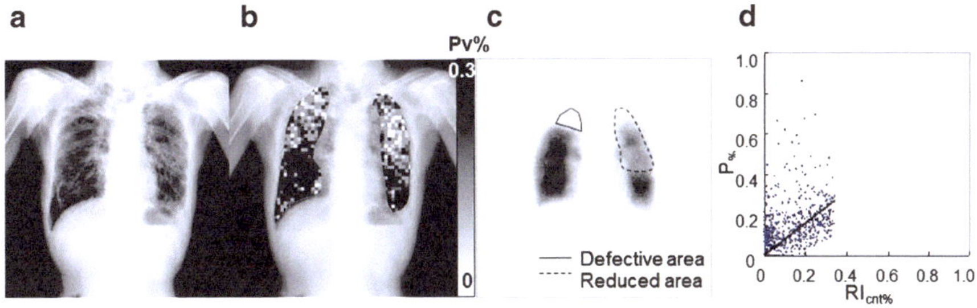

Fig. 12.22 Results in obstructive pulmonary disease (bronchiolitis obliterans with upper-lobe fibrosis and pneumothorax in the right lower lung, 62-year-old man). (**a**) One frame of dynamic chest radiograph. (**b**) Distribution map. (**c**) Lung perfusion scan (^{99m}Tc-MAA). The areas surrounded by *solid* and *broken lines* show reduced blood flow. (**d**) Scatter diagram of $P_{\%}$ – $RIcnt_{\%}$ (r = 0.63). The *regression line* is shown. $RIcnt_{\%}$ was calculated on the basis of RI count using Eq. (12.4)

There was a good correlation between the findings in the distribution map and those in the perfusion scan in ten of the subjects. The results indicated that the distribution map could provide relative measures related to pulmonary blood flow. Although the changes in pixel value do not indicate the absolute blood flow volume, the present method could be utilized for relative or temporal comparison in each patient rather than for inter-subject comparison. The diagnostic criteria and diseases for which the present method is applicable should be determined in further studies in patients with the same diseases.

V/Q Study [41]

Figures 12.13 show the results in a patient with ventilation-perfusion mismatch (hypoxemia, 74-year-old man). The patient had several findings of pleural adhesions in CT images (Fig. 12.23d–g). PFT indicated low vital capacity (VC) and low forced expiratory volume in 1 s (FEV1.0), which meant obstructive abnormality. Figure 12.13 shows resulting V/Q map created from changes in pixel value. Abnormalities were appeared as a reduction of changes in pixel values. For example, the lacks of ventilation and blood flow in the upper and lower left lung were indicated as reduced changes in pixel values. In addition, the area of defective ventilation over the right lung was indicated as remarkably reduced changes in pixel value in the ventilation mapping image. In contrast, the area of reduced blood flow over the right lung was indicated as reduced changes in pixel values. V/Q ratio calculated from the changes in pixel value was consistent with those calculated from RI counts. The results indicated the possibility of V/Q study based on changes in pixel value on dynamic chest radiographs. It is very useful to obtain V/Q ratio as additional information in general chest radiography.

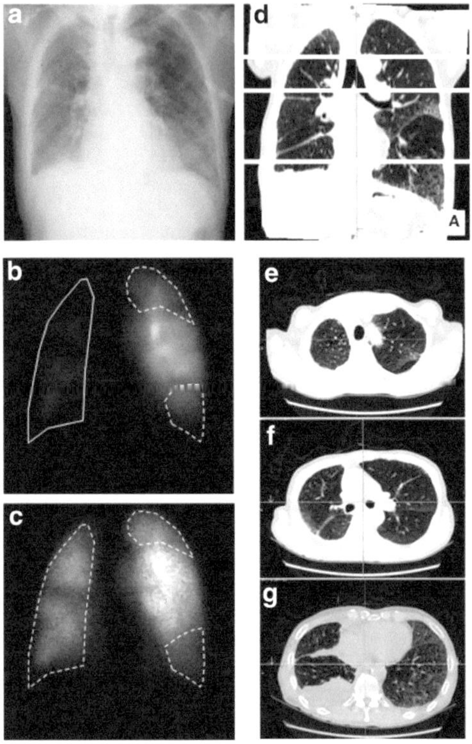

Fig. 12.23 Image findings of the patient evaluated in this study (74-year-old man). (**a**) Chest radiograph, (**b–c**) ventilation and perfusion scintigrams. The area surrounded by *solid* and *broken lines* show defective and reduced blood flow, respectively. (**d–g**) CT images. There were several findings of pleural adhesions

Computer-Aided Diagnosis for Dynamic Chest Radiographs

Computer-aided diagnosis (CAD) for dynamic chest radiographs was only recently introduced; however, two trials have been reported. Tsuchiya et al. developed a CAD system to detect lung nodules using dynamic chest radiographs taken during respiration [42]. Their technique could quantitatively evaluate the kinetic range of nodules and was effective in detecting a nodule on a breathing chest radiograph. Another approach is to detect functional impairments in ventilation and blood circulation in the lungs, as shown in section "Analysis of Ventilation Distribution" in this chapter. In the paper [42], we tested a hypothesis that ventilatory impairment could be detected by comparing respiratory-induced changes in pixel value in symmetrical positions in both lungs. Here, "symmetrical positions" means a pair of locations in the same distance from the axis of thorax on the same level. In the results, abnormalities could not be detected in 50 % of the patients with bilateral abnormalities. However, in many patients, abnormalities could be detected as a deviation from the right and left symmetry of respiratory-induced changes in pixel value. These results indicated that the present method would be useful for detecting unilateral abnormalities. To detect bilateral abnormalities, further studies are required to develop a multilevel detection method combined with several methods of pattern analysis. One of the most potential solutions is machine learning/pattern recognition methods. Abnormalities could be effectively detected based on machine learning/pattern recognition methods using the normal distribution of ventilation and perfusion well-known in pulmonary physiology [19, 40].

Summary

Dynamic FPD allow acquisition of sequential chest radiographs with a large FOV, high image quality, and low patient dose. Dynamic chest radiography with computer analysis is expected to be a new type of functional imaging system that provides measures of cardiopulmonary function, such as diaphragm and heart wall motion, pulmonary ventilation, and blood flow. In the past decade, such functional information has provided additional information for the diagnosis of cardiopulmonary disease. However, it is not easy for a radiologist to interpret cardiopulmonary function on dynamic chest radiographs. Therefore, computerized methods for quantifying cardiopulmonary function are essential for the implementation of dynamic chest radiography. Some recent developments have been discussed in this chapter. Specifically, we used an interframe subtraction technique for the evaluation of pulmonary ventilation and blood flow. Interframe subtraction was useful to quantify and visualize slight changes in pixel value caused by respiration and blood circulation. Functional impairments were indicated as decreased changes in pixel value in the preliminary clinical study. The next step is to develop a CAD system for dynamic chest radiography. It would be more effective for the diagnosis of cardiopulmonary diseases to compare the results in both lungs or evaluate the distribution. Although the present method lacks 3D anatomic information, this method can be used as a rapid substitute for lung perfusion scintigraphy, perfusion CT, and MRI and could be applied to cone beam CT and 4D CT, as an optional means of evaluating cardiopulmonary function.

References

1. Freeman LM, Stein EG, Sprayregen S, Chamarthy M, Haramati LB (2008) The current and continuing important role of ventilation-perfusion scintigraphy in evaluating patients with suspected pulmonary embolism. Semin Nucl Med 38:432–440
2. Zöphel K, Bacher-Stier C, Pinkert J, Kropp J (2009) Ventilation/perfusion lung scintigraphy: what is still needed? A review considering technetium-99m-labeled macro-aggregates of albumin. Ann Nucl Med 23:1–16
3. Goldin JG (2009) Imaging the lungs in patients with pulmonary emphysema. Radiology 24:163–170
4. Salito C, Aliverti A, Gierada DS, Deslée G, Pierce RA, Macklem PT, Woods JC (2009) Quantification of trapped gas with CT and 3 He MR imaging in a porcine model of isolated airway obstruction. Radiology 253:380–389

5. Kiryu S, Loring SH, Mori Y, Rofsky NM, Hatabu H, Takahashi M (2006) Quantitative analysis of the velocity and synchronicity of diaphragmatic motion: dynamic MRI in different postures. Magn Reson Imaging 24:1325–1332
6. Holmes JH, Korosec FR, Du J, O'Halloran RL, Sorkness RL, Grist TM, Kuhlman JE, Fain SB (2007) Imaging of lung ventilation and respiratory dynamics in a single ventilation cycle using hyperpolarized He-3 MRI. J Magn Reson Imaging 26:630–636
7. Ohno Y, Koyama H, Nogami M, Takenaka D, Matsumoto S, Obara M, Sugimura K (2008) Dynamic oxygen-enhanced MRI versus quantitative CT: pulmonary functional loss assessment and clinical stage classification of smoking-related COPD. Am J Roentgenol 190: W93–W99
8. Tokuda J, Schmitt M, Sun Y, Patz S, Tang Y, Mountford CE, Hata N, Wald LL, Hatabu H (2009) Lung motion and volume measurement by dynamic 3D MRI using a 128-channel receiver coil. Acad Radiol 16:22–27
9. Silverman NR (1972) Clinical video-densitometry. Pulmonary ventilation analysis. Radiology 103:263–265
10. Silverman NR, Intaglietta M, Simon AL, Tompkins WR (1972) Determination of pulmonary pulsatile perfusion by fluoroscopic videodensitometry. J Appl Physiol 33:147–149
11. Silverman NR, Intaglietta M, Tompkins WR (1973) Pulmonary ventilation and perfusion during graded pulmonary arterial occlusion. J Appl Physiol 34:726–731
12. Bursch JH (1985) Densitometric studies in digital subtraction angiography: assessment of pulmonary and myocardial perfusion. Herz 10:208–214
13. Liang J, Jarvi T, Kiuru A, Kormano M, Svedström E (1985) Dynamic chest image analysis: model-based perfusion analysis in dynamic pulmonary imaging. J Appl Signal Process 5:437–448
14. Fujita H, Doi K, MacMahon H, Kume Y, Giger ML, Hoffmann KR, Katafuchi T, Ohara K, Chan HP (1987) Basic imaging properties of a large image intensifier-TV digital chest radiographic system. Invest Radiol 22:328–335
15. Suwatanapongced T, Solne RM, Gierada DS, Position D (2000) Shape on standard chest radiographs in patients with normal, obstructive, and restrictive pulmonary function. Med Phys 217:647
16. Fraser RS, Muller NL, Colman NC, Pare PD (1999) Fraser and Pare's diagnosis of diseases of the chest, 4th edn. W.B. Saunders Company, Philadelphia
17. Suga K, Tsukuda T, Awaya H, Takano K, Koike S, Matsunaga N, Sugi K, Esato K (1999) Impaired respiratory mechanics in pulmonary emphysema: evaluation with dynamic breathing MRI. J Magn Reson Imaging 10:510–520
18. Hansen JT, Koeppen BM (2002) Cardiovascular physiology. In: Netter's atlas of human physiology (Netter basic science). Icon Learning Systems, Teterboro
19. West JB (2000) Ventilation – how gas gets to the alveoli. In: Respiratory physiology – the essentials, 3rd edn. Lippincott Williams & Wilkins, Philadelphia, pp 11–19
20. Squire LF, Novelline RA (1988) Fundamentals of radiology, 4th edn. Harvard University Press, Cambridge
21. Tanaka R, Sanada S, Okazaki N, Kobayashi T, Fujimura M, Yasui M, Matsui T, Nakayama K, Nanbu Y, Matsui O (2006) Evaluation of pulmonary function using breathing chest radiography with a dynamic flat-panel detector (FPD): primary results in pulmonary diseases. Invest Radiol 41:735–745
22. Tanaka R, Sanada S, Fujimura M, Yasui M, Tsuji S, Hayashi N, Okamoto H, Nanbu Y, Matsui O (2010) Ventilatory impairment detection based on distribution of respiratory-induced changes in pixel values in dynamic chest radiography: a feasibility study. Int J Comput Assist Radiol Surg 6:103–110
23. Tanaka R, Sanada S, Okazaki N, Kobayashi T, Suzuki M, Matsui T, Matsui O (2008) Detectability of regional lung ventilation with flat-panel detector-based dynamic radiography. J Digit Imaging 21:109–120

24. Heyneman LE (2005) The chest radiograph: reflections on cardiac physiology. Radiological Society of North America. Scientific Assembly and Annual Meeting Program 2005, p 145
25. Goodman LR (2006) Felson's principles of chest roentgenology, a programmed text. W B Saunders Co, Philadelphia
26. Turner AF, Lau FY, Jacobson G (1972) A method for the estimation of pulmonary venous and arterial pressures from the routine chest roentgenogram. Am J Roentgenol Radium Ther Nucl Med 116:97–106
27. Chang CH (1962) The normal roentgenographic measurement of the right descending pulmonary artery in 1,085 cases. Am J Roentgenol Radium Ther Nucl Med 87:929–935
28. Pistolesi M, Milne EN, Miniati M, Giuntini C (1984) The vascular pedicle of the heart and the vena azygos. Part II: acquired heart disease. Radiology 152:9–17
29. Tanaka R, Sanada S, Fujimura M, Yasui M, Nakayama K, Matsui T, Hayashi N, Matsui O (2008) Development of functional chest imaging with a dynamic flat-panel detector (FPD). Radiol Phys Technol 1:137–143
30. International atomic energy agency (1996) International basic safety standards for protection against ionizing radiation and for the safety of radiation sources. International atomic energy agency (IAEA), Vienna
31. Tanaka R, Sanada S, Fujimura M, Yasui M, Tsuji S, Hayashi N, Okamoto H, Nanbu Y, Matsui O (2010) Development of pulmonary blood flow evaluation method with a dynamic flat-panel detector (FPD): quantitative correlation analysis with findings on perfusion scan. Radiol Phys Technol 3:40–45
32. Tanaka R, Sanada S, Fujimura M, Yasui M, Tsuji S, Hayashi N, Okamoto H, Nanbu Y, Matsui O (2009) Pulmonary blood flow evaluation using a dynamic flat-panel detector: feasibility study with pulmonary diseases. Int J Comput Assist Radiol Surg 4:449–454
33. Tanaka R, Sanada S, Tsujioka K, Matsui T, Takata T, Matsui O (2008) Development of a cardiac evaluation method using a dynamic flat-panel detector (FPD) system: a feasibility study using a cardiac motion phantom. Radiol Phys Technol 1:27–32
34. Tanaka R, Sanada S, Okazaki N, Kobayashi T, Nakayama K, Matsui T, Hayashi N, Matsui O (2006) Quantification and visualization of relative local ventilation on dynamic chest radiographs. In: Proceedings of SPIE, medical imaging, The International Society for optical engineering, vol 6143, San Diego, pp 62432Y1–62432Y8
35. Tanaka R, Sanada S, Kobayashi T, Suzuki M, Matsui T, Matsui O (2006) Computerized methods for determining respiratory phase on dynamic chest radiographs obtained by a dynamic flat-panel detector (FPD) system. J Digit Imaging 19:41–51
36. Tanaka R, Sanada S, Kobayashi T, Suzuki M, Matsui T, Inoue H (2004) Breathing chest radiography using a dynamic flat-panel detector (FPD) with computer analysis for a screening examination. Med Phys 31:2254–2262
37. Tanaka R, Sanada S, Kobayashi T, Suzuki M, Matsui T, Hayashi N, Nanbu Y (2003) Automated analysis for the respiratory kinetics with the screening dynamic chest radiography using a flat-panel detector system. In: Proceedings of computer assisted radiology and surgery, pp 179–186
38. Xu XW, Doi K (1995) Image feature analysis for computer-aided diagnosis: accurate determination of ribcage boundary in chest radiographs. Med Phys 22:617–626
39. Li L, Zheng Y, Kallergi M, Clark RA (2001) Improved method for automatic identification of lung regions on chest radiographs. Acad Radiol 8:629–638
40. Tanaka R, Sanada S, Matsui T, Hayashi N, Matsui O (2008) Sequential dual-energy subtraction technique with a dynamic flat-panel detector (FPD): primary study for image-guided radiation therapy (IGRT). Radiol Phys Technol 1:144–150
41. Tanaka R, Sanada S, Fujimura M, Yasui M, Tsuji, S, Hayashi N, Okamoto H, Nanbu Y, Matsui O (2011) Ventilation-perfusion study without contrast media in dynamic chest radiography. In: Proceedings of SPIE, medical imaging, The International Society for optical engineering, vol 7965, pp 79651Y1–79651Y17
42. Tsuchiya Y, Kodera Y, Tanaka R, Sanada S (2009) Quantitative kinetic analysis of lung nodules using the temporal subtraction technique in dynamic chest radiographies performed with a flat panel detector. J Digit Imaging 22:126–135

Chapter 13
Adaptive Noise Reduction and Edge Enhancement in Medical Images by Using ICA

Xian-Hua Han and Yen-Wei Chen

Abstract This chapter focuses on the development of novel image enhancement and robust edge detection methods for practical medical image processing. It is known that the popular transformation-domain shrinkage approach for image enhancement applies a fixed mathematical basis to transform all images to be processed for noise or artifact reduction. However it is not adaptable to processed images, and then easily leads to blurring in the enhanced images. On the other hand, the techniques that are commonly used for edge detection are known as gradient and Laplacian operators (or mask), and smoothed gradient masks are typically used for edge detection in noisy images. However, these methods share a common major drawback wherein the associated masks are always fixed irrespective of the noise level in the images. In this study, we propose a novel learning-based method to adaptively deduce the transforming basis or masks from the processing data for medical image enhancement and robust edge detection. By using independent component analysis (ICA), the proposed learning-based method can extract suitable basis functions or masks for image transformation for processing data, which are adaptable to both the processed image and related noise in the image. The efficiency of the proposed learning-based method for medical image enhancement and edge detection is demonstrated experimentally using positron emission tomography (PET) and magnetic resonance imaging (MRI) medical images.

Introduction

Medical imaging techniques such as positron emission tomography (PET), magnetic resonance imaging (MRI), and computed tomography (CT) provide detailed 3D images of internal organs. The desired information such as the internal organ

X.-H. Han • Y.-W. Chen (✉)
Ritsumeikan University, 1-1-1, Nojihigashi, Kusatsu, Japan
e-mail: chen@is.ritsumei.ac.jp

K. Suzuki (ed.), *Computational Intelligence in Biomedical Imaging*,
DOI 10.1007/978-1-4614-7245-2_13,

structure and shape can be extracted from these images for supporting several medical procedures such as disease diagnosis and surgical planning [1–3]. However, it is difficult to identify different tissues and anatomical structures from the obtained 3D computer-aided diagnosis (CAD) data because of low signal-to-noise or contrast-to-noise ratios [4–6]. In order to accurately extract useful information, image enhancement, which is normally implemented using low-pass filters and transformation-domain shrinkage approaches with fixed basis functions such as a Fourier and wavelet basis, is usually applied to improve the quality of the degraded medical image. In addition, various segmentation techniques, where the extraction or tracking of medical image edges plays a key role, are used to identify the anatomical structure. Recent studies [7–10] have proposed a supervised filter using a neural network to enhance specific structures in medical images, which can realize acceptable performance in emphasizing specific lesions or structures. However, the neural-network-based filter has to first prepare a large amount of training data, which will greatly affect the performance of experimental results, and thus its generalization to real applications. Therefore, this chapter focuses on the development of novel image enhancement and robust edge detection methods for practical medical image processing by using an unsupervised strategy.

As mentioned above, the popular transformation-domain shrinkage approach for image enhancement applies a fixed mathematical basis to transform all processing images for noise or artifact reduction. However, it is not adaptable to the processed images, and then easily leads to blurring in the enhanced images. On the other hand, the techniques that are commonly used for edge detection are known as gradient and Laplacian operators (or mask), and smoothed gradient masks such as Prewitt, Sobel, or Canny are typically used to detect edges in noisy images [11–13]. However, these methods share a common major drawback wherein the associated masks are always fixed irrespective of the noise level in the images. Therefore, in this chapter, we propose a novel learning-based method to adaptively deduce the transforming basis or masks by using a statistical analysis method called independent component analysis (ICA) from the processing data for medical image enhancement and robust edge detection.

ICA [14–17] is a method to find a linear nonorthogonal coordinate system in any multivariate data. The directions of the axes in this ICA coordinate system are determined by not only the second but also higher order statistics of the original data, unlike the principle component analysis (PCA), which considers only the second order statistics and can only deal with the variables that have Gaussian distributions. In computer vision, it is more preferable to extract the source signals produced by independent causes or obtained from different sensors; such signals are easily solved using ICA. This study attempts to decompose a local structure (local patch) of images into a linear combination of an independent basis set, which can be adaptively learned from processing images using ICA. By performing a statistical analysis of ICA, the suitable basis functions or masks for image transformation can be achieved from the processing data, which are adaptable to both the processed image and related noise in the image. Most of the learned basis functions that are obtained by ICA from the images are sparse and similar to localized and oriented receptive fields [18–20]. Similar to transformation-domain shrinkage method, the intensities (components or noisy components) in the transformed domain obtained using the learned ICA basis are either shrunk or removed to enhance image quality; this is called an ICA-domain shrinkage filter [21, 22]. Furthermore, in order to determine the corresponding basis for edge representation, the L p norm is used to estimate the sparseness of the ICA basis functions, and the sparser basis functions were then selected to represent the edge information of an image [23, 24]. In the proposed edge detection method, a test image is first transformed using ICA basis functions, and the high-frequency information can then be extracted with the components of the selected sparse basis functions. In addition, by applying the proposed ICA-domain shrinkage algorithm to filter out the noisy components of ICA, we can readily obtain the sparse components of the noise-free image, thus resulting in a type of robust edge detection, even for a noisy image with a very low signal-to-noise ratio (SNR). The efficiency of the proposed learning-based method for medical image enhancement and edge detection is demonstrated experimentally using PET-CT medical images.

The chapter is organized as follows. In section "Independent Component Analysis and the Image Model", we introduce the basic algorithm of ICA and the image representation model using ICA. Section "Adaptive Noise Reduction for PET Images" explores the shrinkage method for adaptive noise reductions in PET images, and section "Robust Edge Enhancement for Medical Images" discusses a robust edge detection strategy in noisy medical images. The conclusions are summarized in section "Conclusions".

Independent Component Analysis and the Image Model

Basic Concept of Independent Component Analysis

ICA generalizes the technique of PCA and has been shown to be an effective tool for feature extraction [18, 19]. The aim is to express a set of random variables as linear combinations of statistically independent component variables. In the simplest model of ICA, we observe n scalar random variables $x_1, x_2, \cdots, x_n$, which are linear combinations of $k (k \leq n)$ unknown independent sources $s_1, s_2, \cdots, s_k$. We arrange the random variables into a vector $\mathbf{x} = (x_1, x_2, \cdots, x_n)$ and the sources into a vector $\mathbf{s} = (s_1, s_2, \cdots, s_k)$; then, the linear relationship is given by

$$\mathbf{x} = \mathbf{A}\mathbf{s} \tag{13.1}$$

where $\mathbf{A}$ is an unknown mixing matrix. In the application of ICA to feature extraction, the columns of $\mathbf{A}$ represent the basis functions and s_i represent the i-th feature in the observed data $\mathbf{x}$. The aim of ICA is to find a matrix $\mathbf{W}$, such that the resulting vector

$$\mathbf{y} = \mathbf{W}\mathbf{x} \tag{13.2}$$

recovers the independent sources **s**, with its probability permuted and rescaled. Each row of **W** is taken as a filter. To obtain a more unique solution, s_i is usually assumed to have unit variance.

Contrary to PCA, the basis functions of ICA cannot be analytically calculated. The adopted method involves minimizing or maximizing some relevant criterion functions. Several ICA algorithms have been proposed, one of which and its detail implementation will be introduced in section "Basis Functions Learned by ICA".

Before performing ICA, the problem associated with estimating the matrix **A** can be simplified by a prewhitening of the data **x**. The observed vector **x** is first linearly transformed into a vector

$$\mathbf{z} = \mathbf{M}\mathbf{x} \tag{13.3}$$

whose correlation matrix equals unity: $E\{\mathbf{z}\mathbf{z}^T\} = \mathbf{I}$. This can be accomplished by PCA with

$$\mathbf{M} = \mathbf{D}^{-1/2}\mathbf{V} \tag{13.4}$$

where the matrix **V** is the eigenvector matrix and D is the corresponding eigenvalue matrix. At the same time, the dimensionality of the data is reduced. After this transformation, we have

$$\mathbf{z} = \mathbf{M}\mathbf{x} = \mathbf{M}\mathbf{A}\mathbf{s} = \mathbf{B}\mathbf{s} \tag{13.5}$$

where the matrix **B** is the mixing matrix. ICA is performed on the sphered data **z** and the estimated mixing matrix **B** is an orthogonal matrix because $E\{\mathbf{z}\mathbf{z}^T\} = \mathbf{B}E\{\mathbf{s}\mathbf{s}^T\}\mathbf{B}^T = \mathbf{B}\mathbf{B}^T = \mathbf{I}$. The basis function matrix **A** of the original data **x** is

$$\mathbf{A} = \mathbf{V}^T\mathbf{D}^{1/2}\mathbf{B} \tag{13.6}$$

Figure 13.1 presents an example of two non-Gaussian (super-Gaussian) distributed sources (Fig. 13.1a) and the scatter (Fig. 13.1b) of their mixed variables. The basis functions obtained by PCA and ICA are also plotted in Fig. 13.1b, which confirms that PCA transformation cannot capture the main structure of non-Gaussian data. However, ICA can precisely determine the directions of the inherent data structure by maximizing independence.

Image Model

An image patch **x** from an image **I** can be represented by a linear combination of basis functions as in (13.7), where $\mathbf{A}_i$ (size: N' by 1, N' is the dimension of **x**) is the

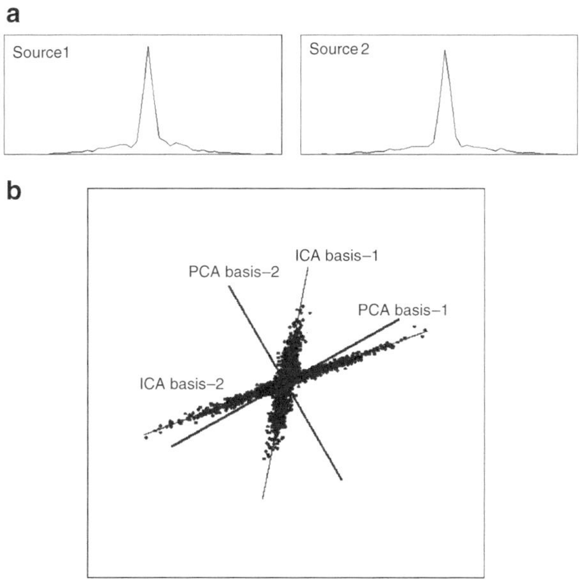

Fig. 13.1 PCA and ICA transformations. (**a**) two components of super-Gaussian data, (**b**) the scatter of the data, and the obtained ICA and PCA basis functions of (**a**)

ith basis function and y_i are the coefficients, which can be used as image features or image coding. Unlike the Fourier transform or wavelet-based methods, in our proposed ICA-based method, the basis functions are learned by ICA from similar structure images with processing images. The advantage of ICA-based method is that we can obtain a set of adaptive basis functions based on images alone.

$$\mathbf{x} = \mathbf{A}\mathbf{y} = \sum_{i=0}^{N-1} \mathbf{A}_i y_i = \mathbf{A}_0 y_0 + \mathbf{A}_1 y_1 + \mathbf{A}_2 y_2 + \cdots + \mathbf{A}_{N-1} y_{N-1} \tag{13.7}$$

Basis Functions Learned by ICA

In (13.7), we attempt to obtain **A** using ICA (size: N' by N, N is the number of ICA basis functions. In our experiments, we retained N' basis functions in ICA learning: i.e., N'=N)) from sample image **x** only, which can also be viewed as a Blind Source Separation (BSS) problem, and can be solved by ICA [10]. The aim of BSS is to find a matrix **W**, called a separator, that results in the estimates of the coefficients of **y** to be as statistically independent as possible for a set of data (**x**), as shown in (13.2)

$$\mathbf{y} = \mathbf{W}\mathbf{x} \tag{13.8}$$

The estimates or independent components $\mathbf{y}$ may be permuted and rescaled. The ICA transformation matrix $\mathbf{W}$ (size: N by N) can be calculated as: $\mathbf{W}=\mathbf{A}^{-1}$. For the reasons given in [18], we orthogonalize $\mathbf{W}$ by $\mathbf{W} = \mathbf{W}(\mathbf{W}^T\mathbf{W})^{-1/2}$, and $\mathbf{A}$ and $\mathbf{W}$ then become square unitary matrices with each row corresponding to a basis function (amounting to a column of mixed matrix $\mathbf{A}$ under the condition of orthogonalized $\mathbf{W}$. In our method, we need to reconstruct images, hence the basis that is used should be orthogonalized and integrated as with the Fourier and wavelet basis).

Bell and Sejnowski proposed a neural learning algorithm for ICA [14, 15]. This approach employs the maximization of the joint entropy by using a stochastic gradient ascent. The updating formula for $\mathbf{W}$ is

$$\Delta\mathbf{W} = (\mathbf{I} + g(\mathbf{y})\mathbf{y}^T)\mathbf{W}, \tag{13.9}$$

where $\mathbf{y} = \mathbf{W}\,\mathbf{x}$ and $g(\mathbf{y}) = \mathbf{1} - \mathbf{2}/(\mathbf{1} + e^{-\mathbf{y}})$ is calculated for each component of $\mathbf{y}$. Before the learning procedure, $\mathbf{x}$ is sphered by subtracting the mean and multiplying by a whitening filter $\mathbf{W}_0 = [(\mathbf{x} - E(\mathbf{x}))(\mathbf{x} - E(\mathbf{x}))^T]^{-1/2}$:

$$\mathbf{x}_0 = \mathbf{W}_0(\mathbf{x} - E(\mathbf{x})), \tag{13.10}$$

where $\mathbf{x}_0$ the whitening data. The aim of the whitening (standardization) by using $\mathbf{W}_0$ is to make the mixture and separator unitary. Therefore, the complete transform is calculated as the product of the whitening matrix and learned matrix:

$$\mathbf{W}_I = \mathbf{W}\mathbf{W}_0. \tag{13.11}$$

To extract the adaptive basis functions by using ICA for image representation, we have to prepare training samples using images that are similar to processed data. In our experiment, more than 10,000 image patches are usually randomly selected as training data samples, which from our experience will be sufficient to obtain reliable basis functions of training images. At the same time, it will not be sufficient for learning over a long time period. The learned ICA basis functions by using natural images are shown in Fig. 13.2. The patch size of each image sample is set as 8×8 and an example regarding the formation of the observation vectors from images is shown in Fig. 13.3.

Adaptive Noise Reduction for PET Images

PET is one of the most important tools for medical diagnostics that has been recently developed. Projection data in PET are acquired as the number of photon counts from different observation angles [13, 25]. Positron decay is a random phenomenon that causes undesirable high variations in measured sinograms, which appear as quantum noise [26]. The reduction of quantum noise or Poisson

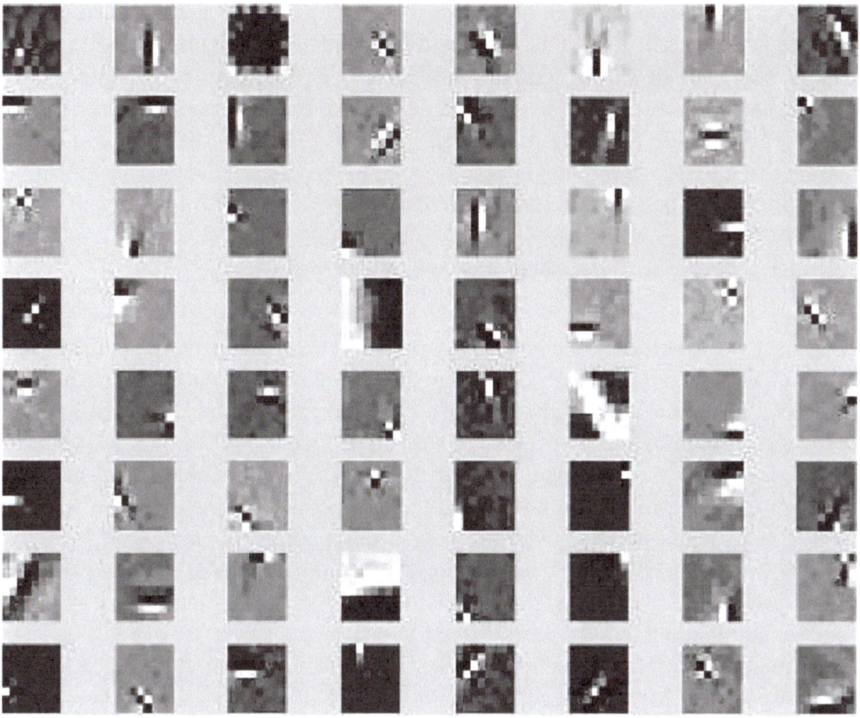

Fig. 13.2 The ICA basis functions obtained using natural images as training samples

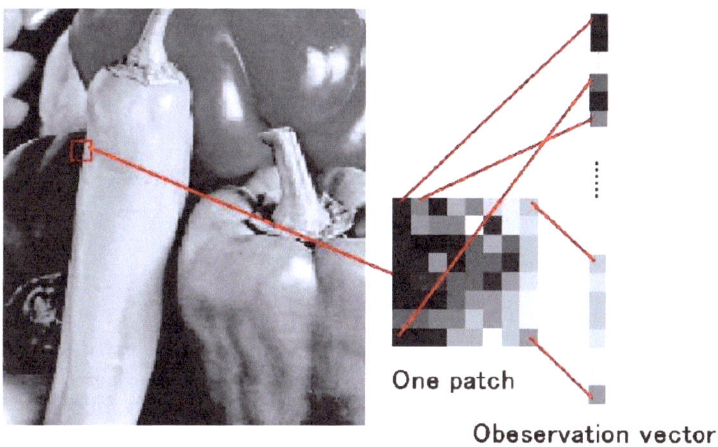

Fig. 13.3 The ICA input observation vector obtained from one sample patch

noise in medical images is an important issue because the quantum noise usually obeys a Poisson law; therefore, it is highly dependent on the underlying intensity pattern being imaged. The contaminated image can therefore be decomposed as the true mean intensity and Poisson noise, and the noise represents the variability of the pixel amplitude about the true mean intensity [27]. It is well known that the variance of a Poisson random variable is equal to the mean: $\sigma^2 = u$. Then, the SNR for an image with a Poisson image is given by

$$SNR = \frac{u}{\sigma} = \frac{u}{\sqrt{\sigma^2}} = \frac{u}{\sqrt{u}} = \sqrt{u} \tag{13.12}$$

Thus, the variability of the noise is proportional to the intensity of the image and is therefore signal dependent [23]. This signal dependence makes it much more difficult to separate the signal from noise. The current methods for Poisson noise reduction include mainly two types of strategies. One would be to work with the square root of a noisy image because the square root operation is a variance stabilizing transformation. However, after preprocessing, Poisson noise will not tend to be a white noise if there are only a few photons present. Thus, it is not entirely suitable to adopt the Gaussian noise reduction algorithm. The other strategy is the method of wavelet shrinkage. However, the basic functions of wavelet transformation are fixed and cannot adapt to different types of sets. In this chapter, we explain the development of an adaptive noise reduction strategy called the ICA-based filter, in the sinogram domain for PET. The shrinkage scheme (filter) adapts to both signal and noise and balances the trade-off between noise removal and excessive smoothing of image details. The filtering procedure has a simple interpretation as a joint edge detection/estimation process. Our method is closely related to the method of wavelet shrinkage; however, compared with other wavelet methods, it has an important benefit that the representation is solely determined by the statistical properties of the data sets. Therefore, ICA-based methods will perform better than the wavelet-based Poisson noise reduction method in denoising applications. At the same time, we also compared the denoising results of different ICA basis functions that are trained from different data sets.

ICA-Based Shrinkage Algorithm

Shrinkage is an increasingly popular method in the wavelet domain for curve and surface estimation. The wavelet shrinkage procedure for statistical applications was developed by Donoho [28]. This shrinkage method relies on the basic idea that the energy of a signal (that is partially smoothed) will often be concentrated within a few coefficients in the wavelet domain, whereas the noise energy is spread among all coefficients. Therefore, the shrinkage function in the wavelet domain will tend to retain a few larger coefficients that represent the signal, whereas the noise coefficients will tend to reduce to zero.

In image decomposition by using ICA, the extracted basis functions represent different properties of training images and those representing clear image information will be almost sparse [21]. Thus, the energy of clear image information will be concentrated in a few coefficients of the ICA components. However, if noise is projected to the ICA basis functions, the energy will uniformly spread in the ICA domain. Hence using the shrinkage method in the ICA domain, we can remove noise in a similar manner as in the wavelet shrinkage procedure.

We assume that an observe an n-dimensional vector is contaminated by noise. We denote the observed noisy vector as $\mathbf{x}$, the original non-Gaussian vector as $\mathbf{P}$, and the noise signal as $\mathbf{v}$. We then have

$$\mathbf{x} = \mathbf{P} + \mathbf{v} \tag{13.13}$$

The goal of signal denoising is to find $\mathbf{P}^{'} = g^{'}(\mathbf{x})$ such that $\mathbf{P}^{'}$ is close to $\mathbf{P}$ in some well-defined sense. The following gives the ICA-based shrinkage procedure:

Step 1 Estimate an orthogonal ICA transformation matrix $\mathbf{W}$ by using the training data (the observed data $\mathbf{x}$ or a set of representative data $\mathbf{z}$).

Step 2 For the observed data $\mathbf{x}$ (corrupted by noise), use the ICA transformation matrix $\mathbf{W}$ to transform into ICA-domain components:

$$\mathbf{y} = \mathbf{W}\mathbf{x} \tag{13.14}$$

where $\mathbf{y}$ can be considered to be a sparse variable, which is also corrupted by noise.

Step 3 Use the ICA-based shrinkage method to estimate noise-free components $\mathbf{y}^{'}$ for the noisy variable $\mathbf{y}$:

$$\mathbf{y}_i^{'} = g_i(\mathbf{y}_i) \tag{13.15}$$

Step 4 Invert the denoised variable $\mathbf{y}^{'}$ and get an estimation of original data $\mathbf{P}$:

$$\mathbf{P}^{'} = \mathbf{A}\mathbf{y}^{'} \tag{13.16}$$

where $\mathbf{A} = [\mathbf{A}_0, \mathbf{A}_1, \cdots, \mathbf{A}_{N-1}] = [\mathbf{W}_0^T, \mathbf{W}_1^T, \cdots, \mathbf{W}_{N-1}^T]^T$ are the ICA basis functions.

In step (3), g(y) is the operator or function of the shrinkage and is used to reduce the noise. In PET images, the noise is signal-dependent Poisson noise; hence, we mainly aim to reduce Poisson noise in the images. In the next subsection, based on Poisson noise's special property, we present an efficient shrinkage scheme with the adaptive ICA basis functions, which can be obtained directly from noisy data, as shown in Fig. 13.4 for PET images. In addition, we select some clean natural images and processed data (observed data) as the training data to estimate the ICA basis functions, and then apply two sets of the ICA basis functions (as shown in

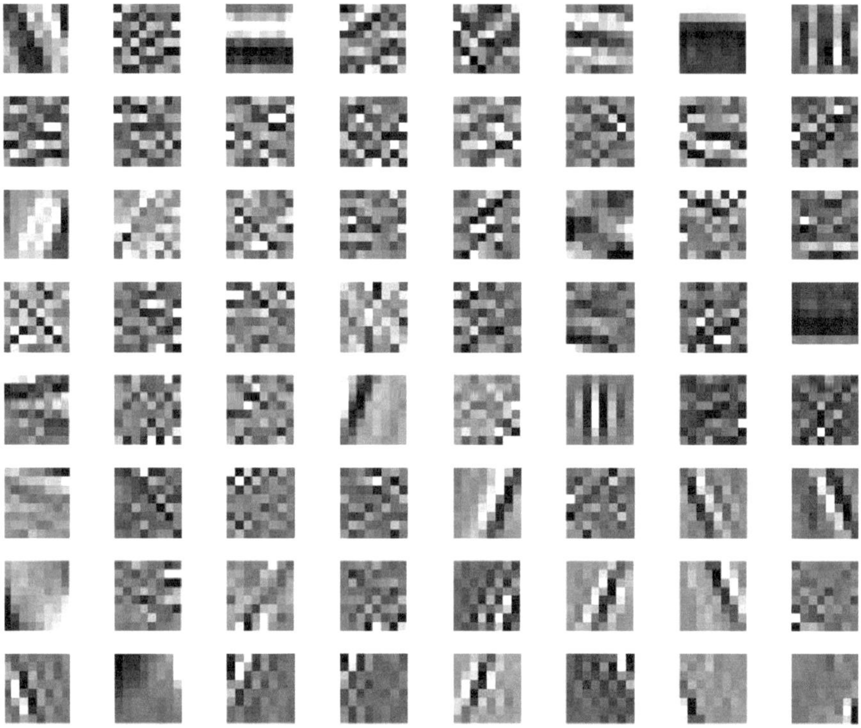

Fig. 13.4 The ICA basis functions obtained using actual PET images as training samples

Fig. 13.2) to the denoising procedure for comparison purposes. The flowchart of the ICA-based filter for actual PET sinograms is shown in Fig. 13.5.

ICA Based Filter for Poisson Noise

In our previous work [17, 18], we proposed a shrinkage function based on the cross-validation algorithm [14] for Poisson noise. The shrinkage function $g(\mathbf{y})$ is given by [17]

$$g(\mathbf{y}) = \mathbf{y}' = \mathbf{y}\frac{\mathbf{y}^2 - \sigma^2}{\mathbf{y}^2} \tag{13.17}$$

where σ^2 is the power of Poisson noise. The noise power of the ith component with ICA basis functions trained from clean natural images can be estimated by [20]

$$\sigma_i^2 = (\mathbf{W}_i.*\mathbf{W}_i)\mathbf{x} \tag{13.18}$$

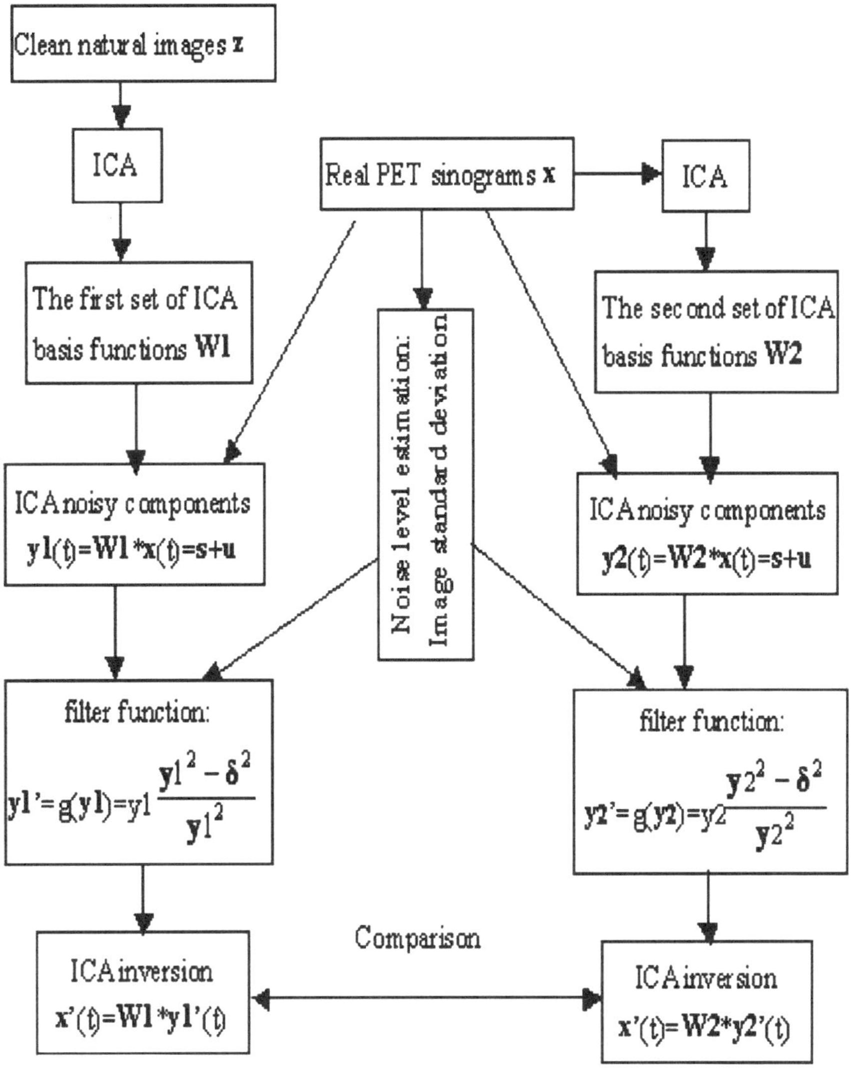

Fig. 13.5 Flowchart of the ICA-based noise reduction strategy using two sets of learned basis functions from natural and PET images, respectively

where the symbol of ".*" represents the multiplication of each entry in vector 1 with its corresponding entry in vector 2, $\mathbf{W}_i$ is the ith row of the ICA transformation matrix $\mathbf{W}$(the ith ICA basis function), and σ_i^2 represents the ith noisy power component in the ICA domain(a row of samples). For clean natural images as the training set, the obtained ICA transform matrix $\mathbf{W}$ can be considered as a local directional filters. The components obtained by ICA transformation would then be the inner product of the image patch and local filters $\mathbf{W}_i$(which is needed to reshape the row vector $\mathbf{W}_i$ into an $l * l$ patch), which is a localized edge or "details." The noise power estimate σ_i^2 equals the projection on the square of the local filters $\mathbf{W}_i$(the ith row of the ICA transformation matrix vector, as in the case of the wavelet basis function [20]), which effectively computes a weighted average of the local intensity in the image. This value will be an approximation of the noise power according to the property of Poisson noise. It is clear that the noise power estimate can adapt to local variations in the signal or noise. However, for the processed PET sinograms that are as training data, only a subset of the estimated ICA basis functions are localized and oriented, whereas the other basis functions appear to be noisy. The noise power estimation mentioned above is not suitable for this set of basis functions. For this type of basis functions, we therefore select a patch of flat ranges in the observed image to estimate their variance as the noise power. This is similar to the estimation of the noise power for small size images. Figure 13.5 shows the process of the ICA-domain shrinkage method.

The above shrinkage function simply weights each noisy ICA coefficient $y(i, j)$ by a factor that is equal to the estimated signal power divided by the estimated signal-plus-noise power. If the ratio of the estimated signal power to the signal-plus-noise power is negative, the shrinkage function just thresholds the ICA-domain coefficients to zero. Hence, this optimal shrinkage function has a very simple interpretation as a data-adaptive ICA-domain Wiener filter.

Experiment Results for Noise Reduction

In this subsection, we apply two sets of the ICA basis functions (the training data are clean natural images and actual PET sinograms, respectively) to the ICA-based filter for actual PET sinograms. The actual PET sinograms were supplied by Shimatsu Corporation of Japan and include 1269 128*128 sinograms scanned from the waist to the head for three persons. For actual PET sinograms, the training data sets include 251 sinograms from all (1269) PET sinograms. We then randomly select 50,000 samples from different sinograms as the ICA input variables.

In our experiments, we used Tony Bell and T.J. Sejnowski's infomax algorithm to learn the ICA transformation matrix $\mathbf{W}$ [14], and 8*8 subwindows were randomly sampled from the training data sets. These subwindows were presented as 64-dimensional vectors. The DC value was removed from each vector as a processing step. The infomax algorithm was performed on these vectors to obtain the transformation matrix $\mathbf{W}$. For the reason given in [18], we orthogonalize $\mathbf{W}$ by

$$\mathbf{W} = \mathbf{W}(\mathbf{W}^T\mathbf{W})^{-1/2} \tag{13.19}$$

After ICA transformation, the denoising algorithm was applied on each subwindow in the image and 64 constructions were obtained for each pixel. The

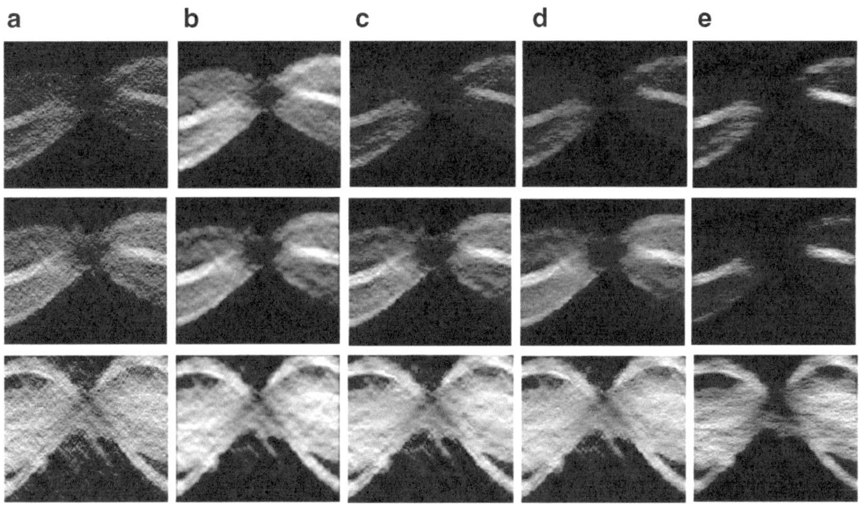

Fig. 13.6 (**a**) The actual PET sinograms, (**b**) denoised images using Gaussian filter, (**c**) denoised images using wavelet shrinkage, (**d**) denoised images using ICA-based filter with natural basis functions, (**e**) denoised images using ICA-based filter with PET basis functions

final result was the mean of these reconstructions. The experimental results are shown in Figs. 13.6 and 13.7. Figure 13.6a represents three actual PET sinograms, Fig. 13.6b shows the denoised images from the Gaussian filter, Fig. 13.6c shows the denoised images from wavelet-domain shrinkage, and Fig. 13.6d, e show the denoised images from the ICA filter with two sets of the ICA basis functions. From Fig. 13.6, it can be seen that the denoised images obtained using our proposed method with the adaptive ICA basis functions (with actual PET sinograms as the training data) can remove all background noise and retain clean information. The original noisy PET images in Fig. 13.6a not only include the random noise (without any structure) but also include the structural noise such as the netlike one which is usually led by the imaging device. Our goal is to reduce not only the random noise but also the structural noise for showing some detail information in reconstructed body images. From Fig. 13.6b, c, the conventional Gaussian and Wavelet-domain filter can reduce most of the random noise but with some blurring in edge regions. However, the netlike noise almost is left. In the other hand, the ICA-based method with the natural basis functions, which is extracted from generic natural images and possibly not adaptive to the processed PET data, can remove not only the random noise without blurring edge region but also a part of netlike noise as shown in Fig. 13.6d. Furthermore, the proposed method with the adaptive ICA basis functions can remove all types of noise with very clean contrast especially for the high-noise level images as shown in Fig. 13.6e. From the experimental results in Fig. 13.6, we can conclude that the ICA-based denoising method usually can

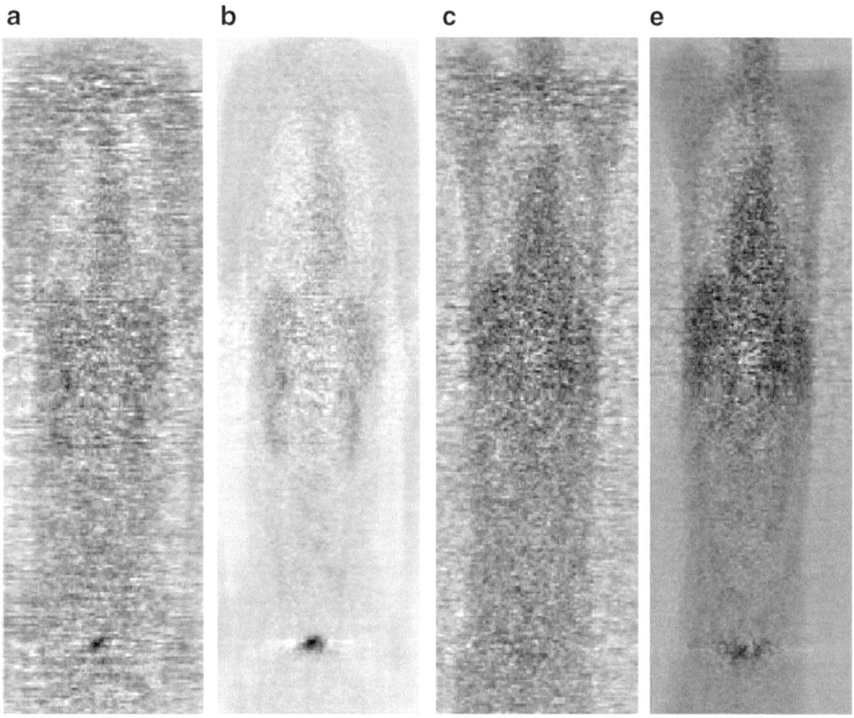

Fig. 13.7 Reconstructed images, (**a**) and (**c**) by using noisy PET images; (**b**) and (**d**) by using denoised PET images with our proposed method. (The displayed body of (**a**) and (**b**) are at the same position; (**c**) and (**d**) are at the same position)

achieve much cleaner and sharper denoised images than the conventional Gaussian and Wavelet-domain filters, and utility of adaptive ICA basis function in the proposed method, which is prospect to learn the specific noise structure in the processed data, can achieve better performance than the learned ones from other data set. Therefore, it can be suggested the suitable basis function is best to be learned from the processed data, which is prospected to learn the detail structure and specific noise structure in the data. In addition, to validate the efficiency of the proposed ICA-based filter, we use the Filtered back-projection (FBP) algorithm to reconstruct body images from sinogram images. The reconstructed results are shown in Fig. 13.7, where we observe that the reconstructed denoised images obtained using the proposed ICA filter remove most of the noise and have a better contrast compared with that of noisy PET images.

Robust Edge Enhancement for Medical Images

Edge detection methods are fundamental to computer vision because they often exist at the first stage of a lengthy image interpretation process. The aim of edge detection is to locate the pixels in the image that correspond with the edges of the objects seen in the image. In medical images, image segmentation is an important issue and the accurate extraction or tracking of medical image edges plays a key role in the active area of medical image segmentation [29, 30]. However, in medical images, distinct boundaries may not exist between the structures to enable the edge detection of organ boundaries because of the similarities between these structures and the presence of noise. Furthermore, the boundaries may be blurred and ambiguous due to partial volume effects, which are caused by the finite resolution of imaging devices. These problems increase the complexity for the segmentation of neighboring structures. In a related research field, gradient masks (or smoothed gradient masks) [11, 12], such as Prewitt, Sobel, or Canny, are typically used for edge detection in noisy images. These methods share a major drawback wherein the associated masks are always fixed irrespective of the noise levels in the images. As a result, the performance of these operators considerably degrades as the noise level increases. This study proposes a robust algorithm for edge detection in noisy medical images by using ICA.

In the proposed robust edge detection strategy, we first need to learn the adaptive ICA basis functions by using images that are similar to processing data. In this subsection, we mainly extract the edge information for the simulated MRI volumes of the brain, which is obtained from the web site (http://www.bic.mni.mcgill.ca/brainweb/selection-normal.html). The parameters describing the database set are Modality=T1, Protocol=ICBM, Phantom_name =normal, Slice_thickness = 3 mm, Noise = 0 %, INU = 20 % (please refer to the BrainWeb homepage for detailed information). Twenty slices of the simulated MRI volumes are selected for composition of the training data, and 11,880 sample patches are then picked up as the input ICA data. The size of patches of each image sample in both training data sets is also set as 8×8. With the prepared training patches, the ICA basis functions can be obtained using the algorithm introduced in the above section, as shown in Fig. 13.8.

In image decomposition using ICA, most independent components have a super-Gaussian distribution and the corresponding basis functions are very sparse and similar to localized and oriented-like receptive fields in the mammalian visual cortex [14, 31]. It is interesting to note that local oriented receptive fields that are similar to the Gaussian derivatives as well as receptive fields that are similar to the Laplacian are found in the human visual cortex. In the proposed ICA-based edge detection method, the target image is first transformed by the ICA basis functions and the edges are then detected or reconstructed with only the sparse basis. However, as shown in Fig. 13.8, not all basis functions are localized and oriented, and some of them clearly show average and low-pass properties. By using all basis functions, we can perfectly reconstruct the original image if we can obtain the

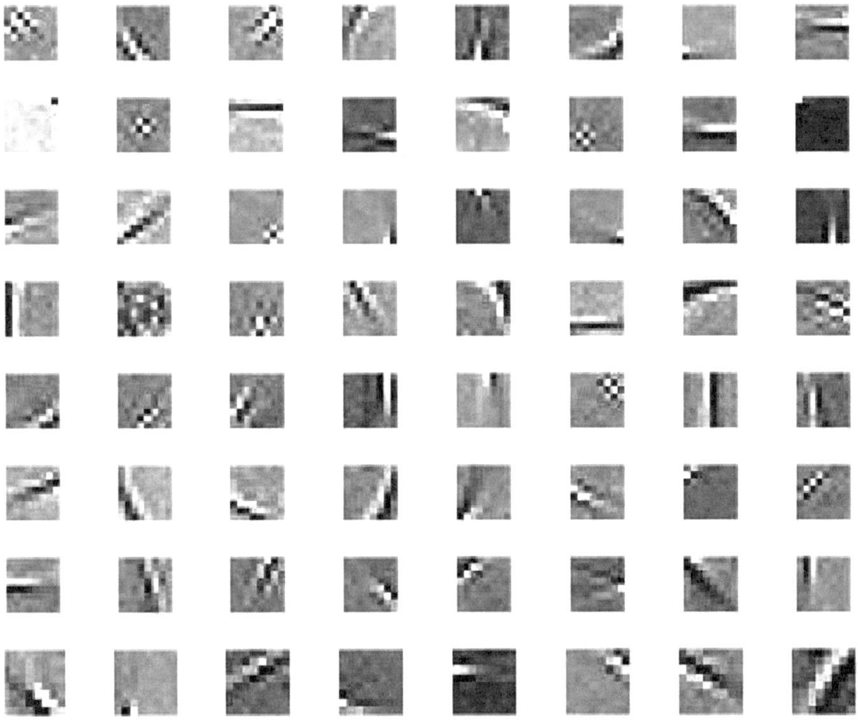

Fig. 13.8 The ICA basis functions obtained from the simulated MRI brain volume

corresponding weighting of the basis functions. Therefore, these basis functions are certain to include the low-frequency region of the image. To represent the edge part of the image with the basis functions, it is necessary to select a subset of them. In the next subsection, we introduce a selection strategy for the sparse basis functions used for edge representation.

Basis Function Selection for Edge Representation

As shown in section "Adaptive Noise Reduction for PET Images", an image patch can be formed by a linear transformation of N basis functions. Because the edges correspond to the sparse components, edge detection can be conducted by carefully choosing the sparse components by excluding the nonsparse basis. Here we use the l^p norm [32] of a basis function as a measure of its sparseness [33], that is

$$||\mathbf{A}_i|| = \left(\sum_{j=0}^{N-1} (|A_{ji}|)^p \right)^{1/p}, \quad \text{with} \quad p < 1 \tag{13.20}$$

where $\mathbf{A}_i$ ($i = 0,1,2,3,\cdots, N-1$) is the ith basis function, and A_{ji} is the jth coefficient of the ith basis function (each basis function has N coefficients). For smaller magnitudes $||\mathbf{A}_i||$, the basis function becomes sparser. If $||\mathbf{A}_i||=0$, the vector $\mathbf{A}_i$ is completely sparse.

To simplify the selection of the sparse components, we rearrange the basis functions according to their sparseness (13.20). Figure 13.9a, b show the rearranged natural and medical basis functions in increasing order of sparseness from Figs. 13.2 and 13.8. As shown in Fig. 13.9, the first few basis functions (at the top left side) appear to be nonsparse, which may represent flat or low-frequency regions of the image. Figure 13.10 shows the sparseness measure magnitude of all 64 basis functions ordered from left to right and top to bottom (here $p = 0.\ 1$, p is the power of the L^p norm). Subjectively observing the two sets of the basis functions in Fig. 13.9, and excluding the first few nonsparse components, we can easily detect or reconstruct the edge image using the sparse components. Figure 13.11 shows three examples of the basis functions and their corresponding images. Figure 13.11a represents the original test image; Fig. 13.11b shows nonsparse basis functions and their reconstructed image only with the basis functions; and Fig. 13.11c, d show two sparse basis functions with different locations and orientations, and their reconstructed images and binary images with simple threshold method. Figure 13.12a, b show the amplitude spatial diagram and 2D contour plot of the ICA natural basis functions (in the same sequence as Fig. 13.9a), respectively. It is observed in Fig. 13.12a that only the value of all elements in the first basis function is positive and have similar intensities (corresponding with the parent wavelet in the wavelet transform). However, the value of other basis elements are varied and may be larger or smaller than zero in a local range; the value of the other place is nearly zero (corresponding to band-pass or high-pass wavelet). They will therefore represent the edge information in images. Based on the integrality and orthogonalization of the basis functions, we can perfectly reconstruct the original image by using all basis functions. In order to represent the edge part of the image with the basis functions, it is necessary to select a subset of them.

The edge image can be reconstructed as

$$\mathbf{Edge}_m = \sum_{i=m}^{N-1} \mathbf{A}_{\beta(i)} y_{\beta(i)} = \mathbf{A}_{\beta(m)} y_{\beta(m)} + \cdots + \mathbf{A}_{\beta(N-1)} y_{\beta(N-1)},\ m \geq 1, \qquad (13.21)$$

where $N - 1 - m + 1$ basis functions are considered to be sufficiently sparse; $\beta i)$ is a permutation of $(0, 1, 2, \cdots, N-1)$. $\mathbf{A}_{\beta(1)}$ is the least sparse basis function and $\mathbf{A}_{\beta(N-1)}$ is the most sparse basis function, i.e., the basis functions were sorted in terms of their sparseness. It should be noted that if $m = 0$, all components are used for image representation resulting in a perfect image reconstruction.

Next, we validate the proposition by a natural image using natural basis functions. Figure 13.13 shows an image representation of all basis functions ($\mathbf{x} = \sum_{i=0}^{N-1} y_i \mathbf{A}_i$) and edge representations of selected sparse basis functions ($\mathbf{edge}_m = \sum_{i=m}^{N-1} y_i \mathbf{A}_i, m > 1$) for a natural sample image. As shown in Fig. 13.13a, we were a

b

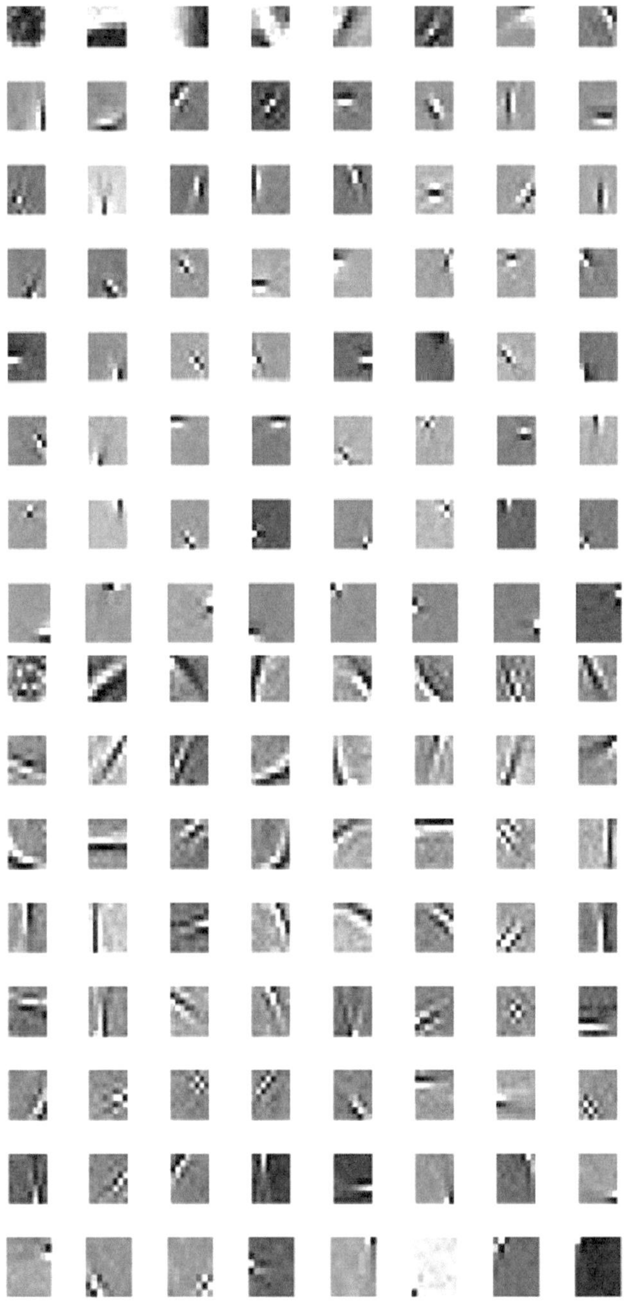

Fig. 13.9 (**a**) Natural basis functions arranged according to sparseness, (**b**) Medical basis functions arranged according to sparseness

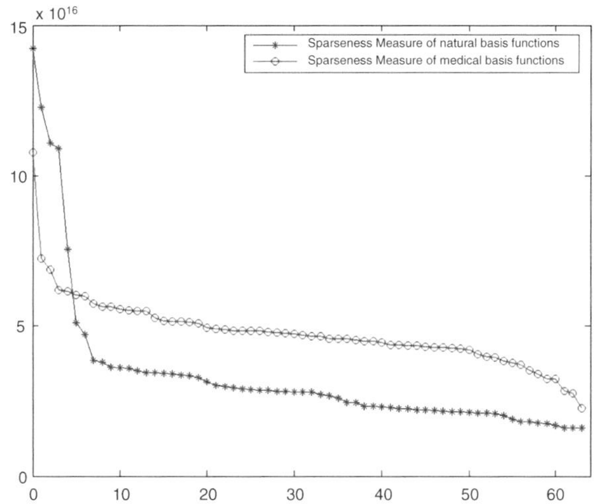

Fig. 13.10 Sparseness vs the number of basis functions

able to perfectly reconstruct or represent the original image by using all basis functions; however, we can also easily obtain edges by excluding the first few nonsparse components (Fig. 13.13b, c). Here the corresponding weighting coefficients of the selected basis functions are required and are given by solving the BSS problem.

In addition, from Fig. 13.9, it is observed that the first basis function of both sets of the basis functions are nonsparse; moreover, the larger the number of basis functions in Fig. 13.9, the sparser the basis functions (see the sparseness measure in Fig. 13.10). We therefore need to determine the smallest number that mainly represents high-frequency information (such as an edge, because an edge appears at the local variation positions and the local variation at the spatial domain will appear at the high-frequency position in the frequency domain). Subsequently, all basis functions after the basis function of the smallest number will mainly represent edge information. It can be shown from Fig. 13.9 that the few selected basis functions from the second basis function for both sets are not very sparse. To determine the suitability of the basis functions for reconstructing the image edges, we conducted experiments by using a single natural basis function to represent a natural image. Here we used the 2nd to 5th basis functions to reconstruct the image. The experimental results are shown in Fig. 13.13d–g. It is apparent that the image resulting from the 2nd basis function has long horizontal edges, the one from the 3rd basis function has long vertical edges, and the images from the 4th and 5th basis functions have the diagonal edges. The resultant images consist of rich edges. To provide numerical and theoretical selection criteria, we calculated the integral area of the amplitude frequency diagram of the ICA basis functions in different regions (low-frequency and high-frequency position). The partition of different frequency regions in the frequency domain is shown in Fig. 13.14a. We denote the frequency amplitude of an ICA basis functions (8×8) as $F(i,j)$ ($i, j=0,1,\ldots,7$). Then the integral

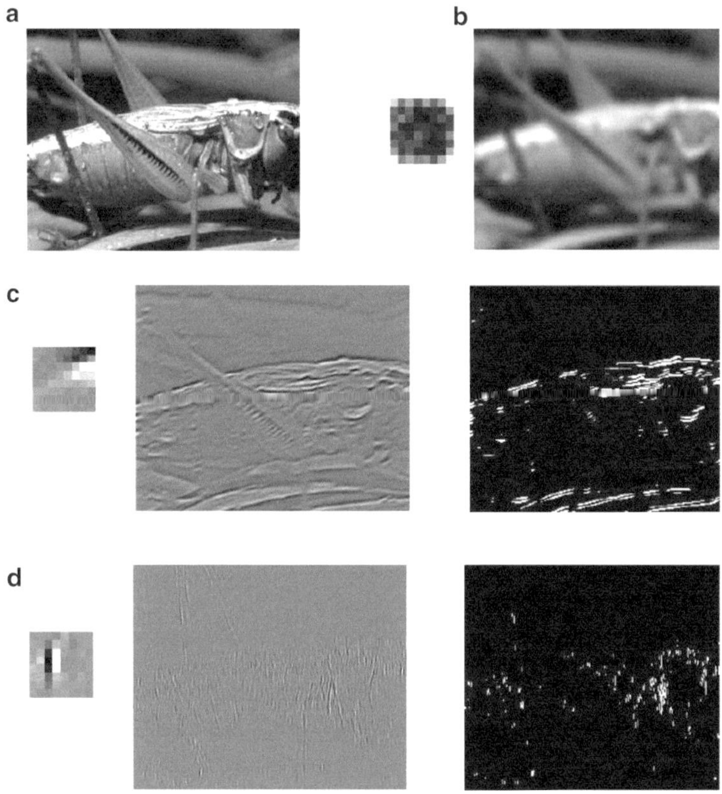

Fig. 13.11 Three samples of the basis functions and their reconstructed images, (**a**) Original image, (**b**) a nonsparse basis function, (**c**) and (**d**) two sparse basis functions with different locations and orientations

magnitude of the low-frequency region is given as $F_l = \sum_{i=0}^{4} \sum_{j=0}^{4-i} F(i,j)$ and that of the high-frequency region as $F_h = \sum_{i=0}^{7} \sum_{j=\max(0,5-i)}^{7} F(i,j)$. Next, we compare F_l and F_h, if $F_l < F_h$. The basis function mainly represents high-frequencies (edge information); otherwise, it will represent low-frequency information. Figure 13.14b shows the integral amplitude of different frequency regions for the ICA natural basis functions. At the same time, we used the same approach to select the ICA medical basis functions that represent edge information. Finally, we can choose $m = 1$ to preserve all information for the two sets of basis functions. It is also evident in Fig. 13.13 that when $m = 6$, the reconstructed edge image has lost some information on the edges. Figure 13.15 shows examples of medical images and the represented images by using a single medical basis function. It also confirmed the validity of the proposed edge representation approach by using sparse basis function.

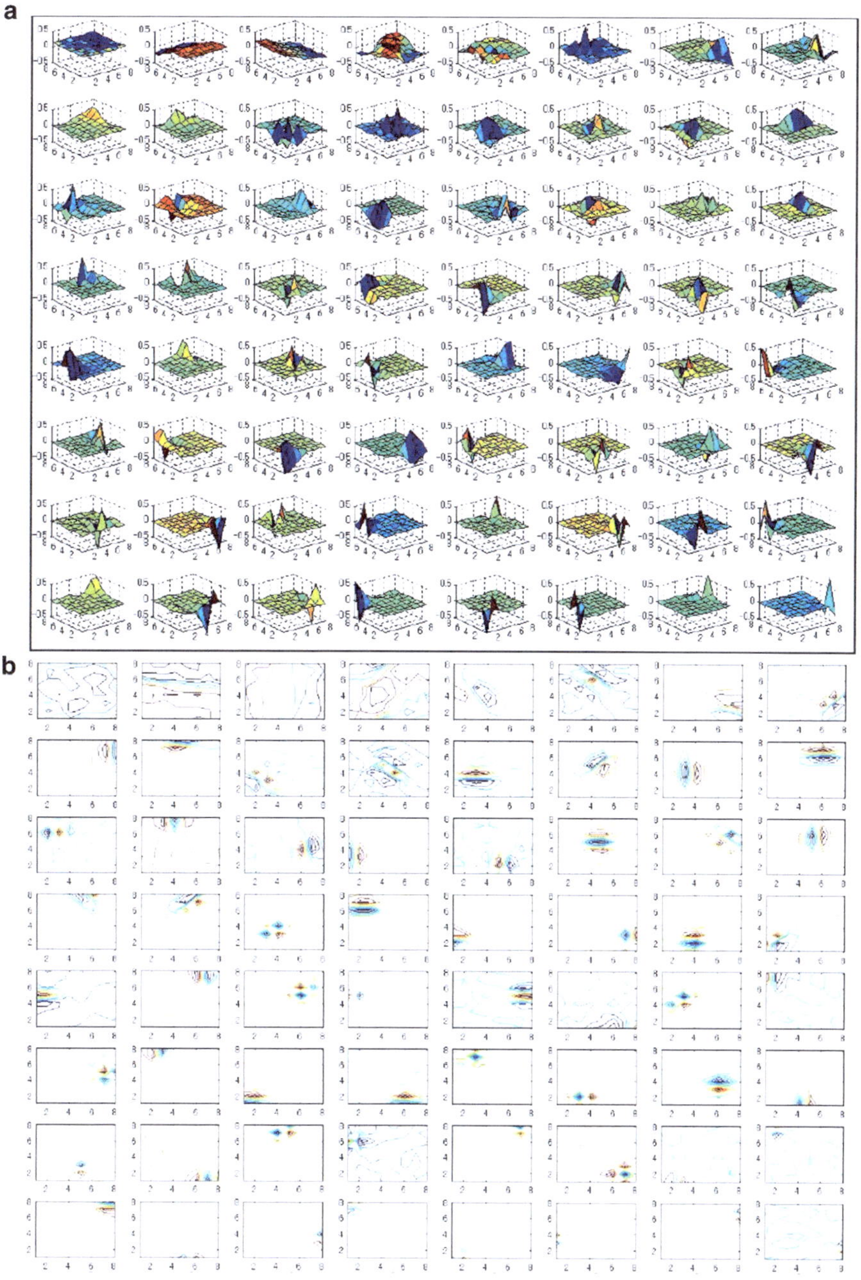

Fig. 13.12 (a) The amplitude spatial diagram of the ICA natural basis functions, (b) 2D contour plots of natural basis functions

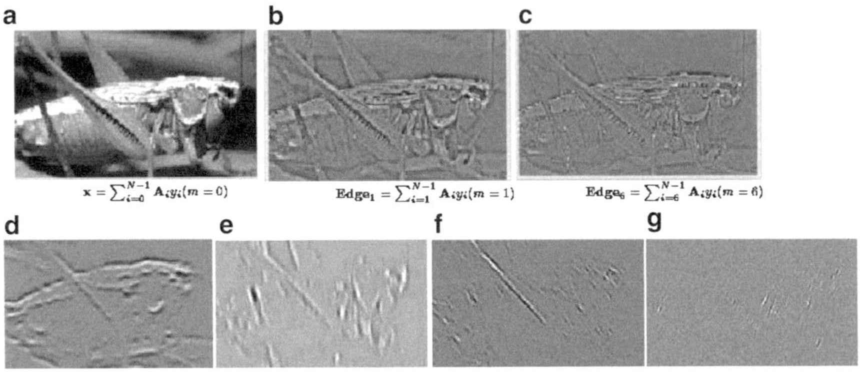

Fig. 13.13 Natural image representation of natural basis functions (Fig. 13.3a). The representation of (**a**) all basis functions, (**b**) the last 63 basis functions, (**c**) the last 58 basis functions ($m = 6$), (**d**) only the 2nd basis function, (**e**) the 3rd basis function, (**f**) the 4th basis function, and (**g**) the 5th basis function

Edge Enhancement by Using Shrinkage ICA Coefficients

For an image patch $\mathbf{x}_0$ from an image $\mathbf{I}_0$ that is corrupted with noise $\mathbf{u}$, the noisy image patch $\mathbf{x}$ from the noisy image $\mathbf{I}$ can be represented as: $\mathbf{x} = \mathbf{x}_0 + \mathbf{u}$. Subsequently, its ICA components will also be composed of both signal and noise components [15]. Thus, it is important to remove the noise components in the ICA domain [14, 15]. In this study, we use a soft thresholding technique, which is known as shrinkage, to reduce the noise. The basic idea is that only a few components are simultaneously active (nonzero) simultaneously in the ICA domain, whereas the components with small absolute values can be considered as noise and can be set to be zero. The basic process for edge detection in noisy images is shown below:

(1) ICA transform $\mathbf{y} = \mathbf{W}\,\mathbf{x}$
(2) Nonlinear shrinkage $\mathbf{y}' = g(\mathbf{y})$
(3) Rearrange basis functions $\mathbf{A}_i (i = 1, 2, \cdots, 64)$ according to their sparseness
(4) Reconstruction of edge images by using the sparse components and shrunken or filtered coefficients $\mathbf{y}'$ (Inverse ICA): $\mathbf{edge}' = \mathbf{A}_{sparse}\mathbf{y}'$

In step (2), $g(\mathbf{y})$ is the operator or the function of the shrinkage, which is used to reduce the noise as designed in section "Adaptive Noise Reduction for PET Images".

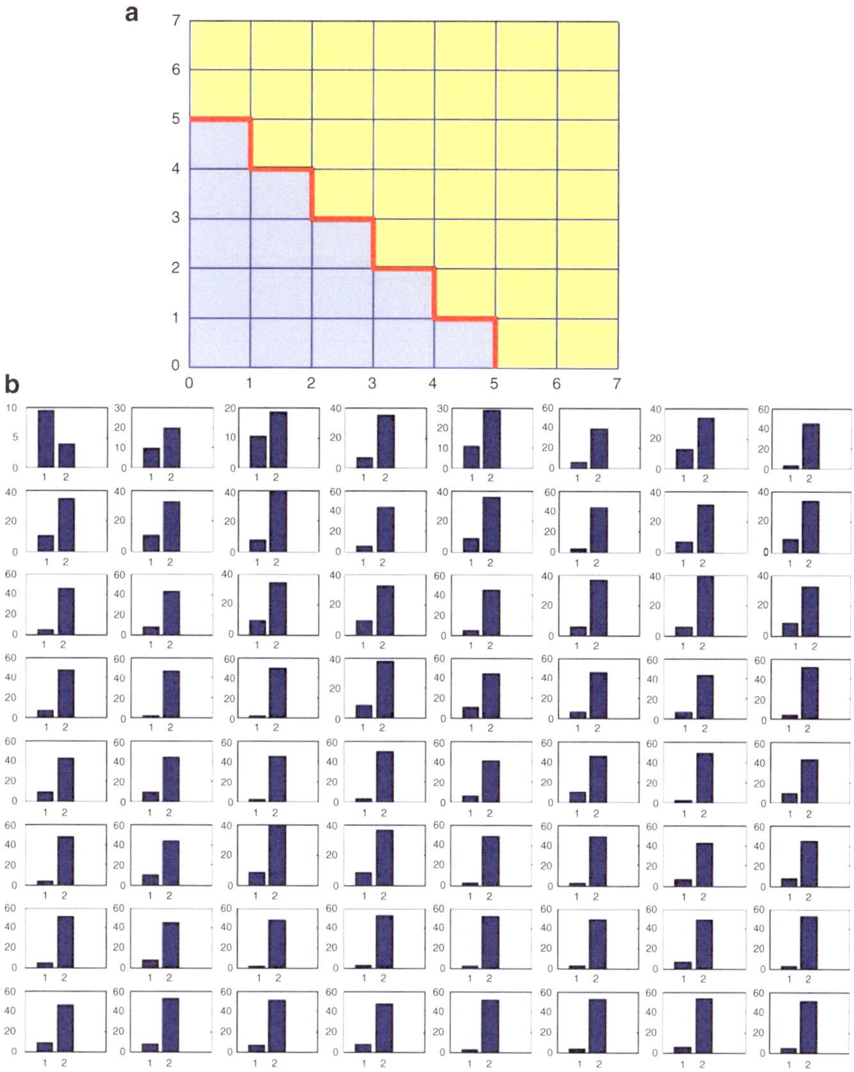

Fig. 13.14 (**a**) Partition of low-frequency and high-frequency regions of the ICA basis function, and (**b**) the integral amplitude of different frequency regions for the ICA natural basis functions

Experimental Results

The test medical data in our experiments are utilized from noisy simulated MRI volumes for a normal brain, which were obtained from the BrainWeb. The parameters describing the database set are: Modality=T1, Protocol=ICBM, Phantom _name=normal, Slice_thickness = 3 mm, Noise = 9 %, INU = 20 % (Please

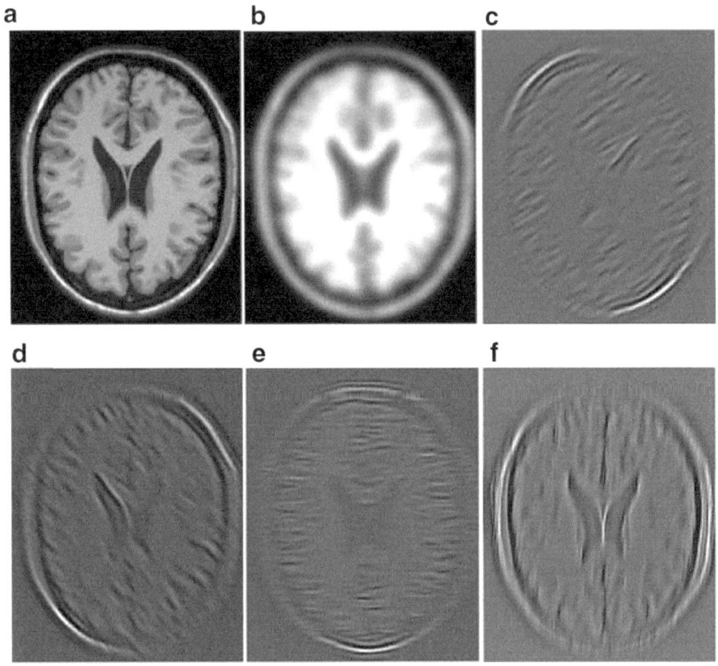

Fig. 13.15 Medical image representation of only one basis function (in Fig. 13.2b). (**a**) The original MRI images. The representation of the (**b**) first basis function, (**c**) 2nd one, (**d**) 3rd one, (**e**) 16th one, (**f**) 18th one

refer to the BrainWeb homepage for detailed information). In other words, the test MRI images are somewhat degraded images of the training MRI groups, from which 20 slices of simulated MRI volumes are selected for the composition of the second set of training data.

To validate the effectiveness of our proposed method compared with the well-known conventional famous Canny method [3], we present one test image with known edge images and their edge detection results in Fig. 13.16. Figure 13.16a shows the original test images, Fig. 13.16b shows the true edge of Fig. 13.16a, c shows the edge extracted by using the Canny method, and Fig. 13.16d shows the edge extracted by our proposed method. In order to give an objective evaluation of the edge detection method, in Fig. 13.16e, we show the pixel numbers (positive) of the true and detected edges obtained using Canny and our method along with the true positive and false positive edges (which indicate the accuracy of detected edge positions) of different methods. At the same time, the effectiveness of our proposed ICA shrinkage filter can be validated using test images with a known reference ground true. Reference [22] shows that the ICA shrinkage method can realize much better results with objective evaluations of PSNR and MSR. For actual applications,

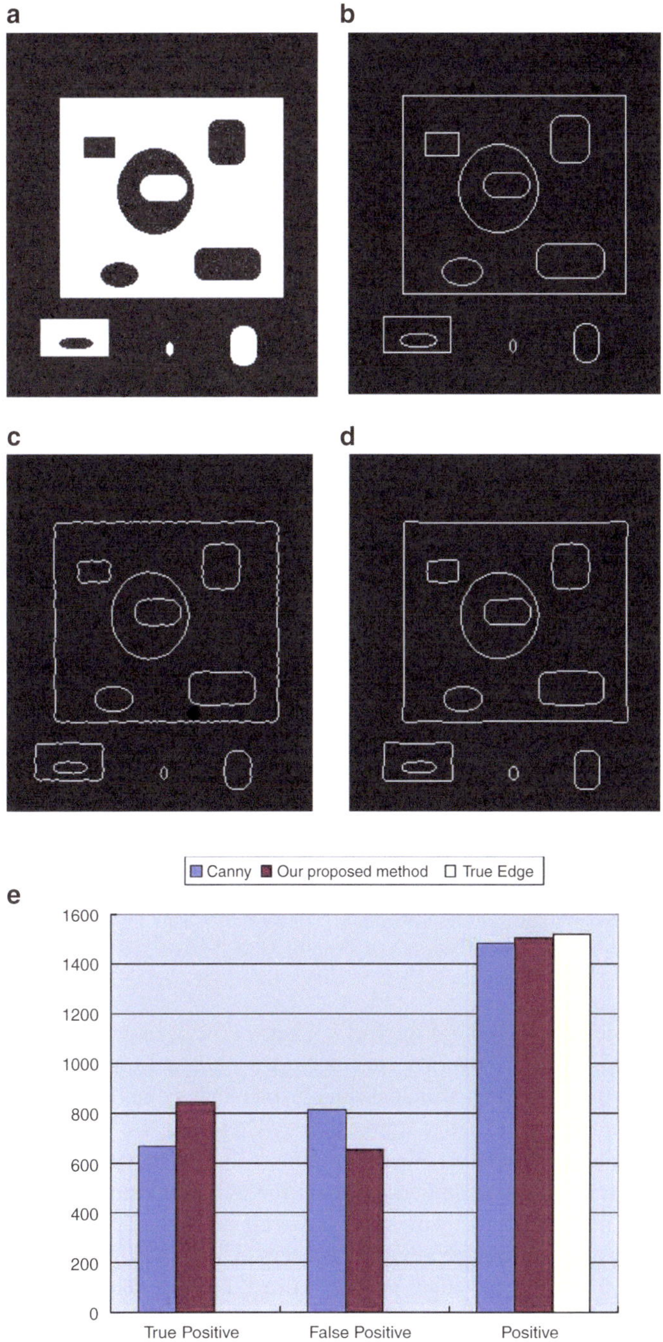

Fig. 13.16 An example of edge detection. (**a**) The test image, (**b**) true edge of the image in (**a**), (**c**) edge detected by Canny, (**d**) edge detected by the ICA-based method, and (**e**) an objective evaluation of the extracted edge by using different methods

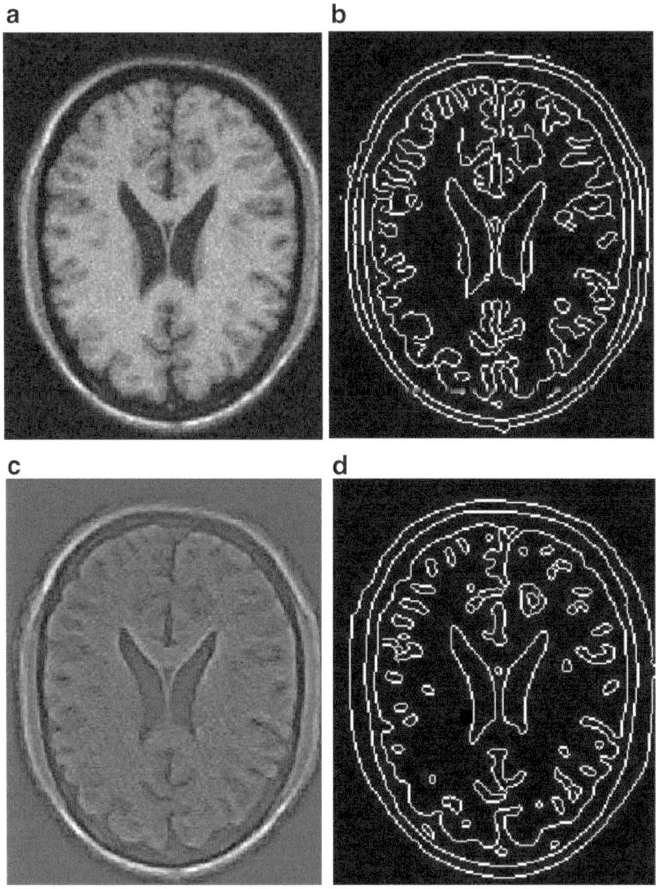

Fig. 13.17 Edge detection. (**a**) The MRI image, (**b**) edge by Canny algorithm, (**c**) preprocessed edge information by ICA, and (**d**) edges extracted by the ICA-based method

typical examples are shown in Fig. 13.17. Figure 13.17a shows the noisy test MRI image, and Fig. 13.17b shows the detected edge obtained using the conventional Canny algorithm. The test medical image has the same statistical properties compared with the second set of training data. Therefore, we select the second set of the basis functions to detect edges for the test image. In the training procedure, the infomax algorithm was applied to obtain the transformation matrix **W** or basis functions **A**. Thus, the sparser part, which was selected according to sparseness, can be used to represent the image edges.

Figure 13.17c shows the edge image obtained using the proposed method with shrinkage. After preprocessing with histogram-based contrast enhancement [34], the binarized edge after the simple gradient is given in Fig. 13.17d. It is evident that most of the edges with the ICA-based method are connected, and at the same

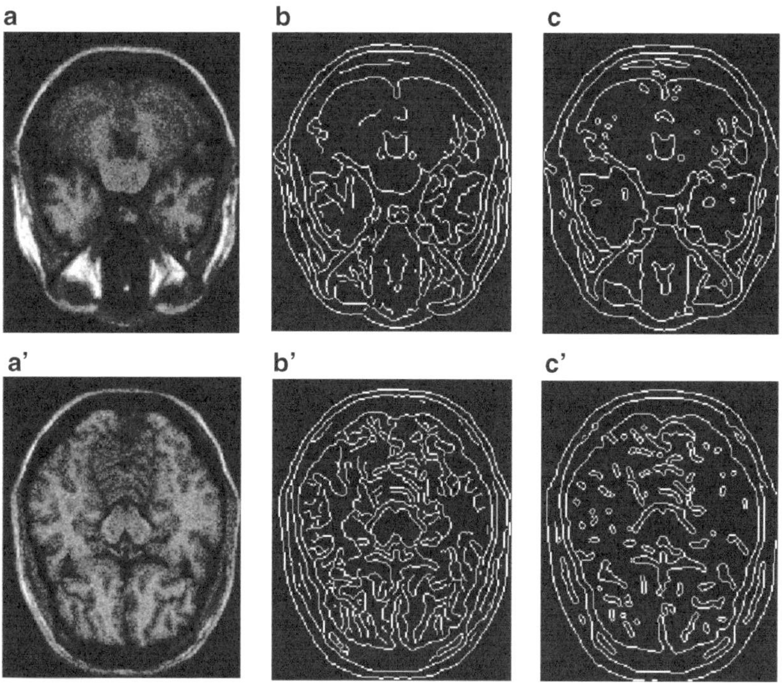

Fig. 13.18 Edge detection of the two test MRI images: (**a**) and (**a'**) The MRI images; (**b**) and (**b'**) edges by Canny algorithm; and (**c**) and (**c'**) edges extracted by the ICA-based method

time, the edges in the blurred part of the test image can also be detected. In order to validate the practicability of our proposed method, we present two additional test images in Fig. 13.18. The validity and connection of the extracted edges obtained using by our method is much better than those obtained using the Canny algorithm.

Conclusions

This chapter proposed an adaptive noise reduction and robust edge enhancement algorithm by using the ICA-domain shrinkage strategy. The proposed method was applied for the reduction of Poisson noise in PET sinograms, and the effectiveness with the adaptive ICA basis functions was demonstrated. Furthermore, we analyzed image edge representation by using the ICA transformed basis functions and demonstrated the selection of the basis functions for image edges. With edge basis functions, we obtained the ICA-domain sparse components of edge information and then explored the robust edge enhancement by the estimation of the ICA-domain edge components that were corrupted by noise using nonlinear shrinkage functions. The experiments proved that the proposed edge enhancement method is very effective for applications involving high noise level medical images, and the performance of the proposed method is much better than the conventional edge detection method, especially for high noise level images.

In the future work, we are going to quantify the adaptive degree of the learned basis function to represent the local structures of processed data and explore the suitability of different basis functions for noise reduction, which can prospect more feasible processing for removing noise. Furthermore, in order to reconstruct more detail structure in the processed images, we also attempt to learn larger number of basis functions using over-complete ICA or the recently popular sparse coding method, which are also proven to be a very effective strategy for noise reduction in natural images.

Acknowledgments This work was supported in part by the Grant-in Aid for Scientific Research from the Japanese MEXT under the Grant No. 2430076, 24103710, 24700179 and in part by the R-GIRO Research fund from Ritsumeikan University. We would also like to thank our co-operating researchers: Keishi Kitamura, Akihiro Ishikawa, Yoshihiro Inoue, Kouichi Shibata, Yukio Mishina and Yoshihiro Mukutaof of Shimadzu Corporation, for providing PET data and valuable discussion.

References

1. Dhawan PA (2003) Medical imaging analysis. Wiley, Hoboken, NJ
2. Freiherr G (2010) Waste not. want not: Getting the most from imaging procedures. *Diagnostic Imaging*, 2010
3. Defrise M, Kinahan P (1998) Data acquisition and image reconstruction for 3D PET. In: Bendriem B, Townsend DW (eds) The theory and practice of 3D PET. Kluwer Academic, Amsterdam, pp 11–53
4. Hohne KH, Fuchs H, Pizer SM (2001) Advanced algorithmic approaches to medical image segmentation: state-of-the-art applications in cardiology, neurology, mammography and pathology. Springer, New York
5. Belaid LJ, Jaoua M, Masmoudi M, Siala L (2005) Image restoration and edge detections by topological asyptotic expansion. *Masmoudi personal communication*
6. Malladi R, Sethian JA (1997) Level set methods for curvature flow, image enhancement, and shape recovery in medical images. In: Conference on Visualization and Mathematics, Springer, Berlin, Heidelberg, pp 329–345
7. Suzuki K, Horiba I, Sugie N (2002) Efficient approximation of a neural filter for quantum noise removal in X-ray images. IEEE Trans Signal Process 50(7):1787–1799
8. Suzuki K (2009) A supervised "lesion-enhancement" filter by use of a massive-training artificial neural network (MTANN) in computer-aided diagnosis (CAD). Phys Med Biol 54 (18):S31–45
9. Suzuki K, Horiba I, Sugie N, Nanki M (2004) Extraction of left ventricular contours from left ventriculograms by means of a neural edge detector. IEEE Trans Med Imag 23(3):330–339
10. Suzuki K, Horiba I, Sugie N (2003) Neural edge enhancer for supervised edge enhancement from noisy images. IEEE Trans Pattern Anal Mach Intell 25(12):1582–1596
11. Canny J (1987) A Computational approach to edge detection. IEEE Trans Pattern Anal Mach Intell 8(6):679–698
12. Haralick RM (1984) Digital step edges from zero crossings of the second directional derivative. IEEE Trans Pattern Anal Mach Intell 6(1):58–68

13. Pratt WK (1978) Digital image processing. Wiley, New York
14. Bell AJ, Sejnowski TJ (1997) The "Independent Components" of natural scenes are edge filters. Vis Res 37:3327–3338.
15. Bell AJ, Sejnowski TJ (1995) An information-maximization approach to blind separation and blind deconvolution. Neural Comput 7:1129–1159
16. Common P (1994) Independent component analysis: a new concept? Signal Process 36:287–314
17. Hyvarinen A, Oja E (1997) A fast fixed-point algorithm for indepepndent component analysis. Neural Comput 9:1483–1492
18. Hyvarinen A, Oja E, Hoyer P (2000) Image denoising by sparse code shrinkage. In: Haykin S, Kosko B (eds) Intelligent signal processing. IEEE Press, New York
19. Hoyer P (1999) Independent component analysis in image denoising. Master's Thesis, Helsinki University of Techonology
20. Hyvarinen A (1999) Sparse code shrinkage: Denoising of nongaussian data by maximum liklihood estimation. Neural Comput 11(7):1739–1768
21. Han X-H, Chen Y-W, Nakao Z (2003) An ICA-based method for Poisson noise reduction. Lecture Notes in Artificial Intelligence, vol 2773. Springer, Heidelberg, pp 1449–1454
22. Han X-H, Nakao Z, Chen Y-W (2005) An ICA-domain shrinkage based Poisson-noise reduction algorithm and its application to penumbral imaging. IEICE Trans Info Syst E88-D (4):750–757
23. Han X-H, Chen Y-W, Nakao Z (2004) Robust edge detection by independent component analysis in noisy images. IEICE Trans Info Syst vol.E87-D(9):2204–2211
24. Han X-H, Nakao Z, Chen Y-W (2006) An edge extraction algorithm based ICA-domain shrinkage for penumbral imaging. Information 9(3):529–544
25. Colsher JG (1980) Fully three-dimensional positron emission tomography. Phys Med Biol 25:103–115
26. Defrise M, Townsend DW, Deconinck F (1990) Statistical noise in three-dimensional positron tomography. Phys Med Biol 35:131–138
27. Ito Y (1988) Poisson analysis and statistical mechanics. Probab Theor Relat Field 77:1–28
28. Donoho DL (1995) De-noising by soft-thresholding. IEEE Trans Inform Theor 41 (3):613–6275
29. Atkins MS, Mackiewich BT (2000) Processing and analysis. Handbook of medical imaging. Academic Press, Orlando, Chap 11, pp 171–183
30. Chalana V, Kim Y (1997) A methodology for evaluation of boundary detection algorithms on medical images. IEEE Trans Med Imag 16(5):642–652.
31. Olshausen BA, Field DJ (1996) Emergence of simple-cell receptive field properties by learning a sparse code for natural images. Nature 381:607–609
32. Julius O. Smith III JO (2003) Mathematics of the discrete fourier transform (DFT). W3K Publishing, http://www.w3k.org/books/. ISBN 0-9745607-0-7.
33. Karvanen J, Cichocki A (2003) Measuring sparseness in noisy signals. Proceedings of ICA 2003, Nara, Japan, pp 125–130
34. Reza AM (2004) Realization of the contrast limited adaptive histogram equalization (CLAHE) for real-time image enhancement. J VLSI Signal Process 33(1):35–44

Chapter 14
Subtraction Techniques for CT and DSA and Automated Detection of Lung Nodules in 3D CT

Takayuki Ishida, Megumi Yamamoto, and Yasuhiko Okura

Abstract The interpretation of a large number of CT images is time consuming and hard work for radiologists. Therefore, we have developed two subtraction techniques based on a 3D morphological filtering technique and a temporal subtraction technique to remove normal structures such as pulmonary vessels and bones.

Digital subtraction angiography (DSA) is inadequate for coronary artery due to the existence of severe motion artifacts. In view of this, we have developed a new DSA technique with an artifact reduction technique based on the time-series image processing. The results indicated a considerable improvement in DSA quality; thus, the coronary arteries, carotid artery, and vein were clearly enhanced.

We have also developed an automated computerized method for the detection of lung nodules in 3D computed tomography (CT) images obtained by helical CT. To enhance lung nodules, we employed 3D cross-correlation method by use of a 3D Gaussian template with zero-surrounding as a template. The average number of false positives was 5.2 per case at the sensitivity of 95.8 %.

T. Ishida (✉)
Department of Medical Physics and Engineering, Osaka University,
Graduate School of Medicine, 1-7, Yamadaoka, Suita, Osaka 565-0871, Japan
e-mail: tishida@sahs.med.osaka-u.ac.jp

M. Yamamoto • Y. Okura
Hiroshima International University, 555-36, Kurose-Gakuendai,
Higashihiroshima, Hiroshima, Japan
e-mail: m-yamamo@hs.hirokoku-u.ac.jp; y-okura@hs.hirokoku-u.ac.jp

K. Suzuki (ed.), *Computational Intelligence in Biomedical Imaging*,
DOI 10.1007/978-1-4614-7245-2_14, © Springer Science+Business Media New York 2014

Background

Subtraction CT Technique

Lung cancer is the leading cause of cancer mortality. Therefore, the detection of small lung nodules is an important task for radiologists. To increase the detection rate of early lung cancer, low-dose helical computed tomography (LDCT) has been employed in screening programs [1, 2]. However, the interpretation of a large number of CT images is time-consuming for radiologists. Thus, we have developed a new subtraction CT technique to remove most of the pulmonary vessels and assist radiologists for the detection of lung nodules on LDCT images.

Temporal Subtraction CT Technique

Lung CT images are commonly interpreted by comparing with previous CT images of the same patient to detect interval changes, such as new lesions or changes in lung nodules, pleural effusions, and interstitial infiltrates. However, it is a difficult task for radiologists to identify very subtle lesions and/or lesions overlapped with vessels. Previously, we have developed the temporal subtraction technique for chest radiographs. Subtle changes and/or newly developed abnormalities on chest radiographs were enhanced and thus the detection accuracy of interval changes in chest radiographs was improved significantly by use of temporal subtraction [3]. In cases with previous CT, subtraction of previous CT image from current CT image can be useful to enhance changes in local opacity. Therefore, we have developed a temporal subtraction CT technique based on a nonlinear geometric warping technique [4, 5].

DSA for Coronary Arteriography

Digital subtraction angiography (DSA) is one of the most important examinations for the diagnosis and treatment of the blood vessels. The radiation dose can be reduced using this examination because the vessels are visualized clearly; however, it is very difficult to apply the DSA technique to the coronary arteries because of the severe motion artifacts caused by cardiac motion and respiration. For the treatment of coronary stenosis, it is important to locate the position of the stenosis and evaluate the effect of interventional radiology (IVR) in real time.

Many methods have been proposed to reduce motion artifacts in DSA based on post-image-processing techniques [6–28]. However, it would be difficult to apply these techniques clinically because most of these image processing methods disable real time.

Therefore, we have developed a real time DSA technique by using a time-series image processing. This method could obtain a high quality DSA image without severe motion artifacts [29].

CAD for the Detection of Lung Nodules in 3D CT

In recent years, the helical CT and multi-detector CT have become popular [30, 31]. The number of slices per examination is increasing from tens to hundreds, and the work load for radiologists is steadily increasing. We have developed a method for the automatic detection of lung nodules in the three-dimensional (3D) computed tomography (CT) images of the lung. For the automated detection of lung nodules in CT images, there are several useful methods [32–45]. A template matching technique employs cross-correlation technique with a ball model obtained from the suspicious cancer and a cylinder model acquired from blood vessels in different directions and sizes [32]. Another cross-correlation technique, the optimal template is selected from the 3D Gaussian distributions of various sizes and lung nodules by using the genetic algorithm [33, 34]. However, these methods require a special technique for the detection of nodules at the area close to chest wall. The rolling ball method facilitates finding of nodules [35]. The selective enhancement based on Hessian matrix is performed for the enhancement of nodule, blood vessels, and airway [36]. Also the nodule enhancement technique by use of difference image technique is effective for the detection of lung nodules based on thresholding technique [37]. In our method, we employed a background trend correction technique based on morphological filtering that can eliminate low spatial frequency components on lung CT. Overall performance could improve the sensitivity and specificity for the detection of the lung nodule in CT [46].

Image Databases

For the development of the subtraction techniques, we used 87 cases with lung nodules due to primary lung cancer from our database of LDCT images, which were obtained from a CT screening program for lung cancer. A total of 17,892 examinations on 7,847 individuals were performed as part of an annual lung cancer screening in Nagano, Japan [1, 2].

An image database for the development of the new DSA technique was used, which consists of 20 cases of intra-arterial coronary angiograms. Each angiogram was acquired at Hiroshima City Hospital using a digital angiography system (Philips Medical Systems, Best, and Netherlands) with a matrix size of 512×512, 8 bits gray-level, and 30 frames/s.

Table 14.1 Imaging system and parameters for CT examination

1.	Hi Speed CT/i(GE MEDICAL SYSTEM) HISPEED-RP, Light Speed16(GE MEDICAL SYSTEM) Light Speed QX/i(GE MEDICAL SYSTEM) GENESIS_FOREIGN(GE MEDICAL SYSTEM)
2.	Reconstruction function: STANDARD, BONE, DETAIL
3.	Matrix size: 512 × 512
4.	Pixel size: 0.570–0.769 mm
5.	Slice thickness: 5–10 mm
6.	Reconstruction interval: 5–14 mm
7.	Contrast enhancement (CE): 8 out of 69

For the development of the nodule detection technique in 3D CT, we used 69 CT cases (73 nodules). The diameters of nodules in this database were in the range of 4.5–15.5 mm. Table 14.1 shows the CT systems and data acquisition parameters.

Methods and Results

Subtraction CT Technique

Overall Scheme

Figure 14.1 shows the overall scheme for the subtraction CT technique.

In this scheme, "mask image" for the subtraction CT is obtained from three CT section images based on a 3D morphological filter applied to two sections, which include the target section image and the upper or lower section image.

The line components of the target section image are detected by using a line enhancement filter. The line components are added to the mask image to reduce artifacts on subtraction CT image.

The subtraction CT image is then obtained by subtracting the warped mask image from the target section image by using the iterative image warping technique [3, 4].

3D Morphological Filtering

We have developed a new method to create a mask image based on morphological filtering with 3D cylindrical and a 2D circular shape kernel. Dilation or erosion corresponds to the replacement of the pixel value with the maximum or minimum value within the kernel, respectively. The 3D opening and the 3D closing operation are illustrated in Fig. 14.2a, b, respectively [47].

Figure 14.3d, e show upper and lower intermediate images obtained by the 3D opening operation on the target section image and two section images immediately

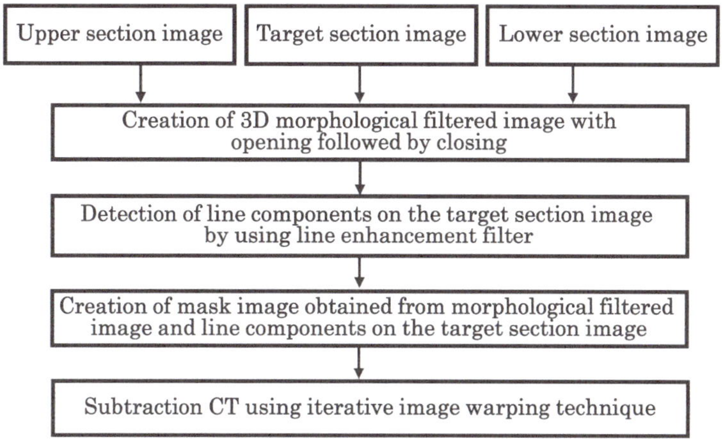

Fig. 14.1 Overall scheme of subtraction CT technique

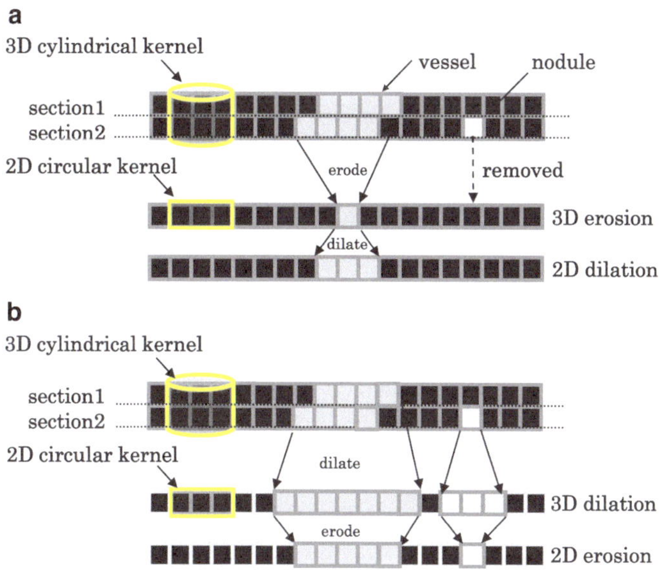

Fig. 14.2 Three-dimensional morphological filtering. (**a**) 3D opening operation, (**b**) 3D closing operation

above and below the target section image (Fig. 14.3a–c), respectively. Figure 14.3f shows the mask image obtained by the 3D closing operation for the two intermediate images.

It should be noted that the mask image, as shown in Fig. 14.3f, can retain vessels, which is basically the same as that on the target section, while removing a small

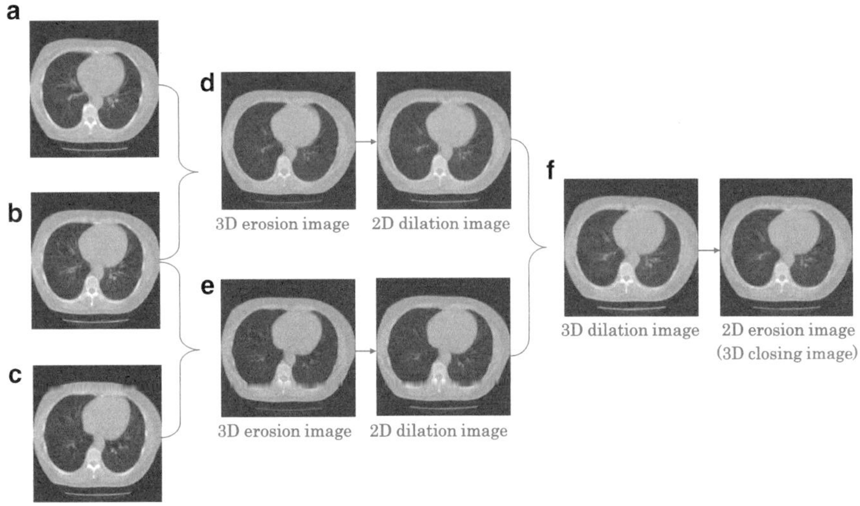

Fig. 14.3 Creation of a mask image with a 3D morphological filter. (**a**) Upper image, (**b**) target image, (**c**) lower image, (**d**) upper intermediate image, (**e**) lower intermediate image, (**f**) mask image

nodule. Therefore, the subtraction of the mask image from the target section can reveal only nodular opacity without the vessels.

Detection of Line Components on Target Image

We extracted line components by using a line enhancement filter on the target image for reduction of misregistration artifacts on subtraction CT image. The line enhancement filter includes eight sets of three templates in eight different directions, as shown in Fig. 14.4 [48, 49]. The output value of the line enhancement filter is defined as follows:

$$\mathrm{Ei} = \begin{cases} 2\mathrm{Bi} - \mathrm{Ai} - \mathrm{Ci} & \text{when } \mathrm{Bi} > \mathrm{Ai} \quad \text{and} \quad \mathrm{Bi} > \mathrm{Ci}, \\ 0 & \text{otherwise} \end{cases}$$

$$\mathrm{E} = \max \mathrm{Ei}, \qquad 1 \leqq \mathrm{i} \leqq 8,$$

where Ai, Bi, and Ci are the summation for all pixel values in each template of a set. The maximum value E, obtained from the outputs of the sets is the final output value.

To detect various diameters of vessels, parameters for the line enhancement filter (i.e., length and width of the templates) and the interval between the templates were varied depending on the distance between the center of the template and the center on the section image.

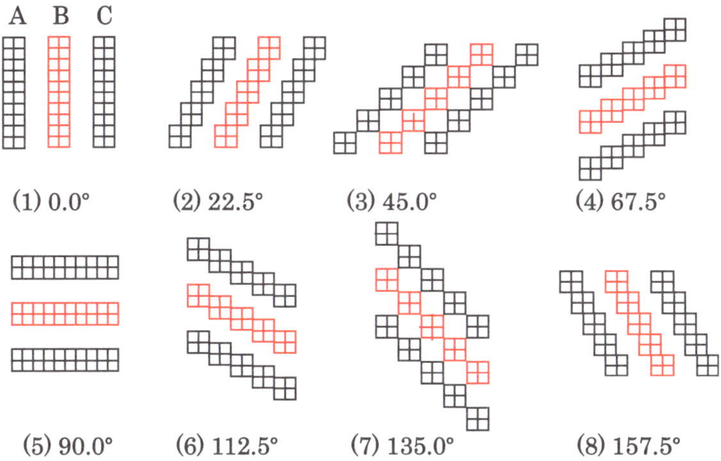

Fig. 14.4 Line enhancement filter

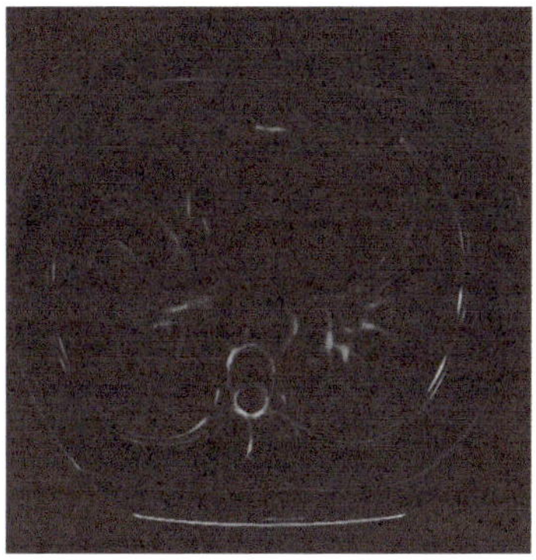

Fig. 14.5 Enhanced line image

An enhanced line image and the extracted line components are shown in Figs. 14.5 and 14.6, respectively. Both vessels at the hilar area and the peripheral area are well enhanced. The line components are added to the mask image obtained by 3D morphological filtering.

Subtraction CT Image by Using 3D Morphological Filtering

Figure 14.7a shows a target image with early lung cancer (arrow). The mask image is obtained by the 3D morphological filtering with the target section image and the sections immediately above and below the target image, as shown in Fig. 14.7b. The mask image can include pulmonary vessels on the target image and thus most vessels can be removed by the subtraction. A nonlinear geometric image warping technique, which is described in the section "Temporal Subtraction CT Technique,"

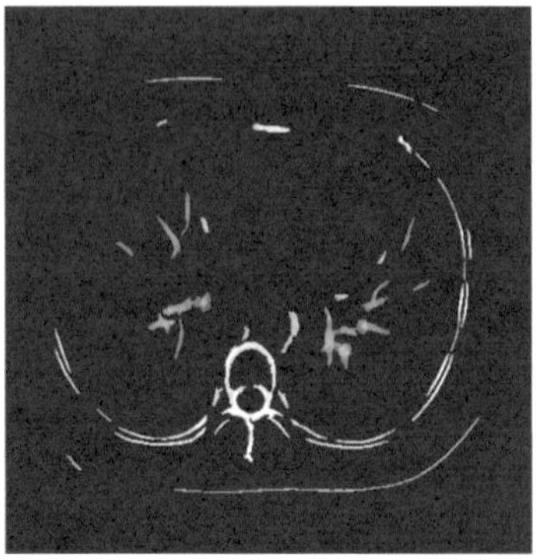

Fig. 14.6 Detected line components

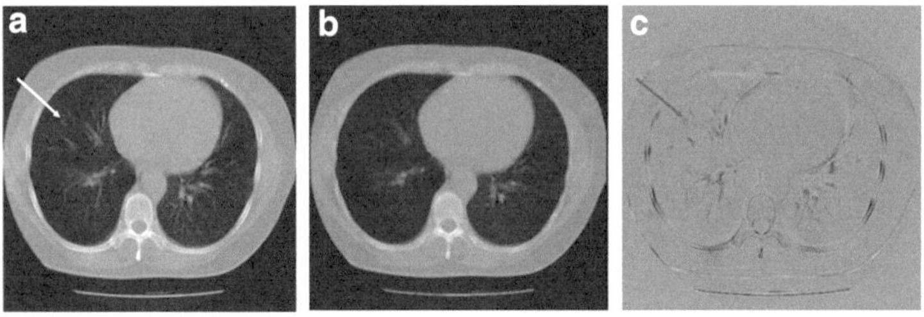

Fig. 14.7 Subtraction CT image by using 3D morphological filtering (case 1). (**a**) Target CT image, (**b**) mask image without line components, (**c**) subtraction CT image

is then performed to the mask image for further reduction of misregistration artifacts on subtraction CT image. The subtraction CT image is obtained by subtracting the warped mask image from the target CT image, as shown in Fig. 14.7c. Subtle nodule is clearly enhanced in the subtraction CT image, although some misregistration artifacts are observed.

Improved Subtraction CT Images by Using Line Enhancement Filter

For further reduction of misregistration artifacts on the subtraction CT image, the pixel values of the target image over the areas of the detected line components are applied to replace the pixel values over the same areas in the mask image, which is obtained by the morphological filtering technique. The mask images with line components are shown in Figs. 14.8b and 14.9b. The subtraction CT images are shown in Figs. 14.8c and 14.9c. It should be noted that the small nodule remains as dark shadows, and the misregistration artifacts in Figs. 14.8c and 14.9c were considerably reduced compared to the subtraction CT image, as shown in Fig. 14.7c.

Image rotation caused by variation in patient positioning between the current and the previous CT images is then corrected by an image rotation technique.

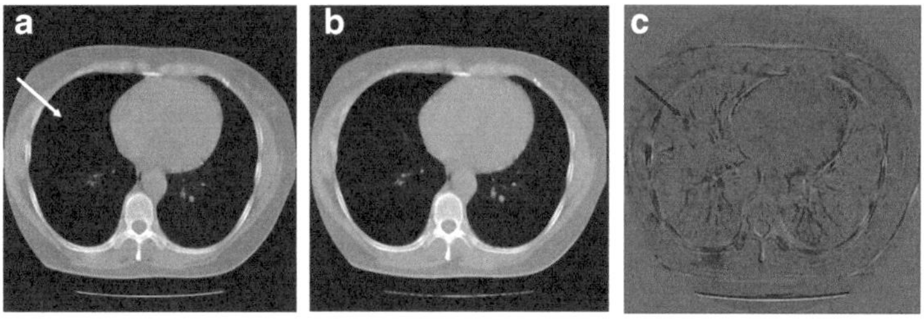

Fig. 14.8 Subtraction CT image by using 3D morphological filtering and line enhancement filtering (case 1). (**a**) Target CT image, (**b**) mask image with line components, (**c**) subtraction CT image

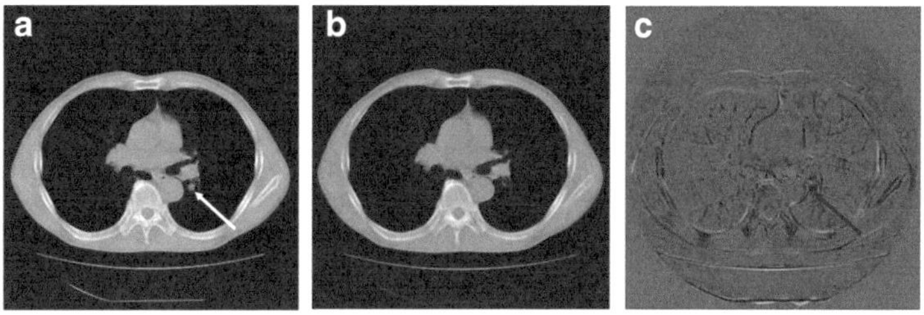

Fig. 14.9 Subtraction CT image by using 3D morphological filtering and line enhancement filtering (case 2). (**a**) Target CT image, (**b**) mask image with line components, (**c**) subtraction CT image

The rotation angles between the current and the previous CT images are determined by use of the template matching technique.

Finally, the temporal subtraction CT image is obtained by subtracting the warped previous CT section image from the current CT section image by using the iterative image warping technique [4, 5].

Temporal Subtraction CT Technique

Figure 14.10 shows the overall scheme for the temporal subtraction CT technique. In this scheme, the corresponding previous section image for each current section image is selected automatically from previous CT images by using a template matching technique.

Automated Selection of Corresponding Section Images

The selection of the corresponding section in the two sets of CT images is performed by a template matching technique. In this method, the current and

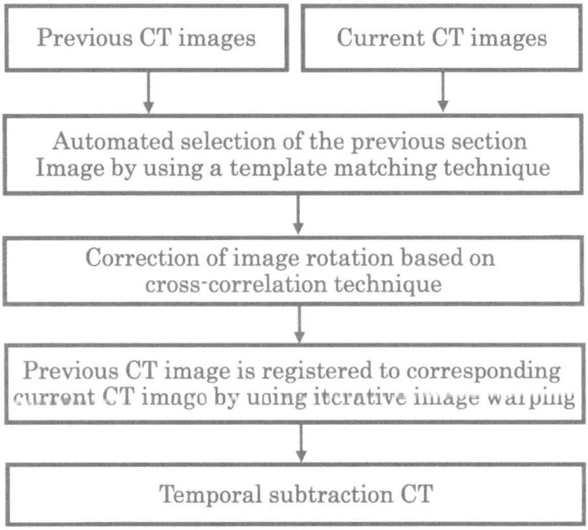

Fig. 14.10 Overall scheme of temporal subtraction CT technique

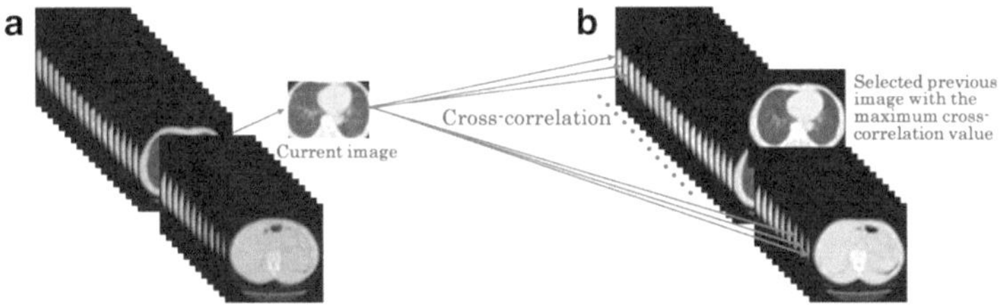

Fig. 14.11 Selection of the best matched previous image. (**a**) Current CT images, (**b**) previous CT images

previous CT images are blurred by a Gaussian filter and then subsampled to low-resolution image (128 × 128 matrix size). A circumscribed rectangular region of interest (ROI) of segmented lung image is selected automatically from each current image. The corresponding image and its best matched location are determined when the cross-correlation value between the current image and previous image becomes the maximum, as shown in Fig. 14.11.

In addition, the image rotation between the current and previous image is corrected based on template matching technique. Thus, the corresponding pairs of the current and previous section images are obtained.

Temporal Subtraction CT

To achieve accurate registration between the current and previous section images, an iterative image warping is applied to the previous CT image. In this method, a

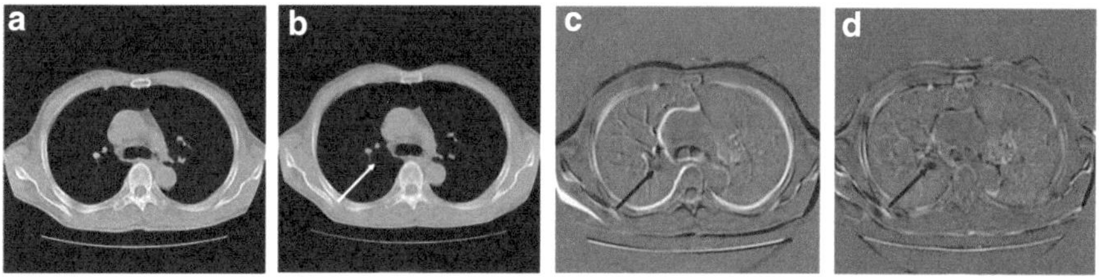

Fig. 14.12 Temporal subtraction CT images (case 1). (**a**) Previous image, (**b**) current images, (**c**) without image warping, (**d**) with image warping

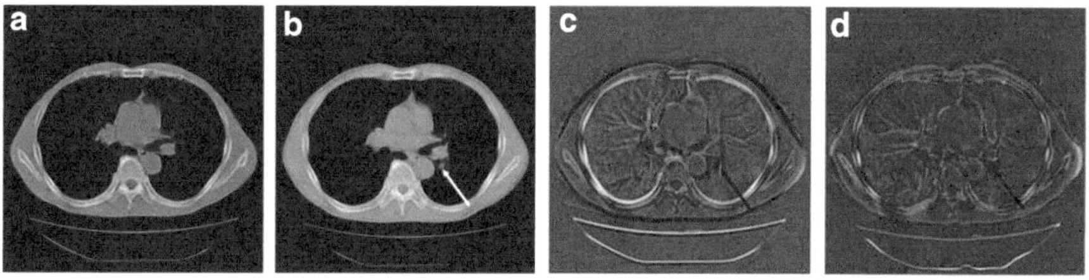

Fig. 14.13 Temporal subtraction CT images (case 2). (**a**) Previous image, (**b**) current images, (**c**) without image warping, (**d**) with image warping

number of template ROIs and the corresponding search area ROIs were selected from the previous and the current CT images, respectively. We determined the shift values for all pairs of selected ROIs by using a template matching technique to find the best matched areas in the search area ROI. A two-dimensional surface fitting using a polynomial function was then applied to each set of mapped shift values for conversion of the coordinates of the previous CT image, i.e., for warping of the image. The warped previous CT image is then subtracted from the current CT image.

Figures 14.12a, b and 14.13a, b show the previous CT images and the current CT images with lung cancer (arrow). The temporal subtraction CT images using global matching but not using iterative image warping technique are shown in Figs. 14.12c and 14.13c. Lung cancers were enhanced as dark shadows on subtraction images; yet, some misregistration artifacts exist. The temporal subtraction CT images with both global matching and the iterative image warping technique, as shown in Figs. 14.12d and 14.13d enhanced clearly the lung cancers. Misregistration artifacts were reduced remarkably compared to the temporal subtraction CT image without iterative image warping technique.

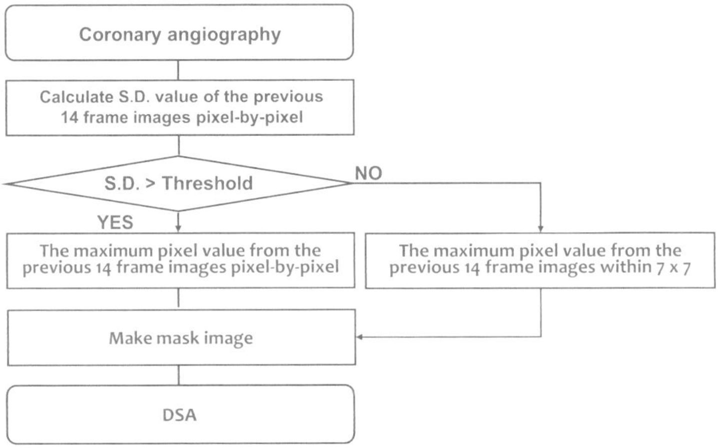

Fig. 14.14 Overall scheme of DSA for coronary artery

Development of DSA for Coronary Arteriography

Method

In this method, "conventional DSA" was obtained as follows. First, we chose a plain image as a mask image. Second, we subtracted the mask image from contrast enhanced images. Then DSA images were obtained and viewed in display.

Figure 14.14 shows the overall scheme of our method. The dynamic range compression technique [26] based on the highest and an average pixel value was applied as a preprocessing to improve the DSA image visibility. To make the mask images, we employed a maximum pixel value selection technique within $1 \times 1 \times 14$ previous frames, as shown in Fig. 14.15. When the pixel is in place of a relatively large vessel without motion, the highest pixel value in the previous 14 frames is employed as pixel value of the mask image. In this mask making method, vessels remain in the obtained mask image occasionally. Therefore, vessel partially disappeared on the DSA image. To avoid this problem, we used a wide search area in selecting the maximum pixel value for the mask image. Because the diameter of large vessel used in this study was around 14 pixels, we applied 7×7 pixels $\times$ 7 frames to a search area (Fig. 14.16).

For the determination of the pixel value of mask image, the standard deviation (SD) of 1×1 pixel $\times$ 14 flames was calculated. The search area is selected according to the following criteria. If the SD was less than or equal to 1.0, the search area was 1×1 pixel $\times$ 14 frames; otherwise, the search area would be 7×7 pixels $\times$ 7 frames. Each pixel value in the mask image was calculated from one of these two search areas. Our method can generate a mask image that excludes vessels. Finally, DSA images were obtained by subtracting the mask images from the live images.

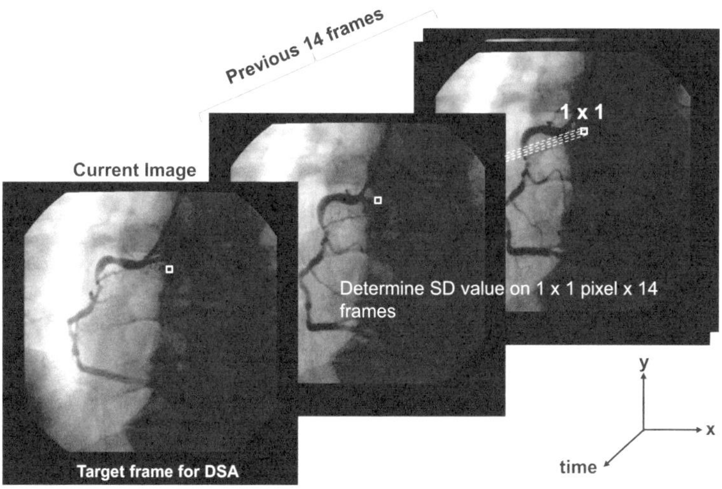

Fig. 14.15 Method for determination of pixel containing vessel

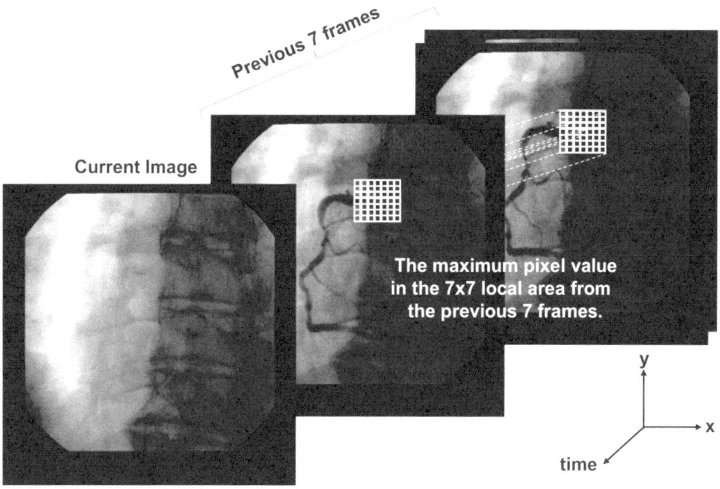

Fig. 14.16 Method for determination of pixel containing vessel

Results of the conventional DSA and our new DSA are shown in Fig. 14.17a, b, respectively. Motion artifacts were reduced remarkably and thus the image quality of the new DSA was improved. For these cases, the calculation time was approximately 0.03 s per frame.

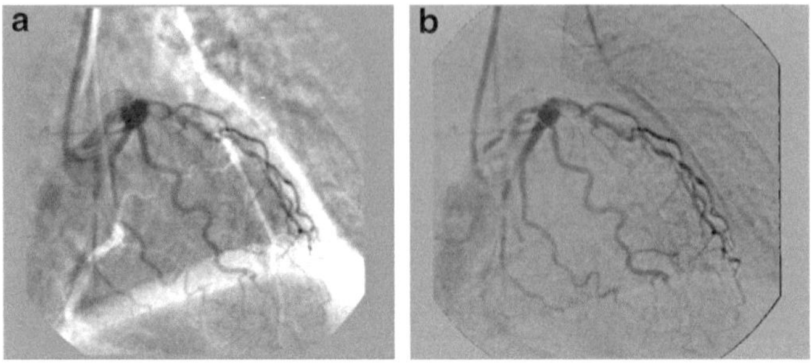

Fig. 14.17 DSA image obtained by conventional DSA and new DSA. (**a**) Conventional DSA, (**b**) new DSA

Table 14.2 Five categories used for subjective study

+2:	Greatly improved
+1:	Slightly improved
0:	Unchanged
−1:	Slightly declined
−2:	Greatly declined

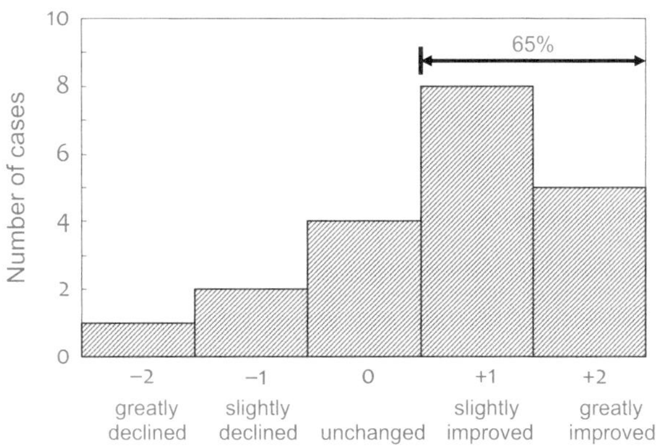

Fig. 14.18 Result of subjective evaluation of motion artifacts in new DSA images

Subjective Evaluation

Three radiological technologists with 9, 10, and 10 years of clinical experience independently classified the DSA images into five categories using a subjective rating scale ranged from +2 to −2, as listed below. Image quality of our new method compared to conventional DSA method was rated as Table 14.2.

Figure 14.18 shows the results of subjective evaluation: motion artifacts were reduced 65 % in the cases obtained by use of our new method compared to conventional DSA.

The average standard deviation of the pixel values calculated by our method was 6.64, in comparison with 10.0 by conventional DSA.

Objective Evaluation

The objective evaluation was performed by the degree of motion artifacts. Three ROIs that included vessels were manually selected for the conventional DSA and the new DSA images. Matrix size of the ROI was 150 $\times$ 150 pixels. We calculated the average and standard deviation of the pixel values of selected ROIs in 30 cases. If there are severe motion artifacts in the DSA images, standard deviation will be a large value.

CAD for the Detection of Lung Nodules

Elimination of Background

Figure 14.19 shows the CAD scheme for the detection of lung nodule in 3D CT. To eliminate the background structures due to the effects of gravity, the original CT image is processed by an opening processing [50] with a circular kernel of the average size of nodule. The opening processing can leave structures larger than the kernel size such as heart, thorax, and low frequency trend components. We subtracted the open processed image from the original lung CT image for the removal of background (Fig. 14.20).

Creation of Template for Simulated Nodule

Since the shape of lung nodule is often spherical, we used the template matching technique with a 3D Gaussian distribution. In order to enhance more effectively the isolated nodules, we used the template including the zero-surrounding as the simulated nodule. The Eq. (14.1) was used for creation of the 3D Gaussian template.

$$G(x,y,z)=\frac{1}{\left(\sqrt{2\pi}\right)^{3}\sigma_x\sigma_y\sigma_z}\exp\left(-\frac{\left\{(x-\overline{x})^2(y-\overline{y})^2(z-\overline{z})^2\right\}}{2\sigma_x^2\sigma_y^2\sigma_z^2}\right) \tag{14.1}$$

where G(x, y, z) is 3D Gaussian distribution at the coordinates $\overline{x},\overline{y},\overline{z}$, is the gravity center position of 3D Gaussian distribution, and σ_x, σ_y, σ_z are standard deviation (SD) at each axis. Figure 14.21 shows the template image used in this method.

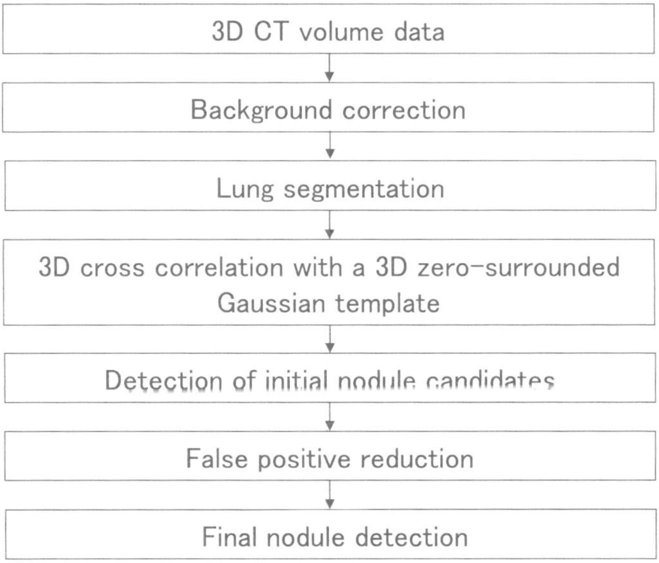

Fig. 14.19 Overall scheme of lung nodule detection

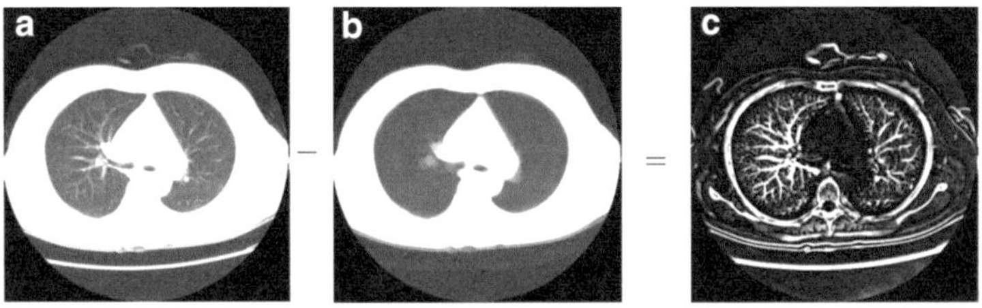

Fig. 14.20 Background correction based on morphological opening filter. (**a**) Original CT image, (**b**) opened image, (**c**) background corrected image

Fig. 14.21 Three-dimensional zero-surrounded Gaussian template as a template of lung nodule

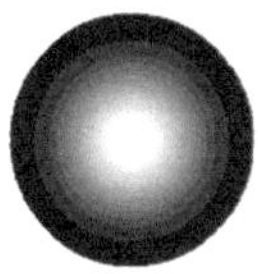

Detection of Nodules Candidate

First, lung segmentation based on a thresholding technique was performed to the 3D CT image. The background suppressed image on the segmented lung area will be lung nodule search area. We then calculated the correlation value by use of the 3D zero-surrounding Gaussian template. Thus, the nodule could be enhanced selectively. The cross-correlation value is obtained by the following Eq. (14.2).

Table 14.3 Features used for the false-positive reduction

1: Volume
2: Sphericity
3: Average of voxel value
4: Standard deviation of voxel value
5: Second-moment of voxel value
6: Third-moment of voxel value
7: Fourth-moment of voxel value
8: Maximum of voxel value
9: Minimum of voxel value
10: Coefficient of variation of voxel value
11: Contrast between maximum value in nodule and average value on circumference of nodule
12: Contrast between average value in nodule and average value on circumference of nodule
13: Overlap ratio on line component
14: Circularity of edge image
15: Average and variance which is average of each angle
16: Vessels reduction to use calculation average and variance each angle

$$C = \frac{1}{XYZ} \sum_{x=0}^{X-1} \sum_{y=0}^{Y-1} \sum_{z=0}^{Z-1} \frac{\left(f(x,y,z) - \overline{f}\right)\left(g(x,y,z) - \overline{g}\right)}{\sigma_f \sigma_g} \tag{14.2}$$

where C is the correlation value and X, Y, Z is the matrix size in x, y, z axis, respectively. σ_f, σ_g is the standard deviation of voxel values of the image and the template image, respectively. $\overline{f}$ is average voxel value of the image, and $\overline{g}$ is the average voxel value of the template image.

For the detection of the initial lung nodule candidates, the threshold technique is applied for the lung nodule enhanced image by use of the template matching technique. Since the sensitivity of the lung nodules was 100 % at the initial detection, there are a huge number of false positives. Therefore, we have to eliminate the false positives without a large loss of sensitivity.

FROC Analysis for the Detection of Lung Nodules

In order to decrease further false positives, we calculated 16 kinds of features as shown in Table 14.3.

Figure 14.22 shows the free response receiver operating characteristic (FROC) curve of final detection of lung nodules after linear discriminant analysis (LDA). We analyzed the 69 clinical cases 10 times by using the jackknife method, which is the common way to estimate classification performance. It is analyzed by splitting the data set at random into training data and validation data each with half the number of cases. The performance of this technique was as follows. When the detection sensitivity was 95.8 %, the number of average false positives was 5.2 in average on the validation test. LDA values were calculated according to the order shown in Table 14.3.

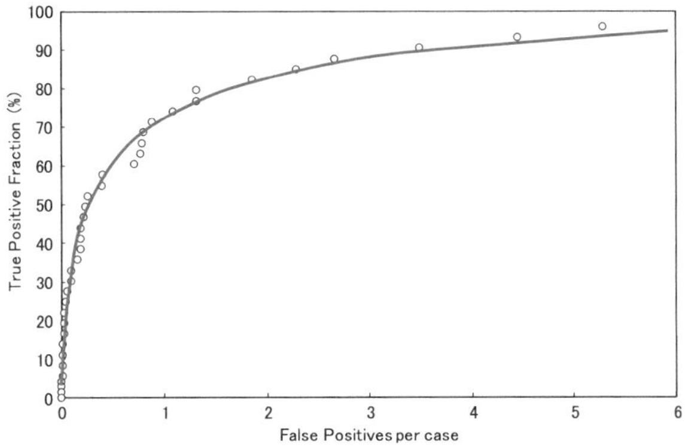

Fig. 14.22 FROC curve for the detection of lung nodule

Conclusions

The subtraction CT and the temporal subtraction CT techniques can remove the majority of normal background structures extended over multiple slices such as ribs, vessels, and heart. Thus, isolated structures such as small nodules, interval changes due to lung lesions were clearly enhanced as dark shadows on subtraction images.

Subtraction CT and temporal subtraction CT images will be useful for the finding of lung cancers on CT images, and so it is able to support radiologists in the early detection of lung cancer.

Our development of new DSA method was for coronary angiography. The motion artifacts in the DSA images were effectively reduced using proposed method. The DSA images could be obtained in almost real time.

We developed the CAD for the detection of the lung nodules in 3D CT. This technique will be useful for the detection of lung nodules on 3D CT image, and thus could assist radiologists in the early detection of lung nodule.

References

1. Sone S, Li F, Yang Z-G et al (2001) Results of three-year mass screening program for lung cancer using mobile low-dose spiral computed tomography scanner. Br J Cancer 84:25–32
2. Sone S, Takashima S, Li F et al (1998) Mass screening for lung cancer with mobile spiral computed tomography scanner. Lancet 351:1242–1245
3. Difazio MC, MacMahon H, Xu XW, Tsai P, Shiraishi J, Armato SG III, Doi K (1997) Digital chest radiography: effect of temporal subtraction images on detection accuracy. Radiology 202:447–452
4. Ishida T, Katsuragawa S, Nakamura K, MacMahon H, Doi K (1999) Iterative image-warping technique for temporal subtraction of sequential chest radiographs to detect interval change. Med Phys 26:1320–1329

5. Ishida T, Ashizawa K, Engelmann R, Katsuragawa S, MacMahon H, Doi K (1999) Application of temporal subtraction for detection of interval changes in chest radiographs: improvement of subtraction image using automated initial image matching. J Digit Imaging 12:77–86
6. Takahashi M, Shinozato J, Korogi Y (1986) Automatic registration for correction of localized misregistration artifacts in digital subtraction angiography of the head and neck. Acta Radiol Suppl Stock 369:281–284
7. Hiroshima K, Nishino J, Odaka T, Ogura H, Fukushima T, Nishimoto Y, Tanaka M, Hayashi N, Komuro H, Ishii Y (1999) New registration method using the local adjustment of ROIs in DSA image of the head and neck. IEICE Trans Inf Syst J82-D-2(3):566–570
8. De Castoro E, Morandi C (1987) Registration of translated and rotated images using finite Fourier transforms. IEEE Trans Pattern Anal Mach Intell 9(5):700–703
9. Lee DJ, Krile TF, Mitra S (1987) Digital Registration Techniques for Sequential Fundus Images, SPIE in Applied Digital Image Processing, vol 829, San Diego, pp 293–300
10. Hiroshima K, Nishino J, Odaka T (2000) Improved registration method for correcting local shifting on DSA images. Jpn Soc Med Imaging Technol 18(1):71–83
11. Brown LG (1992) A survey of image registration techniques. ACM Comput Surv 24 (4):124–145
12. Funakami R, Hiroshima K, Nishino J (2000) Successive approximation algorithm for cancellation of artifacts in DSA images. Jpn Soc Med Imaging Technol 18(3):199–206
13. Meijering EHW, Niessen WJ, Bakker J (2001) Reduction of patient motion artifacts in digital subtraction angiography: evaluation of a fast and fully automatic technique. Radiology 219:288–293
14. Guthaner DF, Wexler L, Bradley B (1985) Digital subtraction angiography of coronary grafts: optimization of technique. AJR Am J Roentgenol 145:1185–1190
15. Katrisis D, Lythall DA, Cooper IC, Crowther A, Webb-Peploe MM (1988) Assessment of coronary angioplasty: comparison of visual assessment, hand-held caliper measurement and automated digital quantitation. Cathet Cardiovasc Diagn 15:237–242
16. Katritsis D, Lythall DA, Anderson MH, Cooper IC, Webb-Peploe MM (1988) Assessment of coronary angioplasty by an automated digital angiographic method. Am Heart J 116:1181–1187
17. Katrisis D, Webb-Peploe MM (1990) Cardiac phase-related variability of border detection or densitometric quantitation of postangioplasty lumens. Am Heart J 120:537–543
18. Booth DC, Nissen S, DeMaria AN (1985) Assessment of the severity of valvular regurgitation by digital subtraction angiography compared to cineangiography. Am Heart J 110:409–416
19. Molloi S, Ersahin A, Tang J, Hicks J, Leung CY (1996) Quantification of volumetric coronary blood flow with dual-energy digital subtraction angiography. Circulation 93:1919–1927
20. Myerowitz PD, Swanson DK, Turnipseed WD (1985) Applications of digital subtraction angiography in cardiovascular diagnosis. Surg Clin North Am 65(3):423–437
21. Hayashi N, Sakai T, Kitagawa M (1998) Nonlinear geometric warping of the mask image: a new method for reducing misregistration artifacts in digital subtraction angiography. Cardiovasc Intervent Radiol 21(2):138–141
22. Dufresne TE, Sarwal A, Dhawan AP (1994) A gray-level thinning method for delineation and representation of arteries. Comput Med Imaging Graph 18(5):343–355
23. Qian Y, Eiho S (2000) Morphological method for automatic extraction of the coronary arteries. Jpn Soc Med Imaging Technol 18(3):231–239
24. Meaney TF, Weinstein MA, Buonocore E, Pavlicek W, Borkowski GP, Gallagher JH, Sufka B, MacIntyre WJ (1980) Digital subtraction angiography of the human cardiovascular system. AJR Am J Roentgenol 135:1153–1160
25. Myerowitz PD, Turnipseed WD, Swanson DK, Lysel MV, Peppler W, Mistretta C, Chopra PS, Berkoff H, Kroncke G, Hasegawa B, Steighorst M, Turski P, Crummy AB (1982) Digital sub-traction angiography as a method of screening for coronary artery disease during peripheral vascular angiography. Surgery 92(6):1042–1048

26. Bellamy GR, Yiannikas J, Detrano R, Simpfendorfer C, Salcedo EE (1986) Detection of multivessel disease after myocardial infarction using intravenous stress digital subtraction angiography. Radiology 161:685–689
27. Bentoutou Y, Taleb N, Mezouar MCE, Taleb M, Jetto L (2002) An invariant approach for image registration in digital subtraction angiography. Pattern Recognit 35:2853–2865
28. Bentoutou Y, Taleb N (2005) A 3-D space-time motion detection for an invariant image registration approach in digital subtraction angiography. Comput Vis Image Underst 97:30–50
29. Yamamoto M, Okura Y, Ishihara M, Kagemoto M, Harada K, Ishida T (2009) Development of digital subtraction angiography for coronary artery. J Digit Imaging 22(3):319–325
30. Ministry of Health, Labour and Welfare, report of medical facility survey (2008), pp 21 (in Japanese)
31. Ministry of Health, Labour and Welfare, report of medical facility survey, (2011), pp 19 (in Japanese)
32. Shigemoto K, Takizawa H, Yamamoto S, Nakazawa T, Matsumoto T, Tateno Y, Iinuma T, Matsumoto M (2003) High-speed recognition of nodule shadow from chest X ray CT images using template matching with third nodule-vessel model. Med Image Technol 21(2):147–156 (in Japanese)
33. Lee Y, Hara T, Fujita H (2000) Evaluation of GA template matching method by simulation using chest helical X-ray CT images. Med Image Inf Sci 17(3):118–129 (in Japanese)
34. Lee Y, Hara T, Fujita H, Itoh S, Ishigaki ST (2001) Automated detection of pulmonary nodules in helical CT images based on an improved template-matching technique. IEEE Trans Med Imaging 20(7):595–604
35. Armato SG 3rd, Giger ML, Moran CJ, Blackburn JT, Doi K, MacMahon H (1999) Computerized detection of pulmonary nodules on CT scans. RadioGraphics 19(5):1303–1311
36. Li Q, Sone S, Doi K (2003) Selective enhancement filters for nodules, vessels, and airway walls in two- and three dimensional CT scans. Med Phys 30(8):2040–2051
37. Arimura H, Katsuragawa S, Suzuki K, Li F, Shiraishi J, Sone S, Doi K (2004) Computerized scheme for automated detection of lung nodules in low-dose computed tomography images for lung cancer screening. Acad Radiol 11(6):617–629
38. Giger ML, Doi K, MacMahon K (1998) Automated detection of nodules in peripheral lung fields. Med Phys 15(2):158–166
39. Yamamoto S, Tanaka I, Senda M, Tateno Y, Iinuma T, Matsumoto T, Matsumoto M (1994) Image processing for computer-aided diagnosis of lung cancer by CT (LSCT). Syst Comput Jpn 25:67–79
40. Jiang H, Yamamoto S, Iisaku S, Mtsumoto M, Tateno Y, Iinuma T, Matsumoto T(1999) Computer-aided diagnosis system for lung cancer screening by CT. In: Doi K, MacMahon H, Giger ML, Hoffmann KR (eds) Computer-aided diagnosis in medical imaging. Excerpta Medica International Congress Series 1182, pp125–130
41. Ukai Y, Niki N, Satoh H, Eguchi K, Mori K, Ohmatsu H, Kakinuma R, Kaneko M, Moriyama N (2000) Computer aided diagnosis system for lung cancer based on retrospective helical CT image. Proc SPIE 3979:1028–1039
42. Armato SG 3rd, Li F, Giger ML, MacMahon H, Sone S, Doi K (2002) Lung cancer: performance of automated lung nodule detection applied to cancers missed in a CT screening program. Radiology 225(3):685–692
43. Wormanns D, Fiebich M, Saidi M, Diederich S, Heindel W (2002) Automatic detection of pulmonary nodules at spiral CT: clinical application of a computer-aided diagnosis system. Eur Radiol 12(5):1052–1057
44. Gurcan MN, Sahiner B, Petrick N, Chan HP, Kazerooni EA, Cascade PN, Hadjiiski L (2002) Lung nodule detection on thoracic computed tomography images: preliminary evaluation of a computer-aided diagnosis system. Med Phys 29(11):2552–2558
45. Brown MS, Goldin JG, Suh RD, McNitt-Gray MF, Sayre JW, Aberle DR (2003) Lung micronodules: automated method for detection at thin-section CT – initial experience. Radiology 226(1):256–262

46. Yamamoto M, Kawashita I, Okura Y, Akiyama M, Fu-jikawa K, Kagemoto M, Mitogawa Y, Ubagai T, Ishine M, Ito K, Ishida T (2008) Improvement of overall performance for lung nodule detection in chest CT images. Jpn J Radiol Technol 64(3):316–324
47. Yoshimura H, Giger ML, Doi K, MacMahon H, Montner SM (1992) Computerized scheme for the detection of pulmonary nodules: nonlinear filtering technique. Invest Radiol 27:124–129
48. Katsuragawa S, Doi K, MacMahon H, Monnier-Cholley L, Morishita J, Ishida T (1996) Quantitative analysis of geometric-pattern features of interstitial infiltrates in digital chest radiographs: preliminary results. J Digit Imaging 9:137–144
49. Ishida T, Katsuragawa S, Kabayashi T, MacMahon H, Doi K (1997) Computerized analysis of interstitial disease in chest radiographs: improvement of geometric pattern feature analysis. Med Phys 24:915–924
50. Yamamoto M, Ishida T, Kawashita I, Kagemoto M, Fujikawa K, Mitogawa Y, Ubagai T, Ishine M, Ito K, Akiyama M (2006) Development of computer-aided diagnostic system for detection of lung nodules in three-dimension computed tomography images. Jpn J Radiol Technol 62(4):555–564

List of Reviewers

The author is grateful to the following reviewers who provided constructive suggestions and improved the chapters.

Professor Hidetaka Arimura, Ph.D., Department of Health Sciences, Faculty of Medical Sciences, Kyushu University, Fukuoka, Japan

Professor Yen-Wei Chen, Ph.D., College of Information Science and Engineering, Ritsumeikan University, Kusatsu, Shiga, Japan

Professor Hiroshi Fujita, Ph.D., Department of Intelligent Image Information, Division of Regeneration and Advanced Medical Sciences, Graduate School of Medicine, Gifu University, Gifu, Japan

Professor Hieu Trung Huynh, Ph.D., Faculty of Information Technology, The Industrial University of Ho Chi Minh City, Ho Chi Minh City, Vietnam

Professor Marius George Linguraru, Ph.D., Sheikh Zayed Institute for Pediatric Surgical Innovation, Children's National Medical Center, Washington, DC, USA

Professor Mia K. Markey, Ph.D., Department of Biomedical Engineering, The University of Texas at Austin, Austin, TX, USA

Professor Dinggang Shen, Ph.D., Department of Radiology and BRIC, University of North Carolina at Chapel Hill, Chapel Hill, NC, USA

Professor Kenji Suzuki, Ph.D., Department of Radiology, The University of Chicago, Chicago, IL, USA

Professor Rie Tanaka, Ph.D., School of Health Sciences, College of Medical, Pharmaceutical and Health Sciences, Kanazawa University, Kanazawa, Japan

Professor Tolga Tasdizen, Ph.D., Department of Electrical and Computer Engineering, Scientific Computing and Imaging Institute, University of Utah, Lake City, UT, USA

Professor Yongyi Yang, Ph.D., Department of Electrical and Computer Engineering, Illinois Institute of Technology, Chicago, IL, USA

K. Suzuki (ed.), *Computational Intelligence in Biomedical Imaging*,
DOI 10.1007/978-1-4614-7245-2, © Springer Science+Business Media New York 2014

Biography

Kenji Suzuki received his B.S. and M.S. degrees in engineering from Meijo University, Japan, in 1991 and 1993, respectively, and his Ph.D. degree (by Published Work) in engineering from Nagoya University, Japan, in 2001. From 1993 to 2001, he worked at Hitachi Medical Corporation, and then at Aichi Prefectural University as a faculty member. In 2001, he joined the Department of Radiology at the University of Chicago, as Research Associate. Since 2006, he has been Assistant Professor of Radiology, Medical Physics, and Cancer Research Center there. Dr. Suzuki's research interests include computer-aided diagnosis, computational intelligence and machine learning in medical imaging, and medical image analysis. He has published more than 240 papers (including 95 peer-reviewed journal papers), 75 scientific abstracts, 9 books, and 18 book chapters, and edited 6 journal special issues. His papers were cited more than 3,000 times by other researchers, and he has an h-index of 28 as of 2013. He is an inventor on 28 patents (including 11 granted patents), which were licensed to several companies and commercialized. He was awarded more than 44 grants including NIH R01 grants. He has served as a grant reviewer for funding agencies, including National Science Foundation (NSF), US Army Medical Research and Materiel Command (USAMRMC), and American Cancer Society (ACS). He has been serving as the Editor-in-Chief and an Associate Editor of 28 leading international journals, including *Medical Physics*, *Academic Radiology*, *International Journal of Biomedical Imaging*, and *Algorithms*. He has been serving as a referee for more than 65 international journals, an organizer of 16 international conferences, and a program committee member of 120 international conferences. He had supervised/co-supervised more than 60 graduate/undergraduate students, post-docs/computer scientists, and visiting professors. He has received numerous awards, including a University of Chicago Paul C. Hodges Award, three Certificate of Merit Awards and Research Trainee Prize from RSNA, Young Investigator Award from Cancer Research Foundation, an IEEE Outstanding Member Award, Honorable Mention Poster Award at SPIE International Symposium on Medical Imaging, and Kurt Rossmann Award for Excellence in Teaching from University of Chicago. He has been a Senior Member of IEEE since 2004.

K. Suzuki (ed.), *Computational Intelligence in Biomedical Imaging*,
DOI 10.1007/978-1-4614-7245-2, © Springer Science+Business Media New York 2014

Index

K. Suzuki (ed.), *Computational Intelligence in Biomedical Imaging*,
DOI 10.1007/978-1-4614-7245-2, © Springer Science+Business Media New York 2014

MIX
Papier aus verantwortungsvollen Quellen
Paper from responsible sources
FSC® C105338

If you have any concerns about our products,
you can contact us on
ProductSafety@springernature.com

In case Publisher is established outside the EU,
the EU authorized representative is:
Springer Nature Customer Service Center GmbH
Europaplatz 3, 69115 Heidelberg, Germany

Printed by Libri Plureos GmbH
in Hamburg, Germany